Handbook of Pediatric Neuro-Ophthalmology

Handbook of Pediatric Neuro-Ophthalmology

Edited by

Kenneth W. Wright, MD
Director, Wright Foundation for Pediatric Ophthalmology
Director, Pediatric Ophthalmology, Cedars-Sinai Medical Center, Clinical Professor of Ophthalmology, University of Southern California—Keck School of Medicine, Los Angeles, California

Peter H. Spiegel, MD
Focus On You, Inc., Palm Desert, California
Inland Eye Clinic, Murrieta, California
Children's Eye Institute, Upland, California

Lisa S. Thompson, MD
Attending Physician, Stroger Hospital of Cook County, Chicago, Illinois

Illustrators
Timothy C. Hengst, CMI
Susan Gilbert, CMI
Faith Cogswell

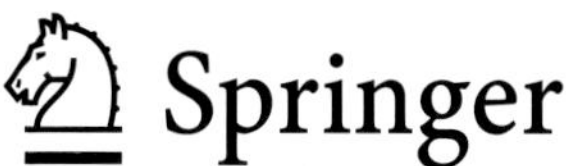

Kenneth W. Wright, MD
Director, Wright Foundation for Pediatric Ophthalmology
Director, Pediatric Ophthalmology, Cedars-Sinai Medical Center,
Clinical Professor of Ophthalmology, University of Southern California—Keck School of Medicine
Los Angeles, CA
USA

Peter H. Spiegel, MD
Focus On You, Inc.
Palm Desert, CA
Inland Eye Clinic
Murrieta, CA
Children's Eye Institute
Upland, CA
USA

Lisa S. Thompson, MD
Attending Physician
Stroger Hospital of Cook County
Chicago, IL
USA

Library of Congress Control Number: 2005932933

ISBN 10: 0-387-27929-6 e-ISBN 0-387-27930-X
ISBN 13: 978-0387-27929-9

Printed on acid-free paper.

Printed in China (BS/EVB)

9 8 7 6 5 4 3 2 1

springer.com

Preface

Pediatric ophthalmology is a broad field encompassing many diverse topics including embryology, chromosomal abnormalities, neurology, craniofacial abnormalities, systemic diseases, retina disease, and strabismus. This variety makes pediatric ophthalmology interesting, and intellectually stimulating, but at the time somewhat daunting. The handbook series is designed to give the practitioner an easy to understand, succinct yet detailed reference on various subjects related to pediatric ophthalmology.

The *Handbook of Pediatric Neuro-Ophthalmology* is a practical resource on the diagnosis and management of neurological disorders with ocular manifestations. A broad range of topics are covered including the pediatric neuro-ophthalmology examination, ocular motility disorders, optic nerve anomalies, nystagmus, and neuro-degenerative disease. Children with neurological disorders often have debilitating disease without viable treatment options. In these cases even the seasoned physician can feel uncomfortable when speaking with the family. A beautifully sensitive chapter is included "Breaking the News" that gives practical points to help the physician communicate with the family.

Chapters in the handbook are reader friendly. They are organized with clear sub-headings that allow the reader to quickly find the area of interest. Excellent color photographs and diagrams illustrate the clinical points and help with disease recognition. Extensive use of tables and information boxes simplify and summarize complex topics. Each chapter is fully referenced to provide evidence-based practice guidelines and further in-depth reading.

Another important use of the *Handbook of Pediatric Neuro-Ophthalmology* is patient and family education. Parents are rightfully concerned about the effects of neurological disease on their child's eyes. Information including diagrams and photographs from the handbook about the eye manifestations of neurological disease can be shared with the families. This important information is often lacking in general texts on ophthalmology and pediatrics.

I hope you will find this book, *Handbook of Pediatric Neuro-Ophthalmology*, to be an invaluable adjunct to your pediatric practice.

Kenneth W. Wright, MD

Contents

Contributors

Brian N. Bachynski, MD

Dean J. Bonsall, MD

Mark S. Borchert, MD

Michael C. Brodsky, MD

Edward G. Buckley, MD

Susan M. Carden, MBBS, FRACO, FRACS

Nancy Chernus–Mansfield

Cynthia S. Cook, DVM, PhD

William V. Good, MD

Richard W. Hertle, MD, FACS

Mitra Maybodi, MD

James W. McManaway III, MD

Ronald M. Minzter, MD

Paul H. Phillips, MD

Michael X. Repka, MD

Kathleen K. Sulik, PhD

Anne Frances Walonker, CO

Kenneth W. Wright, MD

Sarah Ying, MD

Embryology

Cynthia S. Cook, Kathleen K. Sulik, and Kenneth W. Wright

DIFFERENTIATION OF GERM LAYERS AND EMBRYOGENESIS

After fertilization of the ovum within the uterine tube, cellular mitosis results in formation of a ball of 12 to 16 cells, the morula. A fluid-filled cavity within this embryonic cell mass forms, resulting in a transformation into a blastocyst that begins to penetrate the uterine mucosa on approximately the sixth day postfertilization. The cells of the blastocyst continue to divide with the cells of the future embryo proper (embryoblast) accumulating at one pole. The cells of the primitive embryoblast differentiate into two layers, the *epiblast* and the *hypoblast*. These two cellular layers bridge the central cavity of the blastocyst, thus dividing the blastocyst into the amniotic cavity and the yolk sac (Fig. 1-1).

During the third week of gestation, the two-layered embryoblast transforms into a trilaminar embryo as central epiblast cells invaginate between the epiblast and hypoblast layers. Invagination of central epiblast cells creates a longitudinal groove through the midline of the caudal half of the epiblast, the *primitive streak*. This invagination of epiblast cells is termed *gastrulation* (Fig. 1-2A,B). Invaginating epiblast cells differentiate to form the *mesodermal* germ layer, which spreads out to fill the space between the epiblast and hypoblast. Gastrulation proceeds in a cranial to caudal progression and continues through the fourth week of human gestation. These invaginating epiblast cells displace the hypoblast cells to form the *endoderm*. The epiblast cells therefore give rise to all three definitive germ layers: *ectoderm*, *mesoderm*, and *endoderm* (Fig. 1-2C).

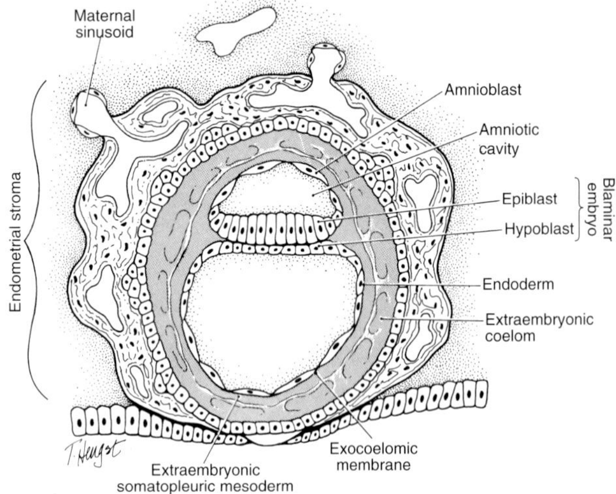

FIGURE 1-1. Drawing of a human blastocyst (12 days gestation) that has penetrated the maternal endometrium. An embryoblast has formed that consists of two cell layers: the epiblast above and the hypoblast below.

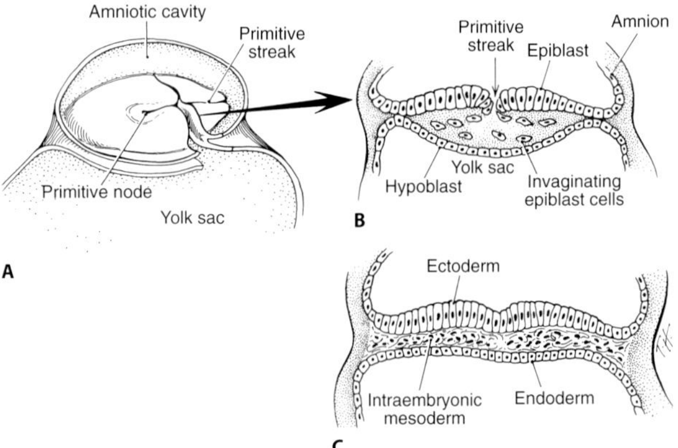

FIGURE 1-2A–C. (A) Drawing of a 17-day-old embryo in gastrulation stage (dorsal view) with the amnion removed. **(B)** Cross section of a 17-day-old embryo through the primitive streak. The primitive streak represents invagination of epiblast cells between the epiblast and hypoblast layers. Note the epiblast cells filling the middle area to form the mesodermal layer. **(C)** Cross section of the embryo at the end of the third week shows the three definitive germ layers: ectoderm, mesoderm, and endoderm.

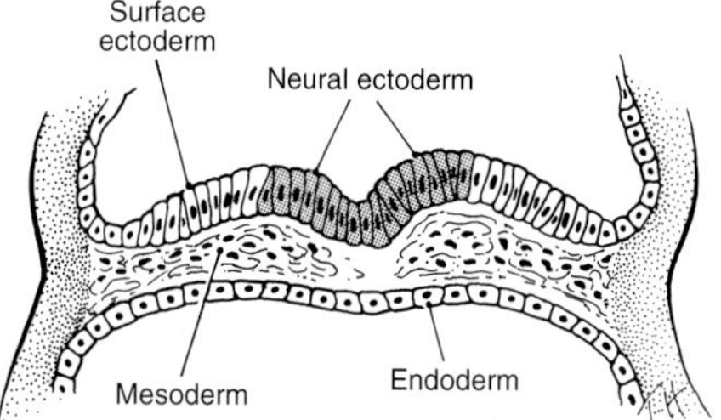

FIGURE 1-3. Drawing of an 18-day-old embryo sectioned through the neural plate. Note that the ectoderm in the area of the neural groove (*shaded cells*) has differentiated into neural ectoderm whereas the ectoderm on each side of the neural groove remains as surface ectoderm (*clear white cells*).

Toward the end of gastrulation, the ectoderm anterior to the primitive streak differentiates into columnar *neural ectoderm*; this expands, forming the *neural plate* from which the brain develops (Figs. 1-3, 1-4). Neural ectoderm on each side of the central neural groove expands to form bilateral elevations called the *neural folds* (Fig. 1-5). A central valley in the enlarging neural plate is called the *neural groove*. Ectoderm at the lateral margins of the neural plate has the flat, hexagonal morphology typical of *surface ectoderm* (Figs. 1-5, 1-6). By 21 days of human

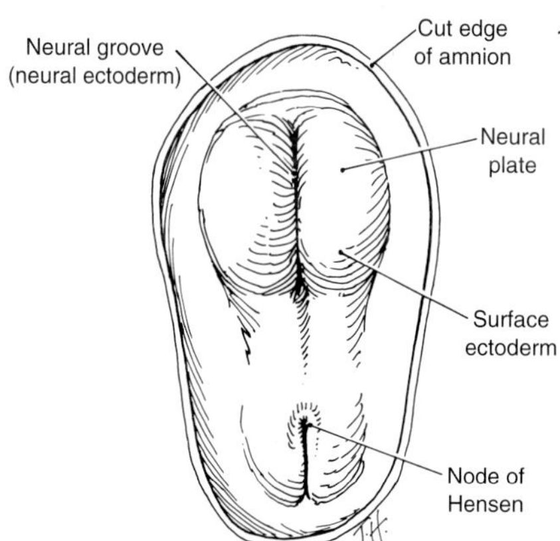

FIGURE 1-4. Drawing of dorsal aspect of embryo at 18 days gestation showing neural groove and enlarging neural plate.

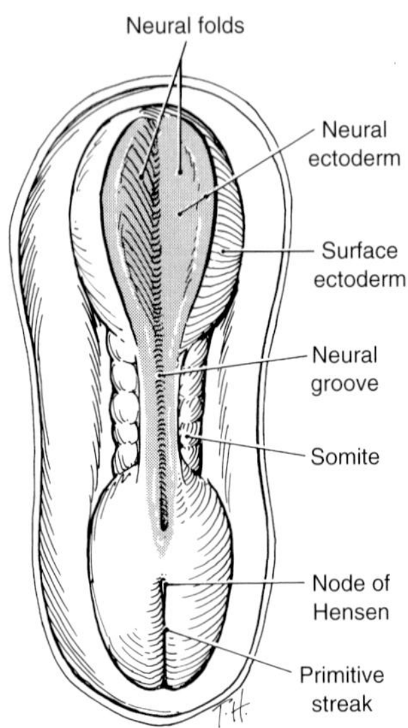

FIGURE 1-5. Dorsal view of a human embryo at 20 days gestation. The neural plate transforms into two neural folds on each side of the neural groove. The neural groove in the middle of the embryo is *shaded* to represent neural ectoderm; the *unshaded* surface of the embryo is surface ectoderm.

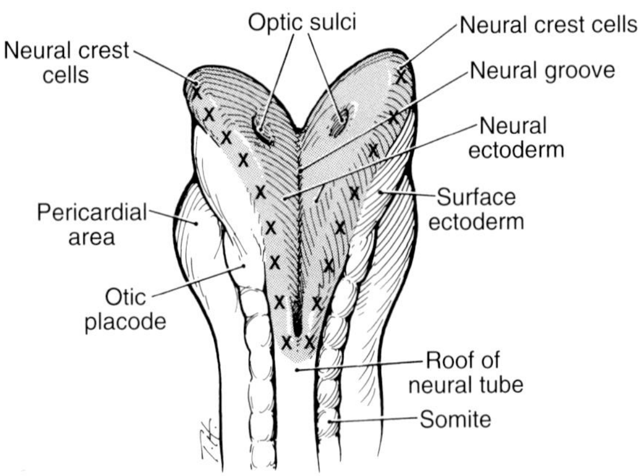

FIGURE 1-6. Drawing of 21-day-old embryo (dorsal view) showing the enlarging cephalic neural folds, which are separate and have not yet fused. The central neural folds have fused to form the neural tube. The neural tube, groove, and facing surfaces of the large neural folds are made up of neural ectoderm; surface ectoderm covers the rest of the embryo. Neural crest cells (*X*) are found at the junction of the neural ectoderm and surface ectoderm. Neural crest cells migrate beneath the surface ectoderm spreading throughout the embryo and specifically to the area of the optic sulci. Neural ectoderm, *dark shading*; surface ectoderm, *white*; neural crest cells, *cross-hatched area*. The neural groove is still open at this point, and somites have formed along the lateral aspect of the neural tube.

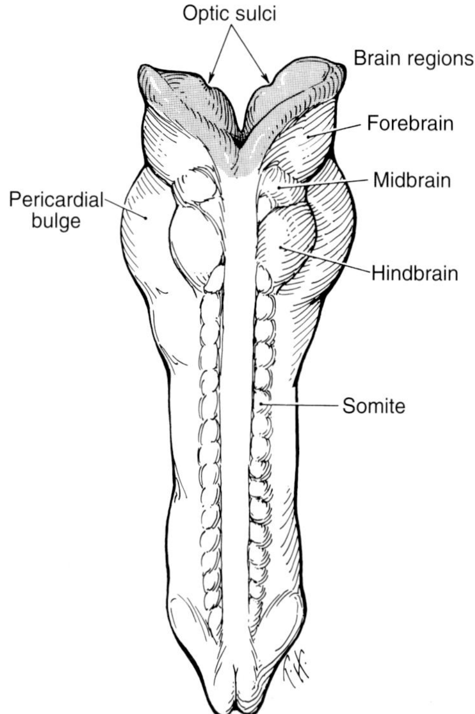

FIGURE 1-7. Drawing of approximately 23-day-old embryo, dorsal view, showing partial fusion of the neural folds. Brain vesicles have divided into three regions: forebrain, midbrain, and hindbrain. Note that the facing surfaces of the forebrain neural folds are lined with neural ectoderm (*shaded cells*) but the majority of the embryo is covered by surface ectoderm (*clear white*). On the inside of both forebrain vesicles is the site of the optic sulci (optic pits). The neural crest cells that will populate the region around the developing optic vesicles originate from the midbrain region.

gestation, while the neural tube is still open, the first sign of the developing eye is seen. The *optic sulci* or *optic pits* develop as invaginations on the inner surface of the anterior neural folds (Figs. 1-6, 1-7, 1-8). During expansion of the optic sulci, the central aspect of the neural folds approach each other and fuse, creating the longitudinal *neural tube.* Fusion of the neural folds

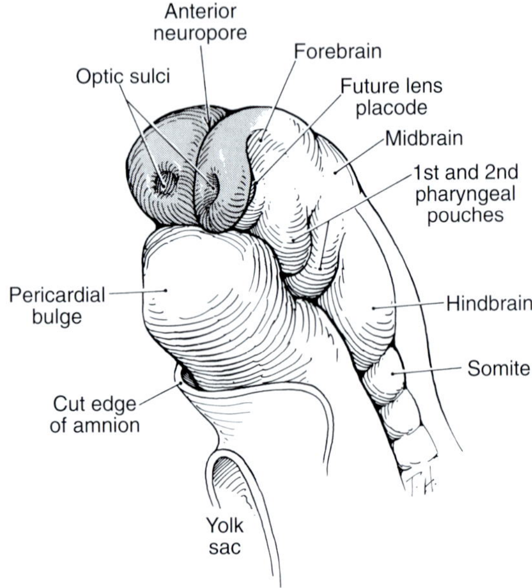

FIGURE 1-8. Drawing of anterior view of embryo at similar stage to Figure 1-7 (23 days) shows the optic sulci on the inside of the forebrain vesicles. *Shaded area*, neural ectoderm. The optic sulci evaginate and expand toward the surface ectoderm as the neural tube closes anteriorly. (From Webster WS, Lipson AH, Sulik KK. Am J Med Genet 1988;31:505–512, with permission.)

is initiated in the region of the future neck and proceeds along the midline in both caudal and cranial directions. Following closure of the neural tube, the neural ectoderm and optic sulci are internalized, and the embryo is then covered by surface ectoderm (Fig. 1-7).

Neural Crest Cell Development

As the neural folds elevate and approach each other, a specialized population of mesenchymal cells, the *neural crest cells*, emigrate from the junction of the neural and surface ectoderm (see Fig. 1-6). Progenitor cells in the neural folds are multipotent, with potential to form multiple ectodermal derivatives, including epidermal, neural crest, and neural tube cells. These cells are induced by interactions between the neural plate and epidermis. The competence of the neural plate to respond to inductive interactions changes as a function of embryonic age.[92] These stellate cells migrate peripherally beneath the surface ectoderm to spread throughout the embryo and surround the area of the developing optic sulci. Neural crest cells play an important role in eye development, as they are the precursors (anlage) to major structures, including cornea stroma, iris stroma, ciliary muscle, choroid, sclera, and orbital cartilage and bone (Table 1-1).[55,64] The patterns of neural crest emergence and emigration correlate with the segmental disposition of the developing brain.[72] Migration and differentiation of the neural crest cells are influenced by the hyaluronic acid-rich extracellular matrix and the optic vesicle basement membrane.[17] This acellular matrix is secreted by a surface epithelium as well as the crest cells and forms a space through which the crest cells migrate. Fibronectin secreted by the noncrest cells forms the limits of this mesenchymal migration.[65] Interactions between the migrating neural crest and the associated mesoderm appear to be essential for normal crest differentiation.[76,77]

TABLE 1-1. Embryonic Origins of Ocular Tissues.

Neural ectoderm (optic cup)	Surface ectoderm (epithelium)
Neural retina	Corneal and conjunctival epithelium
Retinal pigment epithelium	Lens
Pupillary sphincter and dilator muscles	Lacrimal gland
Posterior iris epithelium	Eyelid epidermis
Ciliary body epithelium	Eyelid cilia
Optic nerve	Epithelium of adnexa glands
Neural crest (connective tissue)	Epithelium of nasolacrimal duct
Corneal endothelium	Mesoderm (muscle and vascular endothelium)
Trabecular meshwork	Extraocular muscle cells
Stroma of cornea, iris, and ciliary body	Vascular endothelia
Ciliary muscle	Schlemm's canal endothelium
Choroid and sclera	Blood
Perivascular connective tissue and smooth muscle cells	
Meninges of optic nerve	
Orbital cartilage and bone	
Connective tissue of the extrinsic ocular muscles	
Secondary vitreous	
Zonules	

Somite Development

During the development and closure of the neural groove, paraxial mesoderm increases in the center of the embryo to form *somites* (see Figs. 1-5, 1-6). The somites increase in number to approximately 40, and eventually this paraxial mesoderm becomes mesenchyme that, in turn, develops into connective tissue, cartilage, muscle, and bone for the trunk and extremities. The neural segmentation pattern appears to be dependent on the underlying mesoderm. In the region of the brain rostral to the developing inner ear, the mesodermal segments are called *somitomeres*, whereas segments caudal to this level are somites.[72,75] The somitomeres are mesodermal in origin and give rise to the myoblasts of the extraocular muscles and vascular endothelium in and around the eye. Unlike the trunk and extremities, orbital bone and ocular connective tissue are derived from neural crest cells, not mesoderm.

It is important to point out that *mesenchyme* is a broad term for any embryonic connective tissue, whereas mesoderm specifically relates to the middle embryonic layer. At one time the middle embryonic layer (the mesoderm) was thought to be responsible for most of the ocular and adnexal tissues. Embryologic studies have shown that mesoderm plays a relatively small role in the development of head and neck mesenchyme and is probably responsible only for the striated muscle of the extraocular muscles and vascular endothelium. With respect to the ocular development and development of the head and neck, most of the mesenchyme or connective tissue comes from the neural crest cells (see Table 1-1).

OPTIC VESICLE AND OPTIC CUP

As the neural folds progressively fuse in a cranial direction, dilation of the closed neural tube occurs to form the "brain vesicles." By 3 weeks, these vesicles undergo neural segmentation and form the specific parts of the brain, that is, *forebrain* (prosencephalon), *midbrain* (mesencephalon), and *hindbrain* (rhombencephalon) (see Fig. 1-7). Surface ectoderm covers the outside of the forebrain, and neural ectoderm lines the inner or facing surfaces of the paired forebrain vesicles from which the eyes develop (Figs. 1-8, 1-9). The *optic sulci* develop as bilateral evaginations of neural ectoderm on the facing surfaces of the

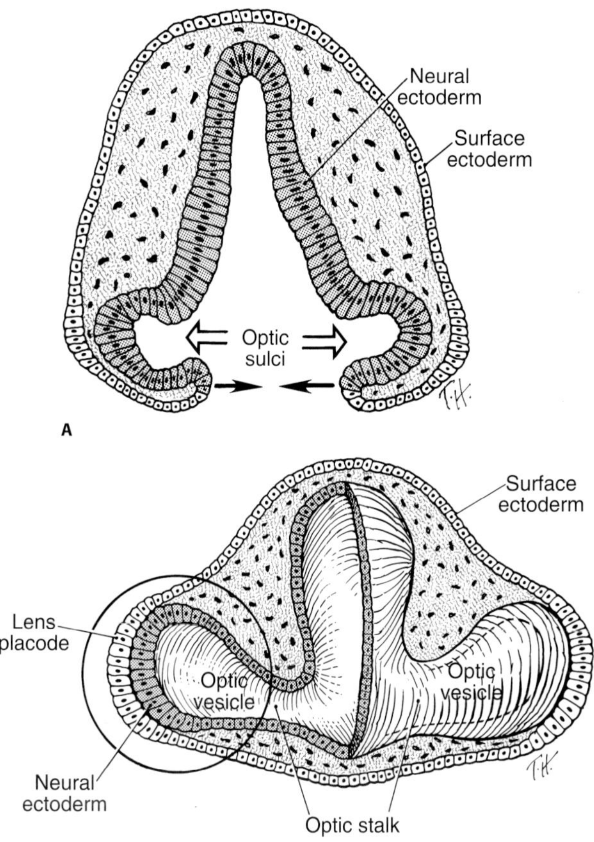

FIGURE 1-9A–B. **(A)** Drawing of a cross section through forebrain and optic sulci of 23- to 26-day-old embryo, during the period of neural tube closure. The optic sulci are lined by neural ectoderm (*shaded cells*); the surface of the forebrain is covered with surface ectoderm (*clear white cells*). As the optic sulci (neural ectoderm) evaginate towards the surface ectoderm (hollow arrows), the edges of the brain vesicles move together to fuse, thus closing the neural tube (*solid arrows*). **(B)** Drawing of a cross section through a 26-day-old embryo at the level of the optic vesicle. The neural tube has closed, the surface ectoderm now covers the exterior of the forebrain, and the neural ectoderm is completely internalized. The surface ectoderm cells overlying the optic vesicles thicken to form the early lens placode. (From Cook CS, Sulik KK. Scanning Electron Microsc 1986;III:1215–1227, with permission).

forebrain vesicles. Expansion of the optic sulci toward the surface ectoderm and fusion of the forebrain vesicles create the *optic vesicles* (Figs. 1-9, 1-10) by approximately day 25 to 26 (embryo size, 3 mm). Closure of the neural tube and expansion of the optic vesicles occur through the mechanical influences of the cytoskeletal and extracellular matrix and localized proliferation and cell growth.[91]

The mesencephalic neural crest cells populate the region around the optic vesicle and ultimately give rise to nearly all the connective tissue structures of the avian eye, and the same can be presumed for the mammalian eye (see Table 1-1).[55,64] An external bulge indicating the presence of the invaginating optic vesicle can be seen at approximately 25 days human gestation (see Fig. 1-9). The optic vesicle appears to play a significant role in the induction and size determination of the palpebral fissure and orbital and periocular structures.[56]

At approximately 27 days gestation, the surface ectoderm that is in contact with the optic vesicle thickens to form the *lens placode* (Figs. 1-9, 1-10, 1-11). The lens placode and underlying neural ectoderm invaginate through differential growth (Fig. 1-10). The invaginating neural ectoderm folds onto itself as the optic vesicle collapses, creating a double layer of neural

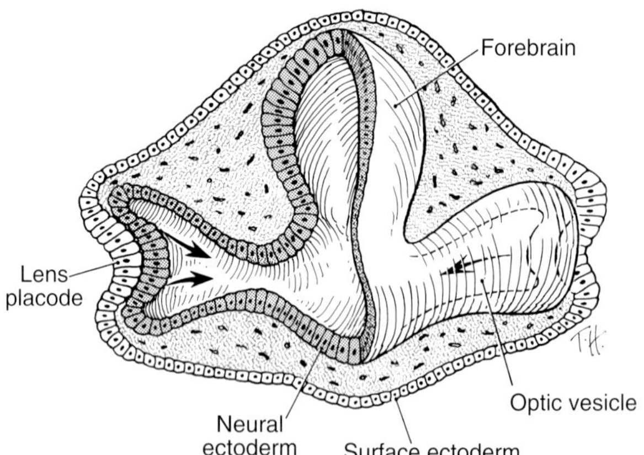

FIGURE 1-10. Drawing of a transection through a 28-day-old embryo shows invaginating lens placode and optic vesicle (*arrows*), thus creating the optic cup. Note the orientation of the eyes 180° from each other; this corresponds to the SEM view shown in Figure 1-12C.

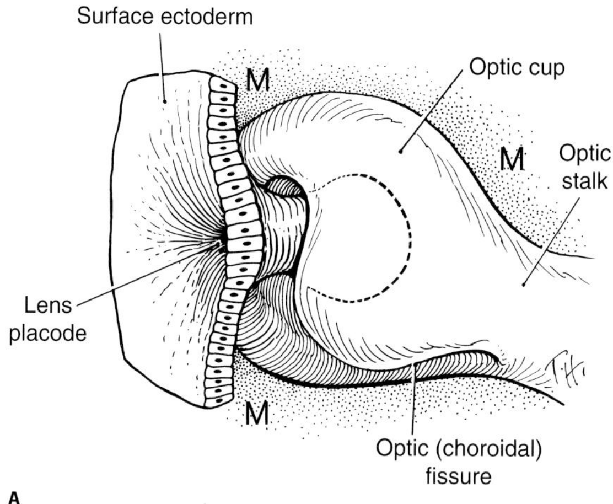

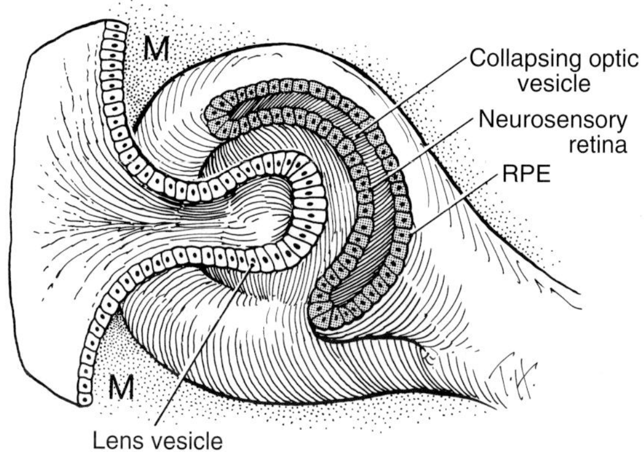

FIGURE 1-11A,B. Drawings show the formation of the lens vesicle and optic cup. Note that the optic fissure is present as the optic cup is not yet fused inferiorly. Mesenchyme (*M*) surrounds the invaginating lens placode. The optic stalk is continuous with the forebrain. Note that the optic cup and optic stalk are neural ectoderm. *RPE,* retinal pigment epithelium.

ectoderm, the *optic cup* (Fig. 1-11). The optic cup will eventually differentiate into *neurosensory retina* (inner layer) and *retinal pigment epithelium* (RPE) (outer layer) (Fig. 1-11). Local apical contraction[112] and physiological cell death[91] have been identified during invagination of the lens placode and formation of the optic cup. In the mouse embryo, Msx2, a homeobox-containing transcription factor, is expressed only in the cells of the optic cup that are destined to become neural retina. In vitro Msx2 has been shown to suppress RPE differentiation and may be involved in the initial patterning of the optic cup.[48] Abnormal differentiation of the outer layer of the optic cup to form aberrant neural retina has been demonstrated in several mutant mouse strains.[21,26,109] The area of future retinal differentiation demonstrates the greatest concentration of vimentin (a cytoskeletal protein) in the optic cup.[53] Regionally, within the optic cup, spatial orientation is predicted by expression of the transcription factor, vax2, which defines the ventral region (area of the optic fissure).[10] The PAX6 gene has been demonstrated within cells of neural ectodermal origin (optic cup and, later, in the ciliary body and retina), surface ectoderm (lens), and neural crest (cornea).[74] The widespread distribution of this gene supports its involvement in many stages of ocular morphogenesis.

The Optic Fissure

Invagination of the optic cup occurs in an eccentric manner with formation of a seam, the *optic fissure*, inferiorly (Figs. 1-11, 1-12). The optic fissure is also known as the *embryonic fissure* or *choroidal fissure*. Mesenchymal tissue (of primarily neural crest origin) surrounds and is within the optic fissure and optic cup, and at 5 weeks the *hyaloid artery* develops from mesenchyme in the optic fissure. This artery courses from the *optic stalk* (precursor to the optic nerve) through the optic fissure to the developing lens (Fig. 1-12). The lens vesicle separates from the surface ectoderm at approximately 6 weeks, the same time as closure of the optic fissure. Closure of the optic cup occurs initially at the equator with progression anteriorly and posteriorly.

Once the fissure has closed, secretion of primitive aqueous fluid by the primitive ciliary epithelium establishes intraocular pressure (IOP), which contributes to expansion of the optic cup.[15,29] Experimental studies have shown that placement of a capillary tube into the vitreous cavity of a chick eye reduces the IOP and markedly slows growth of the eye.[29] Histological

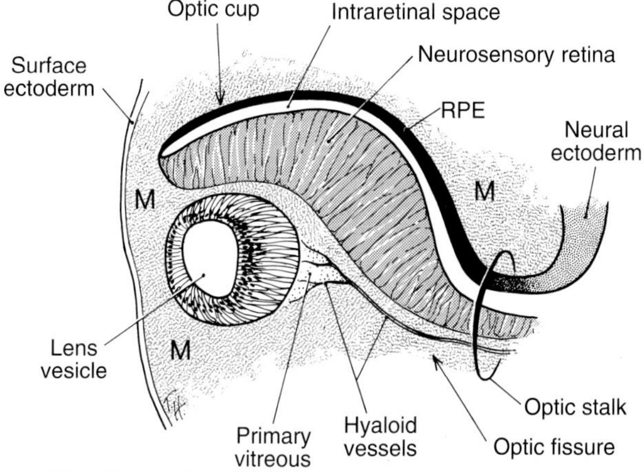

FIGURE 1-12. Drawing of cross section at approximately 5 weeks gestation through optic cup and optic fissure. The lens vesicle is separated from the surface ectoderm. Mesenchyme (*M*) surrounds the developing lens vesicle; the hyaloid artery is seen within the optic fissure. (From Cook CS, Sulik KK. Scanning Electron Microsc 1986;III:1215–1227, with permission.)

examination of these intubated eyes demonstrated proportional reduction in size of all the ocular tissues except the neural retina and the lens, which were normal in size for the age of the eye. The retina in these eyes was highly convoluted and filled the small posterior segment. Thus, it may be concluded that growth of the neural retina occurs independently of that of the other ocular tissues. Experimental removal of the lens in the eye does not alter retinal growth.[30] Growth of the choroid and sclera appear to be dependent upon IOP, as is folding of the ciliary epithelium.[12] Failure or late closure of the optic fissure prevents the establishment of normal fetal IOP and can therefore result in *microphthalmia* associated with *colobomas*, that is, colobomatous microphthalmia (see Ocular Dysgenesis later in this chapter).

Figure 1-13 shows a diagram of the eye at the end of the seventh week and after optic fissure closure. At this stage, the neurosensory retina and pigment epithelium are in apposition, the optic nerve is developing, and the lens has separated from the cornea, thus forming the anterior chamber. Mesenchymal tissue

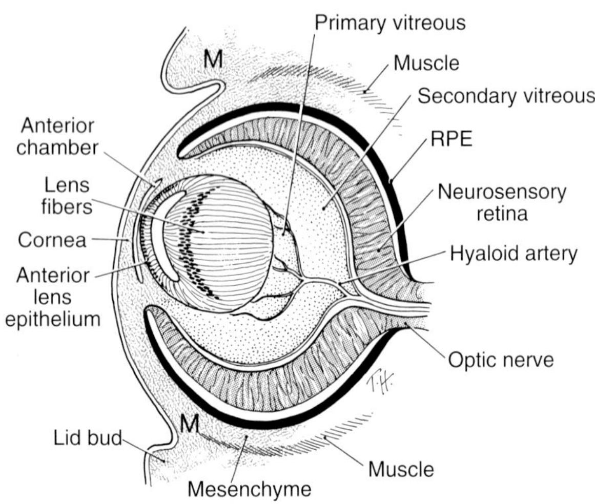

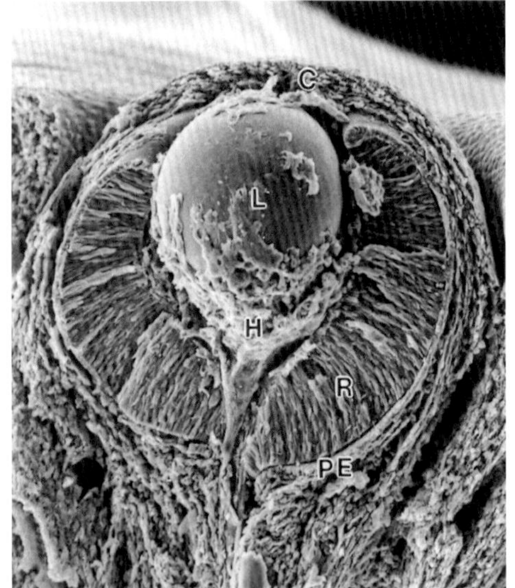

FIGURE 1-13. Overview at the 7th week of gestation. The developing eye is surrounded by mesenchyme of neural crest origin. (From Sulik KK, Schoenwolf GC. Scanning Electron Microsc 1985;IV:1735–1752, with permission.)

(neural crest cell origin) around the primitive retina develops into the choroid and sclera. Peripheral to the developing globe are linear accumulations of myoblasts (mesodermal origin) that are anlagen of the extraocular muscles. The eyelids are small buds above and below the developing eye. The hyaloid vasculature courses from the primitive optic nerve to the posterior lens capsule.

LENS

Thickening of the lens placode can be seen on gestational day 27 in the human (see Fig. 1-10). Before its contact with the optic vesicle, the surface ectoderm must become competent to respond to lens inducers. It then receives inductive signals from the anterior neural plate, so that it gains a "lens-forming bias" specified for lens formation. Complete lens differentiation requires both inductive signals from the optic vesicle and an inhibitory signal from head neural crest to suppress any residual lens-forming bias in head ectoderm adjacent to the lens.[38] In the chick, a tight extracellular matrix-mediated adhesion between the optic vesicle and the surface ectoderm has been described.[47,57,69] This anchoring of the mitotically active surface ectoderm results in cell crowding, cell elongation, and formation of the thickened placode.[119] Adhesion between the optic vesicle and the lens placode is thought to ensure alignment of the lens in the visual axis.[15] Although adhesion between the optic vesicle and surface ectoderm exists, electron microscopic studies have demonstrated that there is no direct cell contact.[22,49,108] The basement membranes of the optic vesicle and the surface ectoderm remain separate and intact throughout the contact period. Experimental studies have demonstrated a requirement for functional PAX6 gene in both the optic vesicle and surface ectoderm to mediate lens placode induction.[23] The BMP4 gene, which is present only in the optic vesicle, is also required for lens induction.[35]

The lens placode invaginates forming the hollow lens vesicle (Figs. 1-11, 1-12). The size of the lens vesicle is determined by the area of contact of the optic vesicle and the surface ectoderm. Lens vesicle detachment from the surface ectoderm occurs on day 33 (7–9 mm) and is the initial event leading to the formation of the chambers of the eye. This process of separation is accompanied by active migration of epithelial cells out of the keratolenticular stalk or junction,[37] cellular necrosis, and basement membrane breakdown.[36] Although apoptosis (programmed cell death) is a normal feature of lens vesicle separation, excessive and persistent cell death is associated with aphakia in the lap mouse mutant.[8]

Induction of a small lens vesicle that fails to undergo normal separation from the surface ectoderm is one of the characteristics of teratogen-induced anterior segment malformations described in animal models.[24,28,81,102] In the mouse mutant (dyl), this failure of lens vesicle separation is caused by a mutation in the FoxE3 gene that promotes survival and proliferation while preventing differentiation of the lens epithelium.[18] AP-2 transcription factors also influence lens vesicle separation as well as causing mis-expression of PAX6 and MIP26 genes.[109] Anterior lenticonus, anterior capsular cataracts, and anterior segment dysgenesis with keratolenticular adhesions (Peters' anomaly) may result from faulty keratolenticular separation. Further discussion of anterior segment dysgenesis follows. Arrest of lens development at the lens stalk stage results in aphakia in mutant mice (*ak* mutation). In addition to aphakia, affected eyes exhibit absence of a pupil and abnormalities in the iris, ciliary body, and vitreous.[40,41]

The hollow lens vesicle consists of a single layer of epithelial cells with cell apices directed toward the center of the sphere. Following detachment from the surface ectoderm, the lens vesicle is surrounded by a basal lamina, the future *lens capsule*. Abnormalities in this basement membrane may result in involution of the lens vesicle, resulting in later aphakia.[8] At approximately 37 days gestation, *primary lens fibers* form from elongation of the posterior lens epithelium of the lens vesicle (Fig. 1-14).[51] The retinal anlage promotes primary lens fiber formation in the adjacent lens epithelial cells. Experimental in vivo rotation of the lens vesicle in the chick eye by 180° results in elongation of the lens epithelial cells nearest the presumptive retina, regardless of the orientation of the transplanted lens.[31] Thus, the retina develops independently from the lens although the lens appears to rely upon the retina for cytodifferentiation. In the mouse, the Prox1 and Maf genes have been demonstrated to mediate lens fiber elongation.[88,110] As these posterior epithelial cells lengthen to fill the lumen of the lens vesicle, they lose their nucleus and most organelles.[14] Upregulation of lens-specific proteins, CP49 and CP95, is demonstrated after closure of the lens stalk.[51] The primitive lens filled with primary lens fibers is the *embryonic lens nucleus*. After the epithelial cells

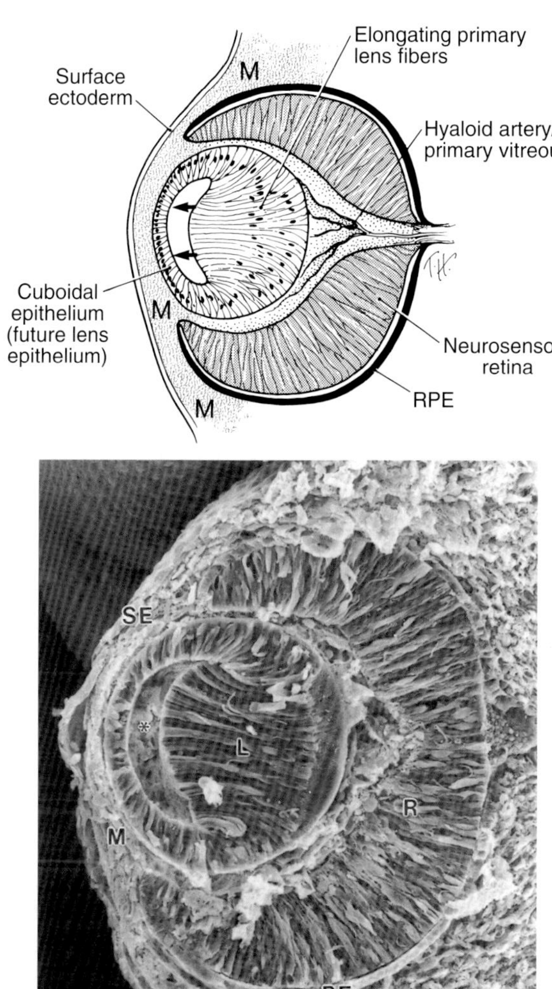

FIGURE 1-14. Formation of the embryonic lens nucleus and primary lens fibers at approximately 7 weeks. Note that mesenchyme (*M*) of neural crest origin surrounds the optic cup. The posterior lens epithelial cells (located nearest the developing retina, *R*) elongate, forming the primary lens fibers (*L*). The anterior epithelium remains cuboidal and becomes the anterior epithelium in the adult. The optic fissure is now closed.

of the posterior lens elongate to form the fibers of the embyronal nucleus, they eventually separate from the posterior capsule; therefore, there is an absence of epithelial cells on the posterior capsule. In the adult, the embryonic nucleus is the central round, slightly dark sphere inside the Y sutures. There are no sutures within the embryonal nucleus. The lens fibers have extensive interdigitations with a relative absence of extracellular space. Anterior lens epithelial cells (nearest the corneal anlage) remain cuboidal and become the permanent lens epithelium, which is mitotic throughout life, giving rise to future secondary fetal and adult cortical lens fibers.

After the embryonic nucleus is formed, *secondary lens fibers* develop from anterior epithelial cells to form the fetal nucleus. The anterior epithelial cells migrate to the periphery of the lens (lens equator), where they elongate and differentiate into lens fibers. This region of the lens is called the *lens bow*. These secondary lens fibers elongate anteriorly and posteriorly around the embryonic nucleus to meet at the anterior and posterior poles of the lens (Fig. 1-15). The lens fibers exhibit surface interdigitations with relative lack of extracellular space. Unlike more mature cortical lens fibers that have tapered ends, these fetal lens fibers (secondary lens fibers) have blunt tips, so when they meet they form a faint adherence or "suture." This meeting of the secondary lens fiber ends results in two Y sutures, the anterior upright Y suture and the posterior inverted Y suture

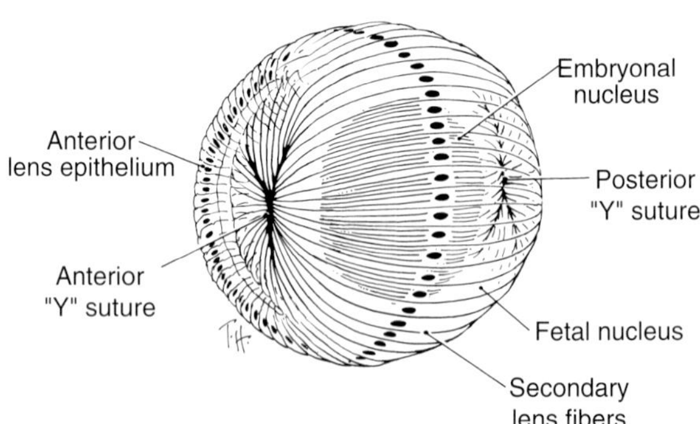

FIGURE 1-15. Diagram of secondary lens fibers and Y sutures. Secondary lens fibers elongate at the equator to span the entire lens, from the anterior Y suture to the posterior Y suture. The anterior Y suture is upright and the posterior Y suture is inverted.

(Fig. 1-15). The fetal nucleus consists of the secondary lens fibers and can be clinically identified as that part of the central lens that is inside the Y sutures but outside the embryonic nucleus. The lens differentiates under the influence of many growth factors, including FGF, IGF, PDGF, and TGF, and genes become active encoding cytoskeletal proteins (filensin, phakinin, vimentin, nestin), structural proteins (crystallins), and membrane proteins.[39,118] Abnormal initiation and differentiation of secondary lens fibers have been demonstrated in the Cat2 and Cat3 mutant mouse strains. These eyes exhibit abnormalities limited to the lens, unlike the aphakia mutant eyes, which have malformations of the anterior segment and vitreous and folding of the retina.[40]

At birth, the lens is almost entirely made up of lens nucleus with minimal lens cortex. Lens cortex continues to develop from the anterior epithelial cells postnatally and throughout life. Congenital cataracts that occur as a result of abnormal formation of primary or secondary lens fibers would be expected to be localized in the nuclear region between the Y sutures. Abnormal lens vesicle separation from the surface ectoderm would be associated with defects in anterior epithelium or lens capsule and may cause anterior polar cataracts. Incomplete regression of the pupillary membrane can be associated with (secondary) anterior lens opacities. A defect of the surface ectoderm or basement membrane could result in cataracts associated with anterior or posterior lenticonus.

Tunica Vasculosa Lentis

The lens receives nutrition and blood supply from the *hyaloid artery*, a branch of the primitive ophthalmic artery. The hyaloid artery first enters the eye through the optic fissure (see Fig. 1-12) and then becomes incorporated into the center of the optic nerve as the optic fissure closes. The hyaloid vessels form a network around the posterior lens capsule and then anastomose anteriorly with the network of vessels in the pupillary membrane (Fig. 1-16). The pupillary membrane consists of vessels and mesenchyme that overlie the anterior lens capsule (see Development of Anterior Segment). This hyaloid vascular network that forms around the lens is called the *tunica vasculosa lentis*. The hyaloid vasculature reaches its greatest development at approximately 10 weeks gestation. The tunica vasculosa lentis and hyaloid artery regress during the end of the fourth month of

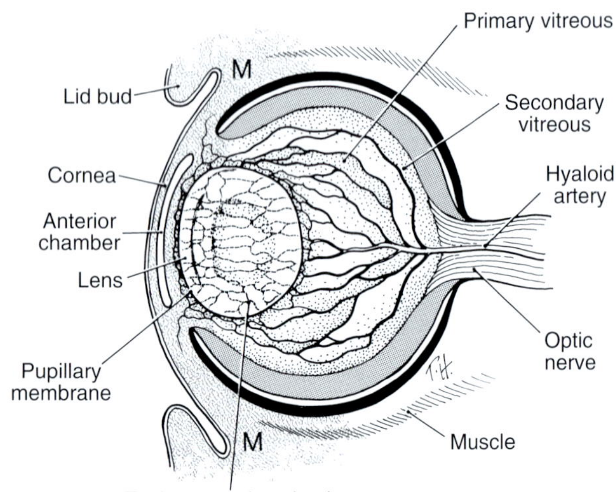

FIGURE 1-16. Drawing of a 2-month-old fetal eye shows the hyaloid vascular system and tunica vasculosa lentis.

gestation. The clinical lens anomaly, *Mittendorf's dot,* is a small (1–2 mm) area of fibrosis on the posterior capsule and is probably a manifestation of incomplete regression of the hyaloid artery where it attaches to the posterior capsule. The regression of the pupillary membrane begins during the sixth month and is usually complete by the eighth month. *Persistent pupillary membranes* result from incomplete regression. These iris strands may connect to an anterior polar cataract (Fig. 1-17) or area of corneal endothelial fibrosis.

CORNEA AND ANTERIOR CHAMBER

The anterior margins of the optic cup advance beneath the surface ectoderm and its subjacent mesenchyme following lens vesicle detachment at approximately day 33 of gestation. The surface ectoderm overlying the optic cup and lens represents the presumptive *corneal epithelium*; it secretes a thick matrix producing the *primary cornea stroma*.[43] This acellular material consists of collagen fibers, hyaluronic acid, and glycosaminoglycans. Neural crest cells migrate between the surface ectoderm and

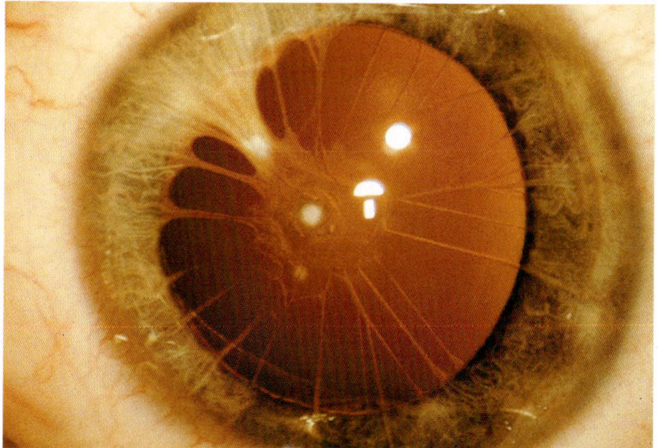

FIGURE 1-17. Photograph of persistent pupillary membrane with small central anterior polar cataract.

optic cup using the basal lamina of the lens vesicle as a substrate or scaffold.[11] Hydration of hyaluronic acid helps to create the space for cellular migration.[105] This loosely arranged neural crest cell-derived mesenchyme initially fills the future anterior chamber and gives rise to the corneal stroma, corneal endothelium, the anterior iris stroma, the ciliary muscle, and most of the structures of the iridocorneal angle. Separation of the corneal mesenchyme (neural crest cell origin) from the lens (surface ectoderm origin) results in formation of the anterior chamber. Mesenchymal tissue surrounds the lens and forms the tunica vasculosa lentis and is continuous anteriorly with the pupillary membrane. Capillaries within the tunica vasculosa lentis anastomose with the hyaloid vascular system. The vascular endothelium appears to be the only component of the anterior segment that is of mesodermal origin, as even the vascular smooth muscle cells and pericytes are of neural crest origin.[55,64]

The anterior corneal stroma remains acellular and gives rise to *Bowman's membrane*, which underlies the corneal epithelium. Although the corneal epithelium is of surface ectodermal origin, Bowman's membrane is a condensation of anterior corneal stroma that is of neural crest cell origin. Type I collagen fibrils and fibronectin secreted by the developing keratocytes (neural crest cell origin) form the secondary corneal stroma. Subsequent dehydration of the corneal stroma results in loss of much of the fibronectin and a 50% reduction in thickness of the stroma.[44,65] The endothelium plays an important role in the dehydration of the stroma. Patches of endothelium become confluent during the early part of the fourth month of gestation and develop zonulae occludentes at their apices by the middle of the fourth month of gestation.[115] By the sixth month of gestation, *Descemet's membrane* and *endothelium* are structurally and functionally present and, at this time, the cornea achieves relative transparency. Proteoglycans containing keratan sulfate chains play a role in generating and maintaining corneal transparency.[34]

IRIS AND CILIARY BODY

The two layers of the optic cup (neural ectoderm origin) consist of an inner nonpigmented layer and an outer pigmented layer. Both the pigmented and nonpigmented epithelia of the iris and ciliary body develop from the anterior aspect of the optic cup whereas the retina develops from the posterior optic cup. The optic vesicle is organized with all cell apices directed to the center of the vesicle (see Figs. 1-10, 1-11). During optic cup invagination, the apices of the inner and outer epithelial layers become adjacent. Thus, the cells of the optic cup are oriented apex to apex.

A thin periodic acid–Schiff-(PAS) positive basal lamina lines the inner aspect (vitreous side) of the nonpigmented epithelium and retina (inner limiting membrane). At approximately 4.5 months, both the pigmented and nonpigmented epithelial cells show apical cilia that project into the intercellular space. There is also increased prominence of Golgi complexes and associated vesicles within the ciliary epithelial cells.[12] These changes and the presence of "ciliary channels" between apical surfaces probably represent the first production of aqueous humor.[113]

The iris develops by an anterior growth of the optic cup. The iris stroma develops from the anterior segment mesenchymal tissue of neural crest cell origin. The iris epithelium, including the pupillary sphincter and dilator muscles, originates from the neural ectoderm of the optic cup.[51,62,63,104] The smooth muscles of the pupillary sphincter and dilator muscles represent the only muscles in the body of neural ectodermal origin. In avian species, however, the pupillary muscles are striated and originate from stromal mesenchymal (neural crest) cells that migrate into the muscle bundles to become skeletal muscle cells.[116,117]

The ciliary body develops as the neuroectoderm of the anterior optic cup folds, and underlying mesenchyme differentiates into the ciliary muscles. Tertiary vitreous in the area of the ciliary body folds develops into lens zonules.

IRIDOCORNEAL ANGLE

Iridocorneal angle maturation begins during the 15th week of gestation through a combination of processes.[85–87] Differential growth of the vascular tunic results in posterior movement of the iris and ciliary body relative to the trabecular meshwork and exposure of the outflow pathways.[4] *Schlemm's canal* is identified during the 16th week.[114] There is gradual cellular rearrangement and mesenchymal atrophy, as well as enlargement of numerous large spaces, until they become confluent with the anterior chamber.[98] The corneal trabeculae enlarges and the corneal endothelium covering the angle recess regresses. The discontinuity of the cellular layer covering the angle and the many lacunae present in late gestation may be correlated with the normal development of an increase in the outflow facility of aqueous humor. It may be speculated that, if the splitting and rebuilding of the endothelial membrane lining of the early iridocorneal angle is arrested, a block to normal outflow may result. Persistence of the endothelial (Barkan's) membrane has been postulated to be of significance in the pathogenesis of congenital glaucoma.[13,42,61,68,70,111] Postnatal remodeling of the drainage angle is associated with cellular necrosis and phagocytosis by macrophages, resulting in opening of the spaces of Fontana (clefts in the trabecular meshwork) and outflow pathways.[86,87]

Studies using staining for neuron-specific enolase (NSE) indicate that, although most of the structures of the iridocorneal angle are of neural crest origin, the endothelial lining of Schlemm's canal (like the vascular endothelium) is mesodermal.[1,78]

CHOROID AND SCLERA

Both the choroid and the sclera are of neural crest origin. The anterior sclera forms as a condensation of mesenchymal tissue that is continuous with the cornea (see Fig. 1-13). This condensation progresses posteriorly toward the optic nerve and, by approximately 12 weeks, the mesenchymal condensation has enveloped the optic nerve. The lamina cribrosa consists of mesenchymal cells that have penetrated the optic nerve. The cornea and sclera are derived from the same mesenchymal tissue, except for the corneal epithelium, which is of surface ectoderm origin.

The choroid is a highly vascular pigmented tissue that develops from mesenchymal tissue (neural crest) surrounding endothelial blood spaces (mesoderm). The blood spaces organize and give rise to the embryonic choriocapillaris at approximately 2 months of gestation.[16,45,80] At approximately 4 months, the choriocapillaris connects with the short posterior arteries and joins with the outer venous layer and the four vortex veins. Outside the choriocapillaris, multiple anastomoses between arterioles and venules occur, thus forming the fetal choroid plexus.

RETINA

The retina develops from neural ectoderm, with the retinal pigment epithelium (RPE) developing from the outer layer of the optic cup and the neurosensory retina developing from the inner layer of the optic cup (Figs. 1-11, 1-12, 1-13, 1-14, 1-18). As with the ciliary epithelium, invagination of the optic vesicle causes the apices of the inner nonpigmented layer to be directed

FIGURE 1-18A–C. **(A)** At approximately 38 days, the hyaloid vasculature surrounds the lens (*L*) with capillaries that anastomose with the tunica vasculosa lentis. Axial migration of mesenchyme forms the corneal stroma and endothelium (*C*). The retina (*R*) is becoming stratified while the pigment epithelium (*PE*) remains cuboidal. **(B)** By day 41, the retina has segregated into inner (*IN*) and outer (*ON*) neuroblastic layers. The ganglion cells are the first to differentiate, giving rise to the nerve fiber layer (*arrowhead*). The pigment epithelium has become artifactually separated from the neural retina in this specimen. (From Cook CS, Sulik KK. Scanning Electron Microsc 1986;III:1215–1227, with permission.) **(C)** Differentiation of the retina progresses from the central to the peripheral regions. At this time, the inner (*IN*) and outer (*ON*) neuroblastic layers are apparent at the posterior pole but, peripherally, the retina consists of outer nuclear and inner marginal zones. Between the inner and outer neuroblastic layers is a clear zone, the transient fiber layer of Chievitz. *PE*, pigment epithelium; *arrowhead*, nerve fiber layer. (From Cook CS, Sulik KK. Scanning Electron Microsc 1986;III:1215–1227, with permission.)

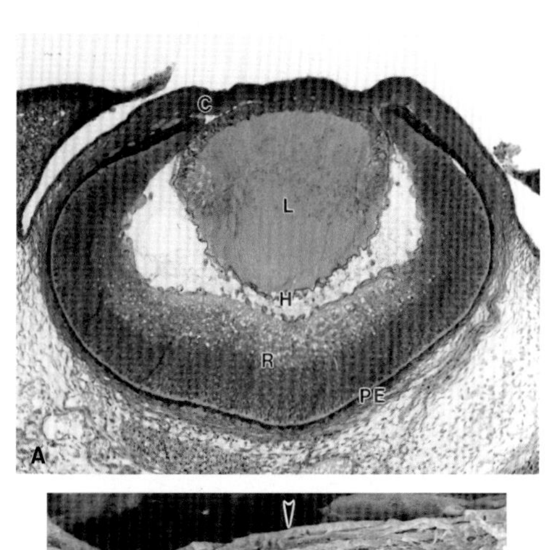
C
L
H
R
PE
A

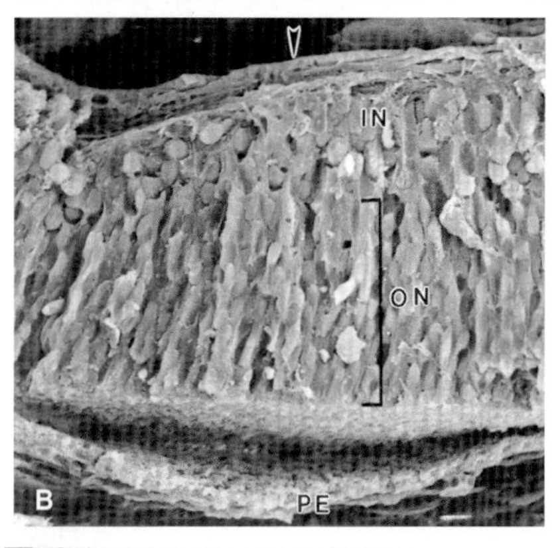
IN
ON
B
PE

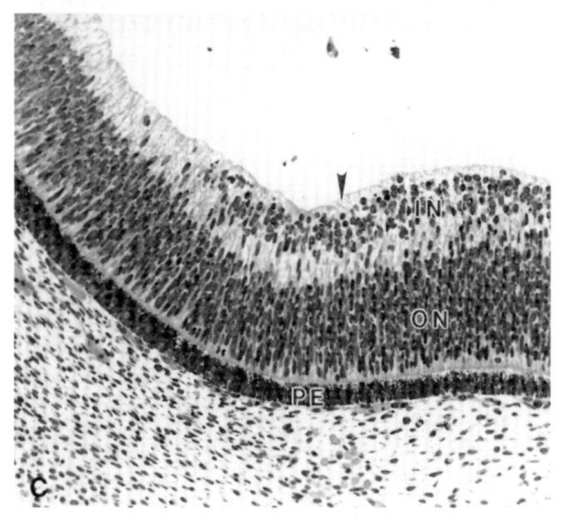
IN
ON
PE
C

outward, to face the apices of the outer pigmented layer, which are directed inward. Thus, the apices of these two cell layers are in direct contact. Primitive RPE cells are columnar, but by 5 weeks they change shape to form a single layer of cuboidal cells that exhibit the first pigment granules in the embryo. Bruch's membrane, the basal lamina of the RPE, is first seen during this time (optic cup stage) and becomes well developed by 6 weeks when the choriocapillaris is starting to form. By 4 months, the RPE cells take on a hexagonal shape on cross section and develop microvilli that interdigitate with projections from photoreceptors of the nonpigmented layer.

By the sixth week postfertilization, the nonpigmented inner layer of the optic cup differentiates into an outer nuclear zone and an inner marginal zone. Cell proliferation occurs in the nuclear zone with migration of cells into the marginal zone. This process forms the inner and outer neuroblastic layers (Fig. 1-18B,C), separated by their cell processes, which make up the transient fiber layer of Chievitz. With further realignment of cells, this layer is mostly obliterated by 8 to 10 weeks gestation. The ganglion cells of the inner neuroblastic layer are the first to differentiate (7th week), giving rise to a primitive nerve fiber layer (Fig. 1-18B,C, arrow).

By the 16th week, mitosis has nearly ceased and retinal differentiation commences, as does synaptic contact between retinal neurons.[99] Cellular differentiation progresses in a wave from inner to outer layers and from central retina to peripheral retina (Fig. 1-18C). The ganglion cells give rise to a more defined nerve fiber layer that courses to the developing optic nerve. Cell bodies of the Mueller and amacrine cells differentiate in the inner portion of the outer neuroblastic layer; bipolar cells are found in the middle of the outer neuroblastic layer, with horizontal cells and photoreceptors maturing last, in the outermost zone of the retina.[99] Early in development, retinal cells demonstrate neurite regeneration in vitro. This regenerative capability decreases with age and is lost postnatally in the rat at a time that corresponds to the time of eye opening and retinal maturation (equivalent to the eighth month of human gestation).[106] Thy-1, the most abundant surface glycoprotein found in the retina, is primarily associated with ganglion cells and appears to regulate neurite outgrowth.[97]

Macular differentiation occurs relatively late, beginning in the sixth month.[46] First, multiple rows of ganglion cells accumulate in the central macular area. At this time, the immature cones are localized in the central macular area while the rods develop in the periphery. At 7 months, the inner layers of the retina (including ganglion cells) spread out to form the central macular depression or primitive fovea. The cones in the foveal area elongate, allowing denser cone populations and enhanced foveal resolution. These changes in foveal cones continue until after birth. At birth, the fovea is fairly well developed and consists of a single row of ganglion cells, a row of bipolar cells, and a horizontal outer plexiform layer of Henle. It is not until several months postpartum that the ganglion cells and bipolar cells completely vacate the fovea centralis.

Retinal Vasculature

The fetal ophthalmic artery is a branch of the internal carotid artery and terminates into the hyaloid artery. The hyaloid artery enters the optic cup via the optic fissures and stalk (developing optic nerve) (see Fig. 1-12). At approximately 6 weeks gestation, the ophthalmic artery becomes entrapped in the optic cup as the optic fissure closes. The portion of the hyaloid artery within the optic stalk eventually becomes the central retinal artery, while the more terminal parts of the hyaloid artery arborize around the posterior aspect of the developing lens. The hyaloid artery gradually atrophics and regresses as branches of the hyaloid artery become sporadically occluded by macrophages.[52,54] Regression of the hyaloid vasculature is usually complete by the fifth month of human gestation. *Bergmeister's papilla* represents a remnant of the hyaloid vasculature that does not regress; this is a benign anomaly consisting of a small fibrous glial tuft of tissue that emanates from the center of the optic disc.

The hyaloid vasculature is the primary source of nutrition to the embryonic retina. Regression of the hyaloid vasculature serves to stimulate retinal vessel angiogenesis. Spindle-shaped mesenchymal cells from the wall of the hyaloid vein at the optic disc form buds that invade the nerve fiber layer during the fourth month of gestation.[6] Subsequently, solid cords of mesenchymal cells within the inner retina canalize and contain occasional red blood cells at approximately 5 months gestation. In situ differentiation of craniofacial angioblasts has been demonstrated in avian species using polyclonal antibodies to quail endothelial cells.[75] Vascular budding and further differentiation form the deeper capillary network in the retina.[73] The primitive capillaries have laminated walls consisting of mitotically active cells secreting basement membrane.[95] Those cells in direct contact with the bloodstream differentiate into endothelial cells while the outer cells become pericytes. Tissue culture experiments have demonstrated that the primitive capillary endothelial cells are multipotent and can redifferentiate into fibroblastic, endothelial, or muscle cells, possibly illustrating a common origin of these different tissue types.[6] Pigment epithelium derived factor (PEDF) has been demonstrated to inhibit angiogenesis of the cornea and vitreous. Inadequate levels may play a permissive role in ischemia-driven aberrant vascularization.[33]

The central retinal artery grows from the optic nerve to the periphery, forming the temporal and nasal retinal arcades. By approximately 5 months, the retinal arcades have progressed to the equator of the eye. At this time, the long and short posterior ciliary arteries are well developed, with the long posterior artery supplying the anterior segment and the short posterior artery supplying the choroid. The retinal arteries grow from the optic nerve toward the ora serrata and reach the nasal periphery first (by 8 months).[73] Even at birth, however, there is usually a crescent of avascular retina in the temporal periphery. The fact that a newborn infant has an immature temporal retina without complete vascularization may explain why there have been scattered cases of retinopathy of prematurity in full-term infants. Oxygen affects angiogenesis and seems to play a role in stimulating and retarding vessel growth.[83] In immature kitten retinas, increased oxygen concentration causes atrophy and regression of capillaries whereas hypoxia increases capillary arborization.[79] Endothelial cell growth is also promoted by low oxygen tension, and endothelial growth is inhibited by high oxygen tension.[7] *Vasoendothelial growth factor (VEGF)* both stimulates and maintains normal vessel growth to the peripheral retina. High oxygen downregulates VEGF, stopping the normal process of peripheral vascularization.[2,58,84] These findings give rise to the hypothesis that retinopathy of prematurity (ROP) is secondary to initial increased oxygen concentration, which results in inhibition or retraction of peripheral capillary networks (*vaso-obliteration*).[5] This lack of peripheral capillary network subsequently results in retinal hypoxia increased VEGF then secondary endothelial cell growth and neovascularization (i.e., ROP).[82] There is evidence that strict curtailment of O_2 dose early in a premature infants course reduces the incidence of severe ROP.[112a]

VITREOUS

The primary vitreous first appears at approximately 5 weeks gestation and consists of the hyaloid vessels surrounded by mesenchymal cells, collagenous fibrillar material, and macrophages (see Fig. 1-12). Most of the mesenchymal cells are of neural crest origin. The secondary vitreous forms at approximately 8 weeks at the time of fetal fissure closure (see Fig. 1-13).[9] It circumferentially surrounds the primary vitreous containing the hyaloid vessels. The secondary vitreous consists of a gel containing compact fibrillar network, primitive hyalocytes, monocytes, and a small amount of hyaluronic acid.[19] Primitive hyalocytes produce collagen fibrils that expand the volume of the secondary vitreous. At the end of the third month, the tertiary vitreous forms as a thick accumulation of collagen fibers between the lens and optic cup (Fig. 1-19). These fibers are called the marginal bundle of Drualt. Drualt's bundle has a strong attachment to the inner layer of the optic cup and is the precursor to the vitreous base and lens zonules. The early lens zonular fibers appear

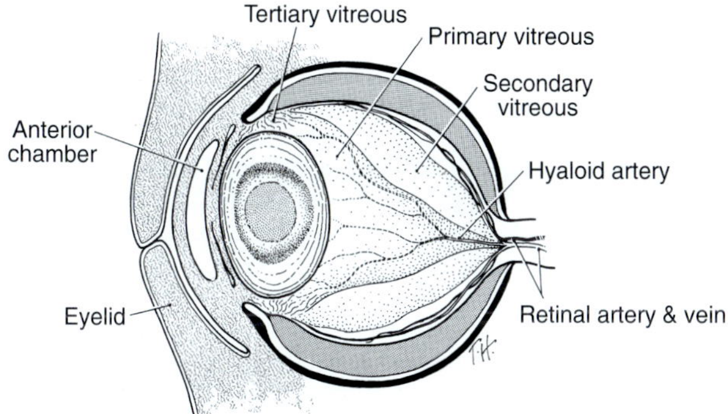

FIGURE 1-19. Drawing of cross section of a 10-week-old eye shows the primary vitreous, secondary vitreous, and tertiary vitreous. The primary vitreous includes the hyaloid artery and associated matrix; it extends centrally from the optic nerve to the retrolental space. The secondary vitreous surrounds the primary vitreous; it has less vasculature and is clearer than the primary vitreous. The tertiary vitreous forms between the lens equator and the area of the ciliary body; the lens zonules develop within the fibrillar matrix in this. Note that eyelids are fused at this stage.

to be continuous with the inner limiting membrane of the nonpigmented epithelial layer covering the ciliary muscle. Toward the end of the fourth month of gestation, the primary vitreous and hyaloid vasculature atrophies to a clear, narrow central zone, *Cloquet's canal.* Apoptosis occurs during hyaloid vessel regression.[51] Persistence of the primary vitreous and failure of the posterior tunica vasculosa lentis to regress can result in *persistent hyperplastic vitreous* (PHPV). PHPV consists of a fibrovascular membrane that extends from the optic nerve along the hyaloid remnant and covers the posterior capsule of the lens. During the fifth month of gestation, an attachment forms between the ciliary body and the lens (*Weiger's ligament,* or capsulohyaloidal ligament). Later in development, at approximately 5 to 6 months, the hyaloid system completely regresses and the hyaloid artery blood flow ceases. At birth, Cloquet's canal persists as an optically clear zone emanating from the optic nerve to the back of the lens. Cloquet's canal is a remnant of primary vitreous. Most of the posterior vitreous gel at birth is secondary vitreous with the vitreous base and zonules representing tertiary vitreous.

OPTIC NERVE

The optic stalk is the initially hollow structure connecting the optic vesicle with the forebrain. At approximately 6 weeks gestation, axons from developing ganglion cells pass through vacuolated cells from the inner wall of the optic stalk. Emanating from the center of the primitive nerve is the hyaloid artery. A glial sheath forms around the hyaloid artery. As the hyaloid artery regresses, a space between the hyaloid artery and the glial sheath enlarges. Bergmeister's papilla represents a remnant of these glial cells around the hyaloid artery. The extent of the Bergmeister's papilla is dependent on the amount of hyaloid and glial cell regression. Glial cells in this area migrate into the optic nerve and form the primitive optic disc. The glial cells around the optic nerve and the glial part of the lamina cribrosa come from the inner layer of the optic stalk, which is of neural ectoderm origin. Later, there is development of a mesenchymal (neural crest cell) portion of the lamina cribrosa. By the third month, the optic nerve shifts nasally as the temporal aspect of the posterior pole enlarges. The *tissue of Kuhnt,* which circumferentially surrounds the intraocular part of the optic nerve and acts as a barrier between the optic nerve and retina, comes from glial tissue in the region of the disc and mesenchyme from nearby developing retinal vasculature. Myelinization of the optic nerve starts at the chiasm at about 7 months gestation and progresses toward the eye. Normally, myelinization stops at the lamina cribrosa at about 1 month after birth. At birth, the myelin is thin, with the layers of myelin increasing into late childhood.

Myelinated nerve fibers occur if the myelinization continues past the lamina cribrosa (Fig. 1-20). The best explanation as to why myelinization passes the lamina cribrosa is the presence of heterotopic oligodendrocytes or glial cells within the retinal nerve fiber layer. This concept contrasts with the theory that there is a congenital defect in the lamina cribrosa that allows myelinization to progress into the retina. Autopsy studies of myelinated nerve fibers have failed to show a defect in the lamina cribrosa; therefore, myelinated nerve fibers most probably represent ectopic myelinization.[100,101] Myelinization of the nerve fibers is often associated with high myopia and amblyopia. Patients with this disorder should be aggressively treated by correcting the refractive error and initiating occlusion

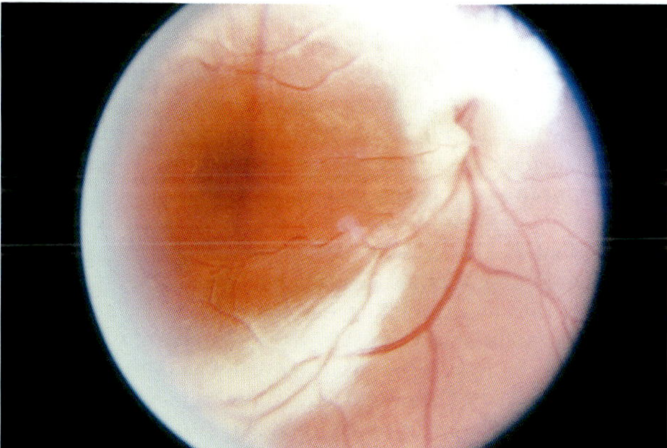

FIGURE 1-20. Photograph of myelinated nerve fibers emanating from the disc. Myelinated nerve fibers will cause a local scotoma; however, in the macular and foveal region, their presence does not usually preclude good central vision.

therapy of the sound eye to treat the amblyopia, as good visual outcome can be achieved even when there is macular involvement.[103]

EYELIDS

The eyelids develop from surface ectoderm that gives rise to the epidermis, cilia, and conjunctival epithelium. Neural crest cell mesenchyme gives rise to deeper structures including the dermis and tarsus. The eyelid muscles, orbicularis and levator, are derived from mesoderm. By 6 weeks of gestation, the upper and lower eyelid buds are visible (see Fig. 1-15). They come from mesenchymal accumulations called frontonasal (upper lid) and maxillary (lower lid) processes. The lid folds grow together and elongate to cover the developing eye. Upper and lower lids fuse together at approximately 10 weeks. By 6 months gestation, glandular structures and cilia develop, and the lids gradually separate.

EXTRAOCULAR MUSCLES

The extraocular muscles arise from mesoderm in somitomeres (preotic mesodermal segments), with the primitive muscle cone first appearing at 5 to 7 weeks gestation (Fig. 1-13). The oculomotor innervated muscles originate from the first and second somitomeres, the superior oblique muscle from the third somitomere, and the lateral rectus muscle from the fifth somitomere.[77] The motor nerves to the extraocular muscles grow from the brain to the muscle and innervate the mesodermal condensation at approximately 1 month.

The extraocular muscles develop from local mesenchyme (mesodermal origin) in situ within the orbit, rather than from anterior growth of surrounding mesoderm, as had been an earlier hypothesis. Additionally, muscles do not grow from the orbital apex anteriorly; rather, the insertion, belly, and origin develop simultaneously.[93,94] The orbital axes rotate from the early stages of optic cup development to adulthood.

OCULAR DYSGENESIS

Syndromes of ocular dysgenesis are summarized in Table 1-2.

Microphthalmia

Studies of ocular malformations induced by teratogen exposure have been helpful in identifying sensitive periods during development. Microphthalmia and anophthalmia may result from insult at a number of developmental stages. Acute exposure to teratogens during early gastrulation stages results in an overall deficiency of the neural plate with subsequent reduction in size of the optic vesicle. This aberration results in microphthalmia, which may be associated with a spectrum of secondary malformations including anterior segment dysgenesis, cataract, and PHPV.[24,27,28] Deficiency in size of the globe as a whole is often associated with a corresponding small palpebral fissure. Because the fissure size is determined by the size of the optic vesicle (most likely during its contact with the surface ectoderm), support is provided for a malformation sequence beginning at the time of formation of the optic sulcus or optic vesicle.

Failure or late closure of the optic fissure prevents the establishment of normal fetal IOP and can result in microphthalmia associated with colobomas, that is, colobomatous microphthalmia (Fig. 1-27). This syndrome may be associated with orbital (or eyelid) cysts (Fig. 1-28). It is important to recognize that delay in closure of the fissure during a critical growth period may result in inadequate globe expansion. However, if the fissure eventually closes, it may be difficult to distinguish between colobomatous and noncolobomatous microphthalmia. In colobomatous microphthalmia, the optic vesicle size is initially normal and a normal-sized palpebral fissure would be expected, whereas with microphthalmia that results from a primary abnormality in the neural plate and optic sulci, the palpebral fissure would be small.

Optic Fissure Closure Anomalies (Coloboma)

Colobomas represent an absence of tissue that may occur through abnormal fusion of the optic fissure, which normally closes at 4 to 5 weeks gestation. Colobomas may occur anywhere along the optic fissure and can affect the iris, choroid,

TABLE 1-2. Summary of Syndromes of Ocular Malformations.

Syndrome	*Microphthalmia*	*Anterior segment dysgenesis*	*Ocular coloboma*	*Glaucoma*
CHARGE	+		+	
Meckel's	+		+ Uveal	
Rubenstein–Taybi			+	
Basal cell nevus syndrome			+ Iris	
Cat's eye	+	+	+	
Axenfeld-Rieger's Autosomal dominant iridogoniodysgenesis		+		+ Gonio-dysgenesis
Nail patella		Iris hypoplasia Ciliary body hypoplasia		
Branchiootorenal		+		Cataract
Microphthalmia	+	+/−	+/−	+/−
Peters' anomaly	+/−	+		

TABLE 1-2. (continued)

Other ocular abnormalities	*Nonocular anomalies*	*Genetics (mice)*	*Genetics (human)*
	Choanal atresia Growth retardation Genital hypoplasia Ear anomalies (deafness) Hypospadias		+/− X-linked autosomal recessive
	Heart defect Renal/hepatic disease Occipital encephaloceles Microcephaly Hydrocephaly Cleft palate		Autosomal recessive condition mapped to chromosome 17q21-q24
Cataract Ptosis	Mental retardation Broad fingers and toes Short stature Cardiac anomalies Renal anomalies		Translocation involving chromosome 2p13.3 and 16p13.3
Strabismus Cataract	Hypertelorism Basal cell nevus Cleft lip/palate Mental retardation		CECR1 on 9q22.3-q31
	Anal atresia Preauricular skin tags Renal anomalies		22q11
Iris hypoplasia	Craniofacial Dental defects Hypertelorism	FoxC1 FoxC2 Mfl (mice)	FKHL7 gene 6p24-p25
		Lmx1B	Chromosome 9
Branchial arch	anomalies Ear anomalies	EYA1	
	Renal anomalies	17 Ccnf	16p13.3 14q32
Anterior lenticonus; cataract	Craniofacial Heart defects Dwarfism Syndactyly	Cat4a on chromosome 8	RIEG1 on chromosome 4q25

(continued)

TABLE 1-2. Summary of Syndromes of Ocular Malformations. (continued)

Syndrome	*Microphthalmia*	*Anterior segment dysgenesis*	*Ocular coloboma*	*Glaucoma*
Renal/coloboma		Optic disc coloboma		
Cyclopia/holo-procecephaly	+/−	+/−	+/−	+/−
Leber's congenital amaurosis				
Septooptic dysplasia				
Rieger's anterior segment dysgenesis		+		
Aniridia	+/−	+	+/−	+
Goldenhar's oculoauriculovertebral	+	Upper lid coloboma		

Source: NIH Online Mendelian Inheritance in Man: www3.ncbi.nlm.nih.gov/

macula, and optic nerve (Figs. 1-21, 1-22, 1-23). Colobomas are often associated with microphthalmia (colobomatous microphthalmia) or, less frequently, orbital or eyelid cysts (Fig. 1-22). Because the optic fissure closes first at the equator of the eye, and then in a posterior and anterior direction, colobomas are most frequently found at the two ends of the optic fissure, that is, iris and optic nerve. When the optic nerve is involved in the coloboma, vision is usually affected, in some cases causing blindness. Optic nerve colobomas may be associated with basal encephaloceles, which also represent a failure of fissure closure.[59,85] Large choroidal colobomas may be associated with posterior pole staphylomas, causing macular disruption and poor vision. Occasionally, a line of choroidal colobomas occur along the fetal fissure area with skip areas (Fig. 1-23). Isolated iris colobomas usually do not affect visual acuity unless there is an associated refractive error. Typical iris colobomas occur infer-

TABLE 1-2. (continued)

Other ocular abnormalities	*Nonocular anomalies*	*Genetics (mice)*	*Genetics (human)*
	Renal anomalies	19 Pax2	PAX2 on 10q24.3-q25.1
Cyclopia	Holoprocencephaly		Sonic hedgehog (SHH) on 7q36 HPE12on 1q22.3
Cataract pigmentary retinopathy Keratoconus	Central blindness Mental retardation	3 Rpe65	CRX Autosomal recessive RPE65 on 1p31
Optic disc hypoplasia	Growth hormone deficiency	14Hesx1	Autosomal recessive HESX1 on 3p21.1-3p21.2
Cataract ± Corneal opacity		Fra-2	Autosomal dominant 4q28-q31(PAX6), PITX3 on 10q25
Cataract Foveal hypoplasia	Wilm's tumor	2Sey	Autosomal dominant PAX6 on 11p13
Epibulbar dermoid	Ear malformations Facial asymmetry Vertebral anomalies		Autosomal dominant GHS on 7p

onasally along the location of the optic fissure whereas atypical iris colobomas are not associated with abnormal fissure closure and can occur elsewhere. Atypical iris colobomas usually have an intact iris root (Fig. 1-24).

Differentiation of choroidal and iris stroma is determined by the adjacent structures of the optic cup: the iris epithelium, anteriorly, and the future retinal pigment epithelium, posteriorly. In animals exhibiting primary abnormalities in differentiation of the outer layer of the optic cup, anterior and posterior segment colobomas are seen in a very specific distribution associated with the iris epithelium or RPE defects,[25,26] and this is the most likely explanation for atypical uveal colobomas. The term lens coloboma is actually a misnomer, as this defect results from a lack of the zonular pull in the region of the coloboma rather than regional hypoplasia of the lens. Ciliary body colobomas are often associated with abnormal lens shape or subluxation or both.

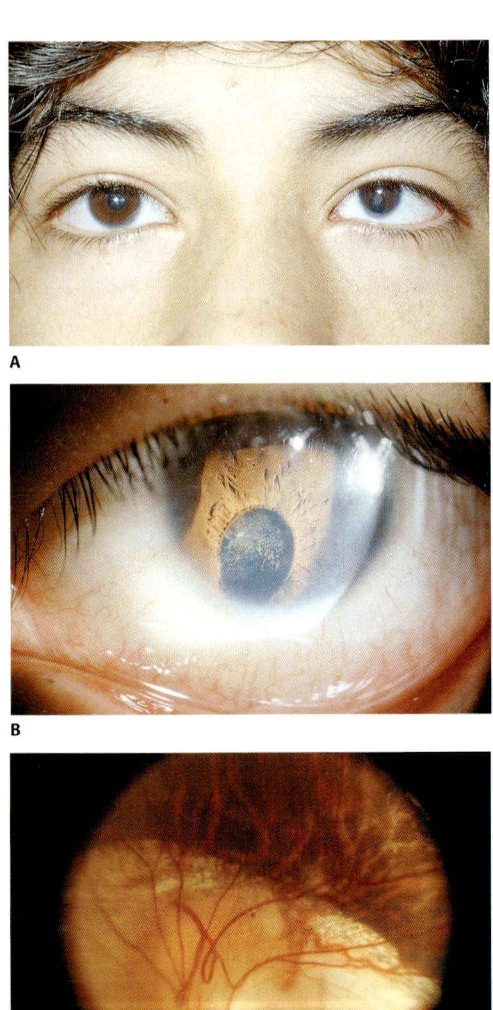

FIGURE 1-21A–C. (**A**) Photograph of patient with left colobomatous microphthalmia and normal right eye. (**B**) Slit lamp view of the iris coloboma left eye. Note the pigment on anterior capsule of the lens. (**C**) Optic nerve coloboma of left eye with inferior choroidal coloboma that extended anteriorly to meet the iris coloboma seen in (**B**).

Colobomatous microphthalmia with eyelid cyst syndrome may be unilateral or bilateral (see Fig. 1-28). Colobomatous cysts form from the inner layer (neuroectoderm) of the optic cup as it grows out of the persistent opening of the optic fissure. The lower lid cyst contains primitive vitreous contents that were not enclosed within the eye because the optic fissure did not close. The cyst has a stalk that connects to the microphthalmic eye. For those who are unaware of the syndrome, the lid cyst is often mistaken as an abnormal eye located in the lid.

Dermoids and Dermolipomas

Dermoids are choristomas (histologically normal tissue in an abnormal location) and are thought to represent arrest or inclusions of epidermal and connective tissues (surface ectoderm and neural crest cells). They may be associated with abnormal closure of the optic fissure. This collection of epidermal and connective tissue can occur at the limbus (limbal dermoid), in the conjunctiva (dermolipoma), and subcutaneously in and around the orbit. The most common location of subcutaneous periorbital dermoid cysts is the superotemporal and superonasal quadrants of the orbital rim. These dermoids are usually found attached to bone, associated with a cranial suture.

Limbal dermoids are similar to subcutaneous dermoid cysts and consist of epidermal tissue and, frequently, hair (Fig. 1-25). Corneal astigmatism is common in patients with limbal dermoids. Astigmatisms greater than +1.50 are usually associated with meridional and anisometropic amblyopia. Removal of limbal dermoids is often indicated for functional and cosmetic reasons, but the patient should be warned that a secondary scar can recur over this area. Limbal dermoids can involve deep corneal stroma, so the surgeon must take care to avoid perforation into the anterior chamber.

Dermolipomas (lipodermoids) are usually located in the lateral canthal area and consist of fatty fibrous tissue (Fig. 1-26). They are almost never a functional or cosmetic problem and are best left alone. If removal is necessary, only a limited dissection should be performed to avoid symblepharon and scarring of the lateral rectus. Unfortunately, restrictive strabismus with limited adduction frequently occurs after removal of temporal dermolipomas.

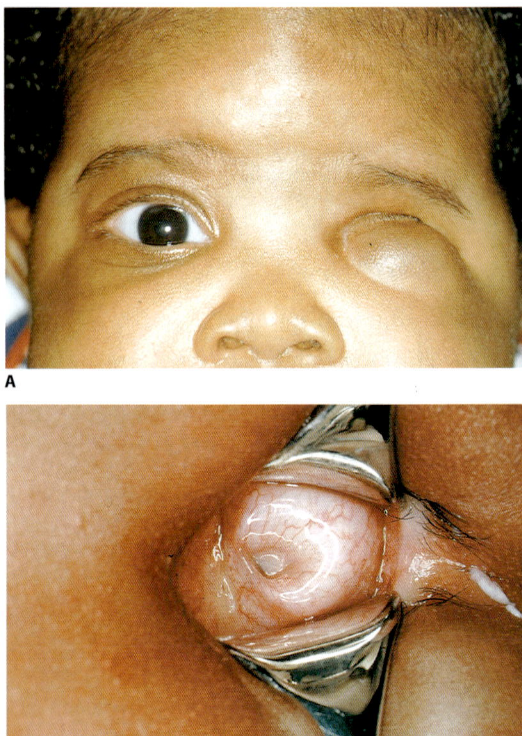

A

B

FIGURE 1-22A–B. **(A)** Photograph of 6-month-old with colobomatous microphthalmia and orbital cyst anomaly. Note the left lower eyelid cyst causing a mass in the lower lid, left blepharophimosis (small lids and narrow lid fissure), and apparently normal right eye. **(B)** Desmarres retractors open the eyelids in an attempt to expose the microphthalmic left eye. The only remnant of eye that could be seen externally was a small dimple just nasal to the lid retractors.

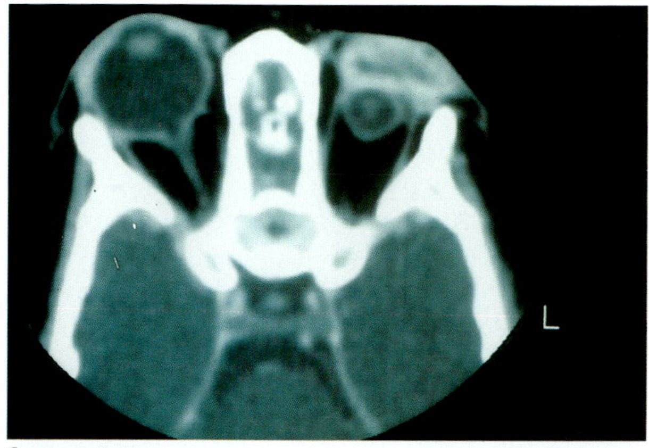

C

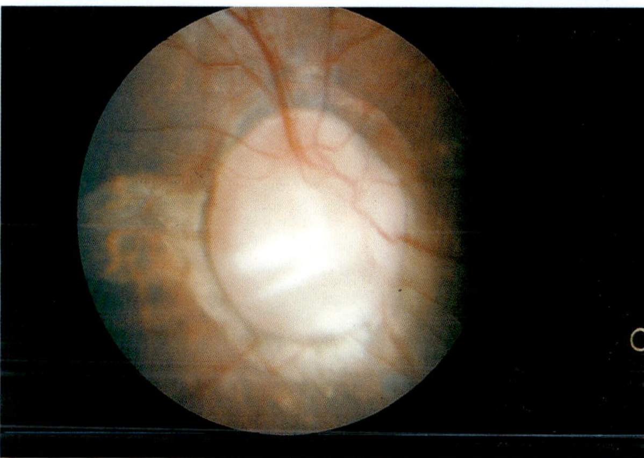

D

FIGURE 1-22C–D. **(C)** CT scan shows the presence of a left microphthalmic eye, left lower lid cyst, and right optic nerve coloboma. At the time of surgery to remove the cyst, a stalk was found connecting the cyst to the microphthalmic eye. **(D)** Fundus photograph of optic nerve, right eye (good eye). Note the presence of a large optic nerve coloboma. This was an isolated optic nerve coloboma; the right eye was otherwise normal.

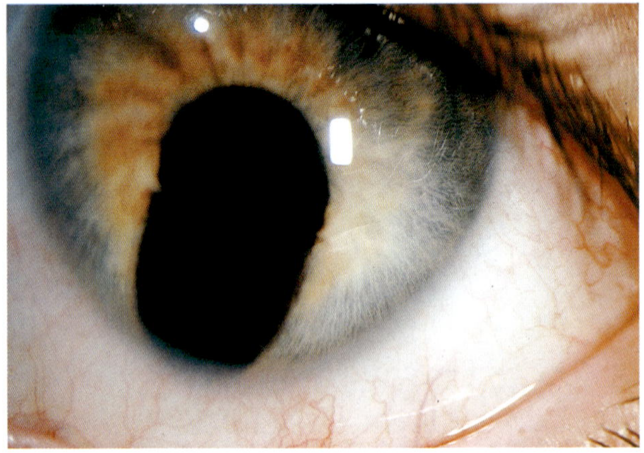

A

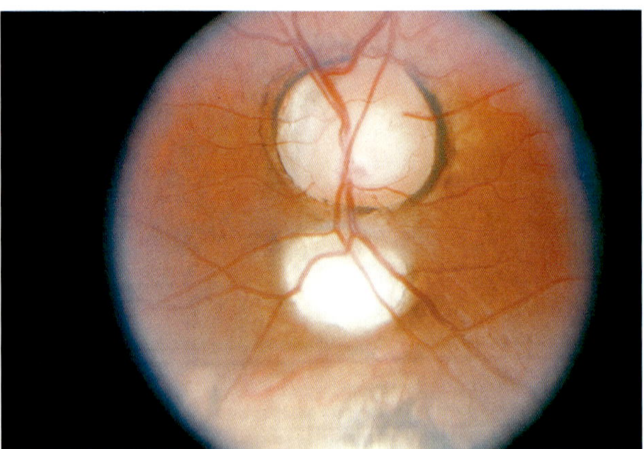

B

FIGURE 1-23A,B. Patient with iris (**A**) and choroidal and optic nerve (**B**) colobomas in typical inferior location. Note the choroidal skip lesion inferior to the disc.

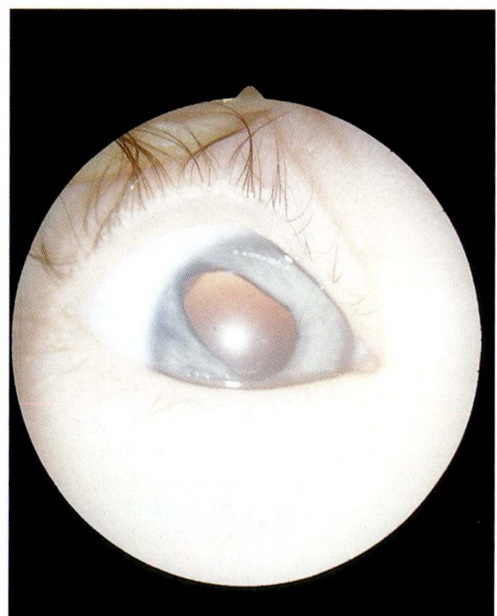

FIGURE 1-24. Photograph of ectropion uvea caused by peripheral anterior stromal membrane pulling the pupillary margin forward, exposing posterior pigment epithelium. Note there is an associated corectopia and dyscoria. The appearance of the eccentric pupil could be classified as an atypical iris coloboma. This is not a true coloboma because of the location and the presence of an intact iris root.

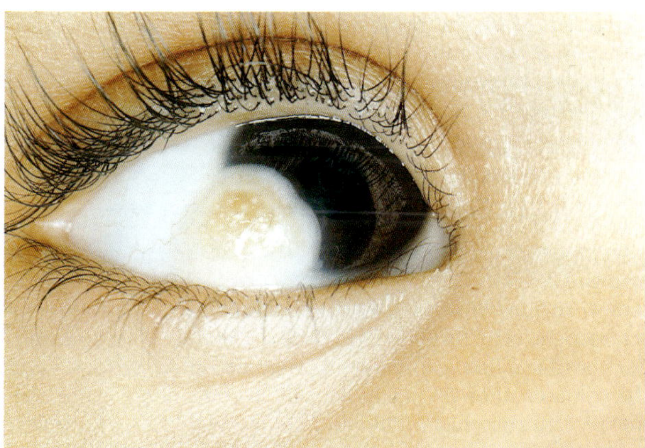

FIGURE 1-25. Isolated limbal dermoid at inferotemporal limbus, right eye. Hair cilia emanates from the center of the lesion. These limbal dermoids are often associated with large astigmatisms and can cause astigmatic, anisometropic amblyopia.

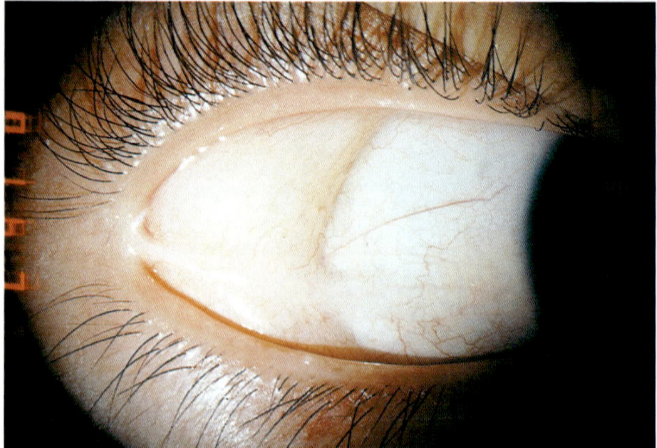

FIGURE 1-26. Dermolipoma in lateral canthal area, right eye. These are benign; however, if removed, can cause restrictive strabismus and fat adherence syndrome.

Goldenhar's syndrome (oculoauriculovertebral dysplasia) is a clefting anomaly of the first brachial arch and is associated with neural crest cell abnormalities. Goldenhar's syndrome is characterized by the combination of epibulbar dermoids (dermolipomas and limbal dermoids), ocular coloboma (Fig. 1-27), incomplete cryptophthalmos or lid colobomas, preauricular skin tags, vertebral anomalies, and, sporadically, with heart and pulmonary defects.

Cryptophthalmos

Cryptophthalmos is a congenital failure of lid and eye separation and development. In most cases, cryptophthalmos is inherited as an autosomal recessive trait, which may include mental retardation, cleft lip or palate, cardiac anomalies, or genitourinary abnormalities. The eyelids may be colobomatous, with the colobomatous lid fusing with the peripheral cornea or conjunctiva (incomplete cryptophthalmos; Fig. 1-27). Complete cryptophthalmos is a total absence of normal eyelids and lid fold, with the eye covered by skin that is adherent to an abnormal cornea. The cornea is often thin, being replaced by a

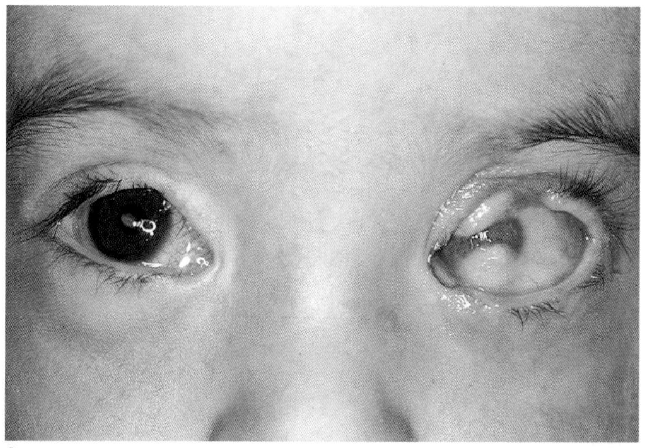

A

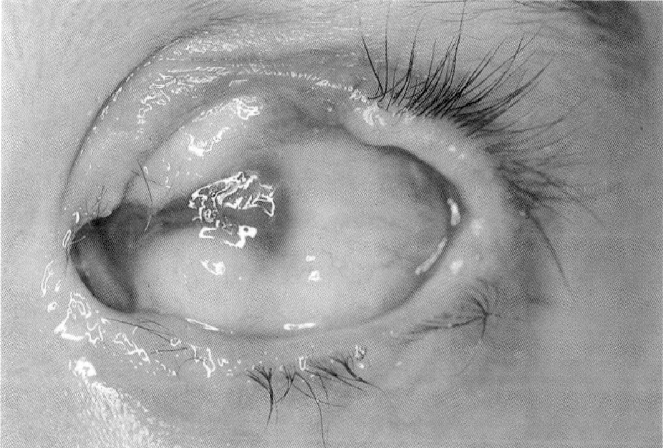

B

FIGURE 1-27A,B. **(A)** Photograph of a patient with Goldenhar's syndrome and incomplete cryptophthalmos of left eye. Cryptophthalmos consists of fusion of the upper lid to the cornea of the left eye. In addition to cryptophthalmos, patient has bilateral upper lid colobomas and left inferior limbal dermoid. **(B)** Close-up view of the left eye shows upper lid coloboma and cryptophthalmos with upper lid adhesion to the cornea and conjunctiva and inferior dermoid cyst.

fibrovascular tissue rather than clear cornea. The anterior segment is often abnormal, having a small or absent lens and anomalies of the iris or ciliary body. When associated with microphthalmia and anterior segment dysgenesis, this developmental abnormality is initiated at the optic vesicle stage with secondary effects on neural crest and surface ectoderm. In the rare cases where the globe and anterior segment are normal, cryptophthalmos could be caused by an abnormality in surface ectoderm.

Cornea Plana

Cornea plana is a failure of the cornea to steepen relative to the curvature of the globe and normally occurs between the third and fourth month of gestation. This failure to steepen results in a relatively flat cornea. Cornea plana can be associated with other anterior segment anomalies (Fig. 1-28) or inherited as an autosomal dominant or recessive trait.

Sclerocornea

Sclerocornea is a condition in which the junction between the cornea and sclera is indistinct. Additionally, the cornea appears

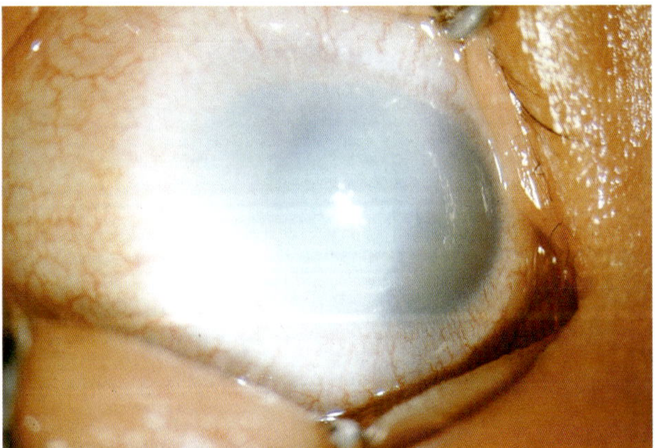

FIGURE 1-28. Photograph of congenital corneal opacity involving the temporal half of the cornea. Handheld slit lamp examination revealed iris strands to the cornea, flat peripheral cornea, and a blending of sclera and cornea in the periphery. The diagnosis is anterior chamber dysgenesis syndrome, including sclerocornea, cornea plana, and Peter's anomaly.

to be relatively small, as the limbal cornea is replaced by a mixture of cornea and scleral tissue.[67] Sclerocornea may be associated with other anomalies such as microphthalmia, coloboma, and anterior chamber dysgenesis (Fig. 1-28).

Anterior Segment Dysgenesis

Human anterior segment dysgenesis encompasses a broad spectrum of malformations including posterior embryotoxon, anterior displacement of Schwalbe's line, Axenfeld's anomaly (anterior displacement of Schwalbe's line associated with peripheral iris strands to Schwalbe's line), Peters' anomaly (central corneal opacity with absence of Descemet's membrane and endothelium in the area of the opacity), Rieger's anomaly (iris stromal hypoplasia with pseudopolycoria and iridocorneal attachments), or other combinations of iridocorneal or iridolenticular adhesions associated with various anterior segment anomalies. Congenital glaucoma is frequently associated with anterior segment dysgenesis syndromes.

Because most of the structures of the ocular anterior segment are of neural crest origin, it is tempting to incriminate this population of cells as being abnormal in differentiation or migration in cases of anterior segment dysgenesis. This theory has received widespread support and has resulted in labeling these conditions as "ocular neurocristopathie," particularly when other anomalies exist in tissues that are largely derived from neural crest cells (e.g., Rieger's syndrome; craniofacial connective tissue and teeth). There are several arguments in opposition to this theory. First, the neural crest is a predominant cell population of the developing craniofacial region including the eye. In fact, the number of tissues that are not neural crest derived is smaller than those which are (see Table 1-1). Thus, most malformations of this region would be expected to involve neural crest tissues, which may reflect their ubiquitous distribution rather than their common origin. The normal development of the choroid and sclera (also of neural crest origin) in anterior segment dysgenesis argues against a primary neural crest anomaly. Second, the neural crest is an actively migrating population of cells that is influenced by adjacent cell populations, and the perceived anomaly of neural crest tissue may be a secondary effect in many cases.

It is also important to recognize that, although much of the maturation of the iridocorneal angle occurs during the third trimester, much earlier events may influence anterior segment development. Anterior segment dysgenesis syndromes that are characterized primarily by axial deficits in corneal stroma and endothelium accompanied by corresponding malformations in the anterior lens capsule and epithelium (Peters' anomaly) most likely represent a manifestation of abnormal keratolenticular separation. The spectrum of malformations included in Peters' anomaly can be induced by teratogen exposure in mice at a time corresponding to the third week postfertilization in the human, just before optic sulcus invagination. Alternative theories for the pathogenic mechanism leading to Peters' anomaly, namely, intrauterine infection or anterior displacement of the lens or iris diaphragm, fail to explain the relatively localized axial defects.

Other anterior segment dysgenesis syndromes are characterized by more peripheral iridocorneal angle malformations and may represent malformations that are initiated somewhat later in gestation. These syndromes are often accompanied by absent or abnormal lining of Schlemm's canal, which is of mesodermal origin. In posterior polymorphous dystrophy and iridocorneal endothelial syndromes, the primary anomalies appear to be associated with the corneal endothelium and its basement membrane, both neural crest derivatives. Abnormal-appearing collagen within the trabecular meshwork has been identified in all these syndromes. Its significance is unknown; however, it may relate to neural crest abnormality.

Gene mutations that affect ocular neural crest cell populations and result in anterior segment dysgenesis have been identified. Of particular note is a genetic form of Rieger's syndrome caused by mutation in a homeobox transcription factor, PITX2.[3] In-situ hybridization in mice has shown that mRNA encoded by this gene is localized in the periocular mesenchyme.

Congenital Glaucoma

Although glaucoma may accompany any of the anterior segment syndromes described previously, elevated intraocular pressure (IOP) is usually not present at birth, in contrast to true congenital glaucoma. Earlier theories described the gonioscopic presence of a "Barkan's membrane" covering the trabecular meshwork in eyes with congenital glaucoma. Most histological examinations of affected eyes have failed to demonstrate such a membrane. Studies have revealed anterior displacement of the ciliary body and iris base, representing the immature conformation seen in fetuses during the second trimester. In the absence of other malformations, these cases of congenital (and juvenile) glaucoma most likely represent arrested maturation and remodeling of the iridocorneal angle, which occur during the last trimester.

Pupillary Anomalies

Corectopia is defined as an eccentric location of the pupil, which may be normal or malformed (Fig. 1-29). The pupil may have an abnormal shape (dyscoria) and not be in line with the lens. Corectopia may be associated with corresponding ectopia of the lens that may or may not be in line with the ectopic pupil. Colobomas can be mistaken as eccentric pupils, but true colobomas lack peripheral iris whereas corectopia has an intact peripheral iris. *Ectopia lentis et pupillae* is the eccentric location of both the lens and pupil, which may be eccentric together and in line or, more commonly, displaced in opposite directions (Fig. 1-29).

Polycoria is a condition in which there are many openings in the iris that result from local hypoplasia of the iris stroma and pigment epithelium. True polycoria actually is a condition in which there is more than one pupil and the multiple pupils all have a sphincter and the ability to contract. Most cases of

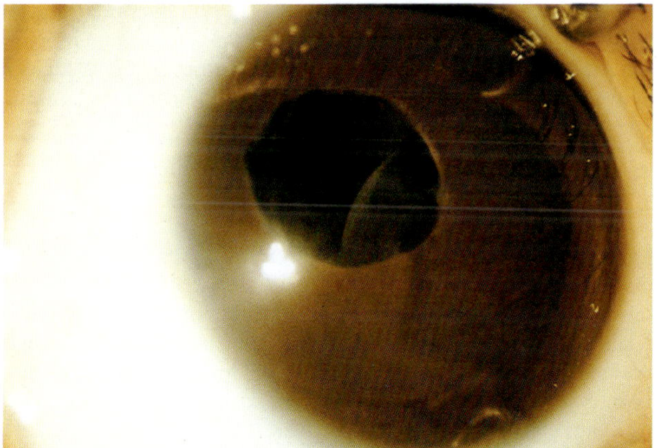

FIGURE 1-29. Photograph of corectopia associated with iris hypoplasia and ectopia lentis. Note that the corectopia is the opposite direction to the ectopia lentis.

polycoria, however, are actually pseudopolycoria as only one of the pupils is the true pupil with an iris sphincter muscle. Therefore, in almost all clinical situations, the correct term is *pseudopolycoria*. Iris stromal hypoplasia, in the absence of an iris epithelium defect, represents a defect in neural crest cell migration and development.

Ectropion uvea (congenital) is iris pigment epithelium that is present at the pupillary margin and on the anterior iris stroma, most likely caused by an exuberant growth of neural ectoderm over the iris stromal mesenchyme. It can also be caused by iris stromal atrophy or congenital fibrosis of the anterior iris stroma that contracts and everts the pupillary margin to expose the pigment epithelium. This last mechanism also results in corectopia (see Fig. 1-24).

Persistent Hyperplastic Primary Vitreous

Persistent hyperplastic primary vitreous (PHPV) relates to an abnormality in the regression of the primary vitreous in the hyaloid artery and is usually associated with microphthalmia. It is also referred to as persistent fetal vasculature. A fibrovascular stalk emanates from the optic nerve and attaches to the posterior capsule. The retrolenticular vascular membrane covers the posterior half of the lens and usually extends to attach to the ciliary processes. With time, the retrolenticular membrane contracts, pulling the ciliary processes centrally. If the lens and membrane are not removed, secondary glaucoma may occur. Early surgery (lensectomy and anterior vitrectomy) is indicated to prevent amblyopia and to maintain integrity of the eye.

Retinal Dysplasia

Disorganized differentiation of the retina is often seen as a component of multiple ocular malformation syndromes. The inner optic cup may continue to proliferate in a microphthalmic eye, leading to folds and rosettes. The retina is dependent on the underlying retinal pigment epithelium for normal differentiation. Expression of cyclin-dependent kinase inhibitor protein, p27(Kip1), precedes withdrawal of retinal cells from the cell cycle, leading to terminal differentiation. Displacement of p27(Kip1)-deficient Müller glia into the photoreceptor layer is associated with experimental retinal dysplasia.[66]

Malformation Complexes Involving the Eye, Brain, and Face

It is not surprising, considering that the eye is an extension of the brain, that developmental abnormalities of the eye and brain frequently are concurrent. Among the most severe brain malformations are those involving abnormal closure of the neural tube or severe forebrain midline reduction abnormalities. These malformations are frequently accompanied by anophthalmia, microphthalmia, anterior chamber cleavage abnormalities, or abnormal ocular placement (hypertelorism or hypotelorism, synophthalmia). Animal models have provided information regarding the developmental basis for a number of these malformation complexes. Because many of the relevant ocular abnormalities have been discussed earlier, the remainder of this chapter focuses on dysmorphogenesis of the brain and face.

Development of the forebrain and the midportion of the face above the oral cavity are intimately related. The olfactory (nasal) placodes become distinguishable on the frontolateral aspects of the frontonasal prominence during the fourth week of gestation. The thickened olfactory ectoderm is initially part of the anterolateral rim of the anterior neural folds. As the frontonasal prominence develops, elevations (termed the medial and lateral nasal prominences) form around the olfactory epithelium. As their name implies, the nasal prominences develop into the nose. The lower portions of the medial nasal prominences also contribute to the upper lip and form the portion of the alveolar ridge that contains the upper four incisors as well as the associated part of the hard palate that is termed the primary palate. On each side of the developing face, fusion of the medial nasal prominence with the lateral nasal prominence and the maxillary prominence of the first visceral arch is required for normal formation of the upper lip. As previously mentioned, neural crest cells are a predominant contributor to craniofacial development and provide, among other components, the skeletal and connective tissues of the face. This function is in contrast to the majority of the skull, whose progenitor populations are mesodermal.

The maxillary prominence, the tissue of which is primarily neural crest derived, is located below the developing eye and contributes to the lower eyelid. The upper lid is associated with the lateral nasal prominence as well as other tissues of the frontonasal prominence. Lid colobomas might be expected to occur at sites between the various growth centers that contribute to the eyelids. In addition to its maxillary component, the first visceral arch is made up of a mandibular subunit that contributes to the lower jaw and part of the external ear. The mandibular portion of the first arch has significant mesodermal progenitor cells in addition to those of neural crest origin.

Holoprosencephaly, Synophthalmia, and Cyclopia

Formation of a single median globe (cyclopia) or two incomplete (and apparently) fused globes (synophthalmia) may occur by two different mechanisms. Experimental studies in amphibian embryos have demonstrated "fate maps" identifying the original location of the ectodermal tissue that will form the globes as a single bilobed area which crosses the midline in the anterior third of the trilaminar embryonic disc. An early failure in separation of this single field could result in formation of a single median globe or two globes that appear to be "fused" which, in reality, have failed to fully separate. Later, in gestation, loss of the midline territory in the embryo could result in fusion of the ocular fields that were previously separated. This loss of midline territory is seen in holoprosencephaly (a single cerebral hemisphere).[96] Mutation in a number of different human genes can cause holoprosencephaly. Among the genes identified are sonic hedgehog (SHH), the protein product that is expressed at early stages of embryogenesis in the ventral midline of the forebrain and the subjacent tissue. SHH mutation results in holoprosencephaly type 3.[90] Mutation in other genes that are conserved in the animal kingdom, including SIX3 (the Drosophila sine oculis homeobox gene) and ZIC2, a homolog of the Drosophila odd-paired gene, are also associated with holoprosencephaly (HPE).[20,107]

Acute exposure of rodent embryos to teratogens at gastrulation stages of embryogenesis can result in the spectrum of malformations associated with holoprosencephaly. Loss of progenitor populations in the median aspect of the developing forebrain epithelium or its underlying mesoderm cause the subsequent dysmorphogenesis. Selective loss of the midline-associated tissues results in abnormally close approximation of the olfactory placodes and tissue deficiencies in the medial nasal prominence derivatives. At the mild end of the spectrum is a facial phenotype characteristic of fetal alcohol syndrome (Fig. 1-30A,B). Midline deficiencies can be so severe that the nose is

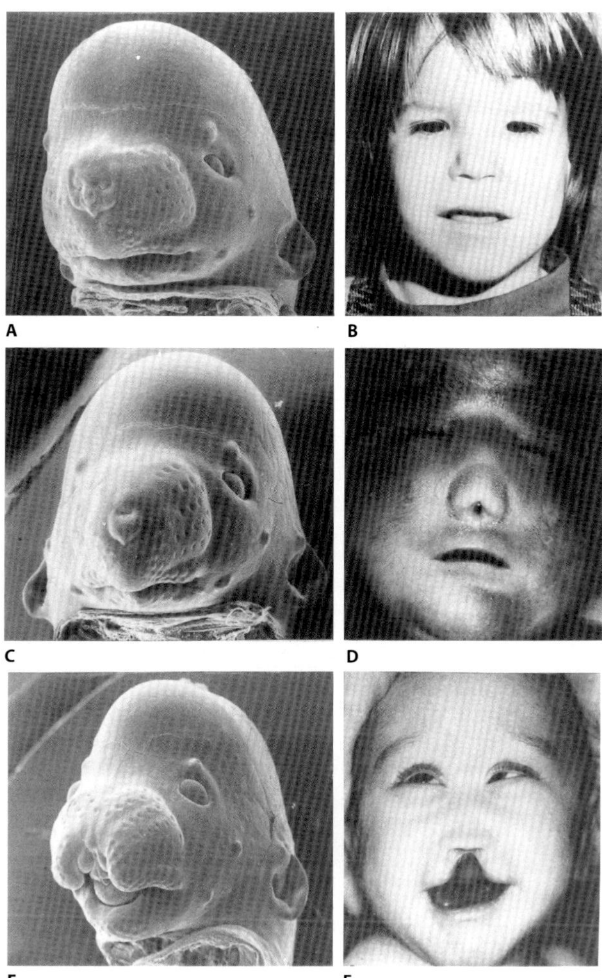

FIGURE 1-30A–F. Abnormally close proximity of the nasal placodes and subsequent deficiency in medial nasal prominence development results in the development of a small nose and a long upper lip (from nose to mouth) with a deficient philtrum. Variable degrees of severity of effect in ethanol-exposed mouse fetuses results in phenotypes comparable to those in humans with fetal alcohol syndrome (**A,B**), cebocephaly (**C,D**), and premaxillary agenesis (**E,F**). (From Siebert JR, Cohen MM Jr, Sulik KK. Holoprosencephaly: an overview and atlas of cases. New York: Wiley-Liss, 1990, with permission.)

derived from two conjoined nasal placodes, and lateral nasal prominences and hypotelorism is marked (Fig. 1-30C,D). Deficiencies that involve not only the anterior midline region but also the neural crest cells that contribute to the maxillary prominences (i.e., the crest cells derived from the mesencephalic neural folds) appear to be the basis for the premaxillary agenesis malformation complex illustrated in Figure 1-30E,F. In some rodent models, as in humans, mandibular deficiencies can also occur in conjunction with upper midface abnormalities, yielding the malformation complex termed *agnathia-holoprosencephaly*.

Exencephaly (Anencephaly) and Encephalocele

Although based on experimental evidence in animal models, most open neural tube defects (exencephaly, or anencephaly) result from failure of the neural tube to close, and some may be accounted for by postclosure rupture. Animal models have also illustrated that encephaloceles may be the result of abnormal closure. For example, delayed closure of the anterior neuropore appears to result in a rather tenuous closure with abnormally thin neuroepithelium and subsequent frontonasal encephalocele.

Because closure of the neural tube depends on a number of factors including the presence of normal neuroepithelium and its underlying mesenchyme and extracellular matrix, the types of and targets for insult that could result in failure of closure are also multiple. One of the most vulnerable periods for insult resulting in exencephaly in rodent embryos occurs before elevation of the cranial neural folds, when the embryos have approximately four to eight somite pairs (corresponding to the end of the third and beginning of the fourth week postfertilization in the human). At this time, premigratory neural crest cells appear to be particularly vulnerable to insult, their loss resulting in mesenchymal deficiency as well as interruption of the neuroepithelial integrity.[60]

Frontonasal Dysplasia

Median facial clefts with accompanying hypertelorism (frontonasal dysplasia) occur in widely varying degrees of severity. Animal models indicate that teratogen-induced distension (resulting from excessive fluid accumulation) of the neural tube shortly after the time of closure can account for some forms of frontonasal dysplasia.[32] Also of interest is an animal model resulting from a transgenically induced mutation.[71] The rather unusual phenotype results from delayed closure of the anterior neural folds and abnormal separation of the olfactory placodes from the rim of the neural plate.

References

1. Adamis AP, Molnar ML, Tripathi BJ, Emmerson MS, Stefansson K, Tripathi RC. Neuronal-specific enolase in human corneal endothelium and posterior keratocytes. Exp Eye Res 1985;41:665–668.
2. Aiello LP. Vascular endothelial growth factor. 20th-century mechanisms, 21st-century therapies. Investig Ophthalmol Vis Sci 1997; 38:1647–1652.
3. Alward WLM, Semina EV, et al. Autosomal dominant iris hypoplasia is caused by a mutation in the Rieger syndrome (RIEG/PITX2) gene. Am J Ophthalmol 1998;125:98–100.
4. Anderson DR. The development of the trabecular meshwork and its abnormality in primary infantile glaucoma. Trans Am Ophthalmol Soc 1981;79:458–485.
5. Ashton N. Oxygen and the growth and development of retinal vessels. In vivo and in vitro studies. Am J Ophthalmol 1966;62: 412–435.
6. Ashton N. Retinal angiogenesis in the human embryo. Br Med Bull 1970;26:103.
7. Ashton N, Tripathi B, Knight G. Effect of oxygen on the developing retinal vessels of the rabbit. I. Anatomy and development of the retinal vessels of the rabbit. Exp Eye Res 1972;14:214.
8. Aso S, Tashiro M, Baba R, Sawaki M, Noda S, Fujita M. Apoptosis in the lens anlage of the heritable lens aplastic mouse (lap mouse). Teratology 1998;58:44–53.
9. Balazs EA, Toth LZ, Ozanics V. Cytological studies on the developing vitreous as related to the hyaloid vessel system. Graefes Arch Klin Exp Ophthalmol 1980;213:71.
10. Barbieri AM, Lupo G, et al. A homeobox gene, vax2, controls the patterning of the eye dorsoventral axis. Proc Natl Acad Sci USA 1999;96:10729–10734.
11. Bard J, Hay E, Meller S. Formation of the endothelium of the avian cornea: a study of cell movement in vivo. Dev Biol 1975;42:334.
12. Bard J, Ross A. The morphogenesis of the ciliary body of the avian eye. Dev Biol 1982;92:87–96.
13. Barkan O. Pathogenesis of congenital glaucoma. Am J Ophthalmol 1955;40:1–11.
14. Beebe D, Compart P, Johnson M, Feagans D, Feinberg R. The mechanism of cell elongation during lens fiber cell differentiation. Dev Biol 1982;92:54–59.

15. Beebe DC. Ocular growth and differentiation factors. New York: Wiley, 1985.
16. Berson D. The development of the choroid and sclera in the eye of the foetal rat with particular reference to their developmental interrelationship. Exp Eye Res 1965;4:102.
17. Blankenship TN, Peterson PE, Hendrickx AG. Emigration of neural crest cells from macaque optic vesicles is correlated with discontinuities in its basement membrane. J Anat 1996;188:473–483.
18. Blixt A, Mahlapuu M, Aitola M, Pelto-Huikko M, Enerback S, Carlsson P. A forkhead gene, FoxE3, is essential for lens epithelial proliferation and closure of the lens vesicle. Genes Dev 2000;14:245–254.
19. Bremer FM, Rasquin F. Histochemical localization of hyal-uronic acid in vitreous during embryonic development. Investig Ophthalmol Vis Sci 1998;39:2466–2469.
20. Brown SA, Warburton D, et al. Holoprosencephaly due to mutations in ZIC2, a homologue of Drosophila odd-paired. Nat Genet 1998;20:180–183.
21. Bumsted KM, Barnstable CJ. Dorsal retinal pigment epithelium differentiates as neural retina in the microphthalmia (mi/mi) mouse. Investig Ophthalmol Vis Sci 2000;41:903–908.
22. Cohen A. Electron microscopic observations of the developing mouse eye. I. Basement membranes during early development and lens formation. Dev Biol 1961;3:297–316.
23. Collinson JM, Hill RE, West JD. Different roles for Pax6 in the optic vesicle and facial epithelium mediate early morphogenesis of the murine eye. Development (Camb) 2000;127:945–956.
24. Cook C. Experimental models of anterior segment dysgenesis. Ophthal Paediatr Gen 1989;10:33–46.
25. Cook C, Burling K, Nelson E. Embryogenesis of posterior segment colobomas in the Australian shepherd dog. Prog Vet Comp Ophthalmol 1991.
26. Cook CS, Generoso WM, Hester D, Peiffer RL Jr. RPE dysplasia with retinal duplication in a mutant mouse strain. Exp Eye Res 1991;52:409–415.
27. Cook CS, Nowotny AZ, Sulik KK. Fetal alcohol syndrome. Eye malformations in a mouse model. Arch Ophthalmol 1987;105:1576–1581.
28. Cook CS, Sulik KK. Keratolenticular dysgenesis (Peters' anomaly) as a result of acute embryonic insult during gastrulation. J Pediatr Ophthalmol Strabismus 1988;25:60–66.
29. Coulombre A. The role of intraocular pressure in the development of the chick eye. J Exp Zool 1956;133:211–225.
30. Coulombre AJ, Coulombre JL. Lens development. I. Role of lens in eye growth. J Exp Zool 1964;156:39.
31. Coulombre JL, Coulombre AJ. Lens development IV. Size, shape and orientation. Investig Ophthalmol 1969;8:251–257.

32. Darab DJ, Minkoff R, Sciote J, Sulik KK. Pathogenesis of median facial clefts in mice treated with methotrexate. Teratology 1987;36: 77–86.
33. Dawson DW, Volpert OV, et al. Pigment epithelium-derived factor: a potent inhibitor of angiogenesis. Science 1999;285:245–248.
34. Dunlevy JR, Beales MP, Berryhill BL, Cornuet PK, Hassell JR. Expression of the keratan sulfate proteoglycans lumican, keratocan and osteoglycin/mimecan during chick corneal development. Exp Eye Res 2000;70:349–362.
35. Furuta Y, Hogan BLM. BMP4 is essential for lens induction in the mouse embryo. Genes Dev 1998;12:3764–3775.
36. Garcia-Porrero JA, Collado JA, Ojeda JL. Cell death during detachment of the lens rudiment from ectoderm in the chick embryo. Anat Rec 1979;193:791–804.
37. Garcia-Porrero JA, Colvee E, Ojeda JL. The mechanisms of cell death and phagocytosis in the early chick lens morphogenesis. A scanning electron microscopy and cytochemical approach. Anat Rec 1984;208:123.
38. Grainger RM, Henry JJ, Saha MS, Servetnick M. Recent progress on the mechanisms of embryonic lens formation. Eye 1992;6:117–122.
39. Graw J. Genetic aspects of embryonic eye development in vertebrates. Dev Genet 1996;18:181–197.
40. Graw J. Cataract mutations and lens development. Prog Retin Eye Res 1999;18:235–267.
41. Grimm C, Chatterjee B, et al. Aphakia (ak), a mouse mutation affecting early eye development: fine mapping, consideration of candidate genes and altered Pax6 and Six3 gene expression pattern. Dev Genet 1998;23:299–316.
42. Hansson HA, Jerndal T. Scanning electron microscopic studies on the development of the iridocorneal angle in human eyes. Investig Ophthalmol 1971;10:252–265.
43. Hay E. Development of the vertebrate cornea. Int Rev Cytol 1980; 63:263.
44. Hay ED, Revel JP. Fine structure of the developing avian cornea. In: Wolsky A., Chen P (eds) Monographs in developmental biology. Basel: Karger, 1969.
45. Heimann K. The development of the choroid in man. Choroidal vascular system. Ophthalmol Res 1972;3:257.
46. Hendrickson A, Kupfer C. The histogenesis of the fovea in the macaque monkey. Investig Ophthalmol 1976;15:746.
47. Hendrix RW, Zwaan J. Changes in the glycoprotein concentration of the extracellular matrix between lens and optic vesicle associated with early lens differentiation. Differentiation 1974;2: 357.
48. Holme RH, Thomson SJ, Davidson DR. Ectopic expression of Msx2 in chick retinal pigmented epithelium cultures suggests a role in patterning the optic vesicle. Mech Dev 2000;91:175–187.

49. Hunt H. A study of the fine structure of the optic vesicle and lens placode of the chick embryo during incubation. Dev Biol 1961;3: 175–209.
50. Imaizumi M, Kuwabara T. Development of the rat iris. Investig Ophthalmol 1971;10:733.
51. Ireland ME, Wallace P, et al. Up-regulation of novel intermediate filament proteins in primary fiber cells: an indicator of all vertebrate lens fiber differentiation? Anat Rec 2000;258:25–33.
52. Ito M, Yoshioka M. Regression of the hyaloid vessels and pupillary membrane of the mouse. Anat Embryol 1999;200:403–411.
53. Iwatsuki H, Sasaki K, Suda M, Itano C. Vimentin intermediate filament protein as differentiation marker of optic vesicle epithelium in the chick embryo. Acta Histochem 1999;101:369–382.
54. Jack RL. Regression of the hyaloid vascular system. An ultrastructural analysis. Am J Ophthalmol 1972;74:261.
55. Johnston M, Noden D, Hazelton R, Coulombre J, Coulombre A. Origins of avian ocular and periocular tissues. Exp Eye Res 1979;29: 27–43.
56. Jones K, Higgonbottom M, Smith D. Determining the role of the optic vesicle in orbital and periocular development and placement. Pediatr Res 1980;14:703–708.
57. Karkinen-Jaaskelainen M. Permissive and directive interactions in lens induction. J Embryol Exp Morphol 1978;44:167–178.
58. Klagsbrun M, Moses MA. Molecular angiogenesis. Chem Biol 1999;6:217–224.
59. Koenig S, Naidich T, Lissner G. The morning glory syndrome associated with sphenoidal encepyhalocele. Ophthalmology 1982; 89:1368–1373.
60. Kotch LE, Sulik KK. Experimental fetal alcohol syndrome: proposed pathogenic basis for a variety of associated facial and brain anomalies. Am J Med Genet 1992;44:168–176.
61. Kupfer C, Kaiser-Kupfer M. New hypothesis of developmental anomalies of the anterior chamber associated with glaucoma. Trans Ophthal Soc UK 1978;98:213–215.
62. Lai YL. The development of the dilator muscle in the iris of the albino rat. Exp Eye Res 1972;14:203.
63. Lai YL. The development of the sphincter muscle in the iris of the albino rat. Exp Eye Res 1972;14:196.
64. Le Lievre C, Le Dourin N. Mesenchymal derivatives in the neural crest. Analysis of chimaeric quail and chick embryos. J Embryol Exp Morphol 1975;34:125.
65. LeDourin N. The neural crest. Cambridge: Cambridge University Press, 1982.
66. Levine EM, Close J, Fero M, Ostrovsky A, Reh TA. p27(Kip1) regulates cell cycle withdrawal of late multipotent progenitor cells in the mammalian retina. Dev Biol 2000;219:299–314.
67. March W, Chalkley T. Sclerocornea associated with Dandy–Walker cyst. Am J Ophthalmol 1974;78:54–57.

68. Maumenee A. The pathogenesis of congential glaucoma: a new theory. Am J Ophthalmol 1959:827–859.
69. McKeehan M. Cytological aspects of embryonic lens induction in the chick. J Exp Zool 1951:31–64.
70. McMenamin PG. Human fetal iridocorneal angle: a light and scanning electron microscopic study. Br J Ophthalmol 1989;73:871–879.
71. McNeish JD, Thayer J, Walling K, Sulik KK, Potter SS, Scott WJ. Phenotypic characterization of the transgenic mouse insertional mutation, legless. J Exp Zool 1990;253:151–162.
72. Meier S. The distribution of cranial neural crest cells during ocular morphogenesis. Prog Clin Biol Res 1982;82:1–15.
73. Michaelson IC. The mode of development of the vascular system of the retina with some observations on its significance for certain retinal diseases. Trans Ophthalmol Soc UK 1948;68:137–180.
74. Nishina S, Kohsaka S, et al. PAX6 expression in the developing human eye. Br J Ophthalmol 1999;83:723–727.
75. Noden D. Vertebrate craniofacial development: the relation between ontogenetic process and morphological outcome. Brain Behav Evol 1991;38:190–225.
76. Noden D. Periocular mesenchyme: neural crest and mesodermal interactions. In: Tasman W, Jaeger E (eds) Duane's foundations of clinical ophthalmology. Hagerstown: Lippincott, 1993:1–23.
77. Noden DM. The embryologic origins of avian craniofacial muscles and associated connective tissues. Am J Anat 1983;168:257–269.
78. Nucci P, Tredici G, Manitto MP, Pizzini G, Brancato R. Neuron-specific enolase and embryology of the trabecular meshwork of the rat eye: an immunohistochemical study. Int J Biol Markers 1992;7:253–255.
79. Oshima K, Ishikawa T. Effects of oxygen on developing vessels in the kitten retina. Nippon Ganka Gakkai Zasshi 1975;79:813.
80. Ozanics V, Rayborn ME, Sagun D. Observations on the ultrastructure of the developing primate choroid coat. Exp Eye Res 1978;26:25.
81. Ozeki H, Shirai S. Developmental eye abnormalities in mouse fetuses induced by retinoic acid. Jpn J Ophthalmol 1998;42:162–167.
82. Patz A. Current concepts of the effects of oxygen on the developing retina. Curr Eye Res 1984;3:159–163.
83. Patz A, Hoeck L, DeLaCruz E. Studies on the effect of high oxygen administration in retrolental fibroplasia: nursery observations. Am J Ophthalmol 1952;27:1248–1253.
84. Pierce EA, Foley Ed, Smith LE. Regulation of vascular endothelial growth factor by oxygen in a model of retinopathy of prematurity. Arch Ophthalmol 1996;114:1219–1228.
85. Pollock J, Newton T, Hoyt W. Transsphenoidal and transethmoidal encephaloceles: a review of clinical and roentgen features in 8 cases. Radiology 1968;90:442–452.

86. Reme C, D'Epinay SL. Periods of development of the normal human chamber angle. Doc Ophthalmol 1981;51:241.
87. Reme C, Urner U, Aeberhard B. The development of the chamber angle in the rat eye. Graefe's Arch Clin Exp Ophthalmol 1983;220: 139–153.
88. Reme C, Urner U, Aeberhard B. The occurence of cell death during the remodelling of the chamber angle recess in the developing rat eye. Graefe's Arch Clin Exp Ophthalmol 1983;221:113–121.
89. Ring BZ, Cordes SP, Overbeek PA, Barsh GS. Regulation of mouse lens fiber cell development and differentiation by the Maf gene. Development (Camb) 2000;127:307–317.
90. Roessler E, Belloni E, et al. Mutations in the human Sonic Hedgehog gene cause holoprosencephaly. Nat Genet 1996;14:357–360.
91. Schook P. A review of data on cell actions and cell interactions during the morphogenesis of the embryonic eye. Acta Morphol Neerl Scand 1978;16:267–286.
92. Selleck MA, Bronner-Fraser M. The genesis of avian neural crest cells: a classic embryonic induction. Proc Natl Acad Sci U S A 1996;93:9352–9357.
93. Sevel D. Reappraisal of the origin of human extraocular muscles. Ophthalmology 1981;88:1330.
94. Sevel D. The origins and insertions of the extraocular muscles: development, histologic features, and clinical significance. Trans Am Ophthalmol Soc 1986;84:488–526.
95. Shakib M, De Oliveira F. Studies on developing retinal vessels. X. Formation of the basement membrane and differentiation of intramural pericytes. Br J Ophthalmol 1966;50:124–133.
96. Siebert JR, Cohen MM Jr, Sulik KK, Shaw C, Lemire R. Holoprosencephaly: an overview and atlas of cases. New York: Wiley-Liss, 1990.
97. Simon PD, McConnell J, et al. Thy-1 is critical for normal retinal development. Brain Res Dev Brain Res 1999;117:219–223.
98. Smelser GK, Ozanics V. The development of the trabecular meshwork in primate eyes. Am J Ophthalmol 1971;71:366.
99. Spira AW, Hollenberg MJ. Human retinal development. Ultrastructure of the inner retinal layers. Dev Biol 1973;31:1–21.
100. Straatsma B, Foos R, Heckenlively J, Christensen R. Myelin-ated retinal nerve fibers: clinicopathologic study and clinical correlations. Excerpta Med 1978;32:36.
101. Straatsma B, Foos R, Heckenlively J, Taylor G. Myelinated retinal nerve fibers. Am J Ophthalmol 1981;91:25–38.
102. Stromland K, Miller M, Cook C. Ocular teratology. Surv Ophthalmol 1991;35:429–446.
103. Summers C, Romig L, Lavoie J. Unexpected good results after therapy for anisometropic amblyopia associated with unilateral peripapillary myelinated nerve fibers. J Pediatr Ophthalmol Strabismus 1991;28:134–136.

104. Tamura T, Smelser GK. Development of the sphincter and dilator muscles of the iris. Arch Ophthalmol 1973;89:332.
105. Toole B, Trelstad R. Hyaluronate production and removal during corneal development in the chick. Dev Biol 1971;26:28.
106. Tsai RK, Sheu MM, Wang HZ. Capability of neurite regeneration of rat retinal explant at different ages. Kao Hsiung I Hsueh Ko Hsueh Tsa Chih 1998;14:192–196.
107. Wallis DE, Roessler E, et al. Mutations in the homeodomain of the human SIX3 gene cause holoprosencephaly. Nat Genet 1999;22: 196–198.
108. Weiss P, Jackson S. Fine structural changes associated with lens determination in the avian embryo. Dev Biol 1961;532–554.
109. West-Mays JA, Zhang J, et al. AP-2alpha transcription factor is required for early morphogenesis of the lens vesicle. Dev Biol 1999; 206:46–62.
110. Wigle JT, Chowdhury K, Gruss P, Oliver G. Prox1 function is crucial for mouse lens-fibre elongation. Nat Genet 1999;21:318–322.
111. Worst J. Congenital glaucoma. Remarks on the aspect of chamber angle, ontogenetic and pathogenetic background, and mode of action of goniotomy. Investig Ophthalmol 1968;7:127–134.
112. Wrenn JT, Wessels NK. An ultrastructural study of lens invagination in the mouse. J Exp Zool 1969;171:359.
112a. Hong PH, Wright KW, Fillafer S, Sola A, Chow LC. Strict Oxygen Management is Associated with Decreased Incidence of Severe ROP, Presented ARVO, 2002.
113. Wulle K. The development of the productive and draining system of the aqueous humor in the human eye. Adv Ophthalmol 1972: 296–355.
114. Wulle KG. Electron microscopic observations of the development of Schlemm's canal in the human eye. Trans Am Acad Ophthalmol Otolaryngol 1968;72:765.
115. Wulle KG, Ruprecht KW, Windrath LC. Electron microscopy of the development of the cell junctions in the embryonic and fetal human corneal endothelium. Investig Ophthalmol 1974;13:923.
116. Yamashita T, Sohal G. Development of smooth and skeletal muscle cells in the iris of the domestic duck, chick and quail. Cell Tissue Res 1986;244:121–131.
117. Yamashita T, Sohal G. Embryonic origin of skeletal muscle cells in the iris of the duck and quail. Cell Tissue Res 1987;249:31–37.
118. Yang J, Bian W, Gao X, Chen L, Jing N. Nestin expression during mouse eye and lens development. Mech Dev 2000;94:287–291.
119. Zwaan J, Hendrix RW. Changes in cell and organ shape during early development of the ocular lens. Am J Zool 1973;13:1039–1049.

2

Pediatric Neuro-Ophthalmology Examination

Edward G. Buckley

This chapter highlights the areas of the eye examination that are of significance in assessing pediatric neuro-ophthalmic disorders. Before beginning the formal examination, spend a few moments interacting with the child in a nonthreatening way. Gaining the child's confidence early in the exam will be rewarded later when cooperation is imperative. A great deal of information can be gathered by simple observation and, therefore, surveillance for subtle findings should be maintained during the exam. After establishing rapport with the child, the order in which information is collected depends on the conditions of the examination and the cooperation of the child. Rigid adherence to a particular regimen may lead to a frustrating experience. It is fruitless to begin taking a long, detailed history if it is obvious that the child is already somewhat fussy and rapidly losing attention. In such circumstances, the exam will have to be goal directed. By prioritizing the examination to fit the "problem," the maximum amount of information can be obtained in what often turns out to be a very limited amount of time.

HISTORY

The past medical history plays an important role in diagnosis and often dictates which portions of the examination are the most important to accomplish. Because pediatric neuro-ophthalmic problems are often secondary to central nervous system damage at birth, special areas to explore include maternal infections, prematurity, birth trauma, and suspected brain damage such as hydrocephalus and cerebral palsy. Special emphasis should be placed on visual and neurological development and details of similar problems in other family members. Information about previous evaluations and the results of past neuroradiologic studies (MRI/CT) are also helpful in understanding the current issues.

VISUAL ACUITY

Parental assessment of the child's visual activity is helpful in determining the degree of impairment. Ask such questions as: "Does the child appear to see?" "Does the child respond to light, faces, and toys?" and "Does the child fix on the parent's face, bottle, hands, and feet?" Does the child smile appropriately? If the child does display visually guided behavior, an effort should be made to get some idea as to the degree of visual function. How far away can the child see? Does the child follow movement across the room, pick up small objects, or reach for things? This approach is helpful not only in determining the etiology of visual loss but also in predicting future visual performance.

Rarely, the parent will indicate that no visual function is present. In this circumstance the parent is usually correct because the normal tendency is to be optimistic and overestimate visual function. Caution must be exercised in dismissing parental observations of visual function in a child who is apparently blind from cortical damage. In this circumstance, visual function can fluctuate significantly and can be intermittently present.

Visual Acuity Measurement

The accurate assessment of visual function is an important part of the neuro-ophthalmic exam. Many of the entities in subsequent chapters have decreased visual acuity as the presenting symptom. Special techniques are required to obtain an objective assessment of visual function in the young child. Table 2-1 contains a summary of the methods applicable to the various age groups.

Binocular visual acuity should be evaluated first because it is often superior to monocular function and the manipulation

TABLE 2-1. Visual Acuity Testing by Age.

Age	*Acuity*	*Test*
Birth to 2 months	20/200–20/60	Observation Blink to light Fix and follow objects OKN drum
2–6 months	20/50+	Observation Blink to threat Reach for objects Preferential looking OKN drum VER
6–18 months	20/40+	Preferential looking OKN drum Reach for candy beads (1 cm–1 mm) VER
18–36 months	20/30+	Preferential looking OKN Reach for candy beads (1 cm–1 mm) VER Allen cards HOTV
3–5 years	20/30+	Reach for candy beads (1 cm–1 mm) Allen cards HOTV "E" game Snellen chart

OKN, optokinetic nystagmus; VER, visual evoked response; HOTV, matching of Snellen characters.

required to test the vision monocularly may result in loss of cooperation. Near visual function testing should also be attempted because in most neuro-ophthalmic disorders visual acuity will be better at near than at distance. This point is extremely important when trying to assess whether the child will be able to attend regular schools and whether large-print books or other visual aids will be necessary.

OKN Testing

Optokinetic nystagmus (OKN) testing is especially useful in assessing visual function in infants. The optokinetic response elicits a jerk nystagmus, which, if present, is indicative of visual function. This nystagmus was first described by Helmholtz, who observed the eyes of passengers gazing out of train windows.[9] He noted a slow following phase in the direction of target movement and a rapid jerk return in the opposite direction to pick up fixation. Because the slow phase is initiated by vision, optokinetic nystagmus may be used as a parameter of visual function and, by varying the size of the optokinetic target, to assess the degree of visual acuity.[13] If a vertical optokinetic nystagmus can be superimposed on an already present horizontal nystagmus, this is usually indicative of visual function good enough to attend normal schools with some assistance (Fig. 2-1). The absence of an optokinetic response, however, is not helpful and does not necessarily imply a lack of visual function.

Low-Illumination Acuity Testing

Testing visual acuity under reduced illumination can be used to distinguish amblyopia (strabismic or anisometropic) from retinal or optic nerve dysfunction.[14] If the illumination to a normal eye is decreased using a neutral density filter (no. 96 2-Log filter; Kodak), the vision will be mildly reduced from 20/20 to 20/40. In an eye with a retinal or optic nerve lesion, the vision will be reduced dramatically (20/40 to 20/200) whereas an eye with amblyopia will exhibit little or no reduction (20/40 to 20/50). (Neutral-density filters can be obtained in most camera shops.) Newer electrophysiological methods of assessing

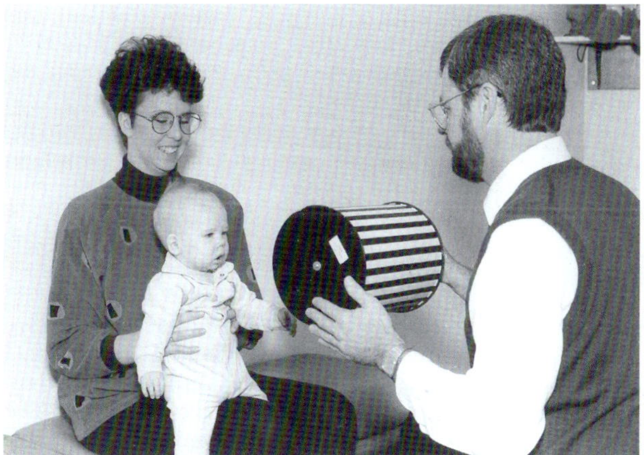

FIGURE 2-1. Vertical optokinetic nystagmus testing using an OKN drum. If a vertical nystagmus can be elicited, vision is 20/400 or better.

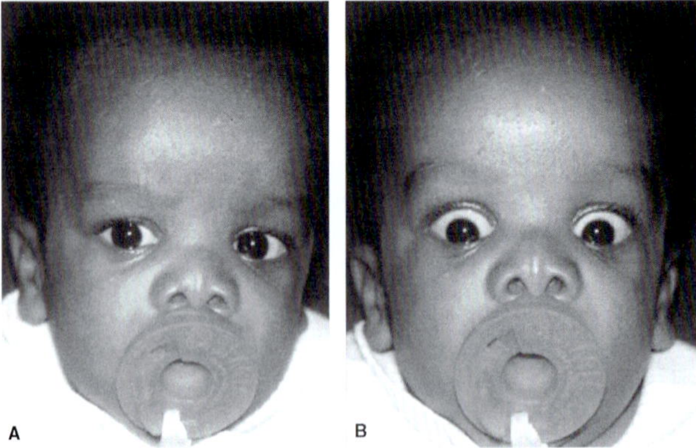

FIGURE 2-2A,B. **(A)** Child with lights on. **(B)** Same child immediately after lights are turned down. Note marked retraction of the upper lids. This reflex indicates some visual function.

visual function include visual evoked potentials and pattern electroretinography.

Very young children (1–3 months of age) will exhibit marked lid retraction when the lights are suddenly turned off (Fig. 2-2). This primitive reflex can be used to assess function in the apparently blind infant. If little or no visual function is present, this reflex will not occur. However, if visual acuity is 20/400 or better, marked lid retraction will occur immediately after the room lights are turned off. The lids may stay retracted for 20 to 30 s but will eventually return to the normal position. This reflex will occur repeatedly every time the lights are turned off. The presence of this reflex offers reassurance that some visual function exists.

Visual Evoked Potential

With the advent of computer technology, the ability to analyze brain electrical activity (EEG) during repetitive visual stimulation has evolved. By averaging 200 to 300 such tracings, a waveform results that has been termed the visual evoked potential (VEP). The VEP is commonly used to detect disorders of the visual pathway, and the two main characteristics are the wave amplitude and latency. The latency is a measure of optic nerve conduction and is delayed in such entities as optic neuritis. When using a patterned visual stimulus the amplitude can be a measure of visual acuity. A recent modification called the sweep VEP may prove promising in assessing visual acuity in preverbal infants.

PUPILLARY EXAMINATION

A wealth of information can be learned from examination of the pupils. An attempt should first be made to determine whether the pupils react to light and, if so, how briskly? A brisk constriction to light usually indicates good ocular and optic nerve function. A sluggish response, or no response at all, implies retina, optic nerve, or third nerve dysfunction. This assessment of pupil response to light can be helpful in localizing the site of visual loss, which is especially helpful in the child with possible cortical visual impairment (Fig. 2-3). Brisk pupillary reactions in a child with profound visual loss indicate a cortical etiology (Table 2-2).

Afferent Pupillary Defect (Marcus Gunn Pupil)

A specific sign for optic nerve dysfunction is the presence of an afferent pupillary defect (Marcus Gunn pupil). In testing for an afferent pupillary defect, room illumination should be decreased, the patient should be fixating at a distant target, and a bright light source should be used. The test compares the pupillary constriction, and hence optic nerve function, of the two eyes. The eye with the optic nerve dysfunction perceives the light source as being less bright and the pupils constrict less as compared to when the same light is shown in the "normal" eye. Therefore, the direct response to light (light shown into the involved eye) is less than the consensual response (light shown into the uninvolved eye). Clinically, the test is performed by swinging a flashlight between the two eyes, resting approximately 2 s at each eye.[12] During the swinging flashlight test it appears to the observer as if the involved eye is exhibiting pupillary dilation to the light source (see Fig. 2-3). This seemingly "paradoxical dilatation to light" is the hallmark of an afferent pupillary defect, and the eye with the pupil that "dilates" to light has either an optic nerve or retinal abnormality.

Performing the swinging flashlight test on young children is often troublesome because distance fixation cannot be

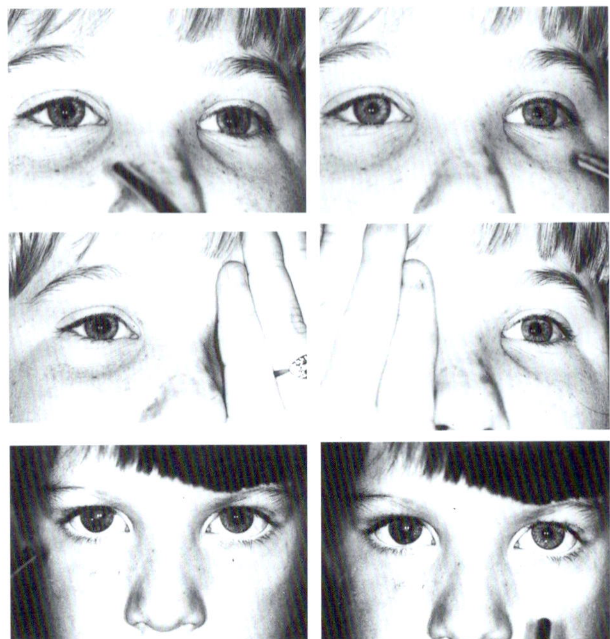

FIGURE 2-3. Testing for an afferent pupillary defect. The "swinging flashlight test" is performed by shining a light in the right eye (*top right*) and noting the pupil size of both eyes. The light is then "swung" to the left eye and both pupils observed (*top left*). The poorer response when shining the light in the right eye indicates a right afferent pupillary defect. The test can also be performed using room illumination by alternatively covering each eye (*middle left and right*). The larger pupil on the right eye indicates a right afferent defect. *Bottom*: testing for an afferent defect with a fixed right pupil. Compare the size of the left pupil when light is shone in the right eye (*bottom left*) as compared to the left eye (*bottom right*). The better response from the left eye indicates a right afferent defect.

TABLE 2-2. Pupil Evaluation in Low-Vision Infant.

	Location of disorder	
	Anterior pathway	***Cortical***
Pupil reactivity to light	Sluggish	Brisk
Afferent defect	Possible	Never
Paradoxical pupil	Possible	Never
Iris defects	Possible	Never

maintained and, with near fixation, accommodative miosis makes interpretation difficult. In such circumstances, normal room illumination can be used to assess optic nerve function[10] (Fig. 2-3 demonstrates this technique). This approach is especially helpful in the infant or toddler who invariably fixates on the light source, making traditional testing impossible. An afferent pupillary defect can even be detected if one of the pupils is non-reactive secondary to trauma, pharmacological dilation, or ocular inflammation (Fig. 2-3). In such cases, the direct and consensual responses of the single reactive pupil must be compared. If the consensual response is less than the direct response there is an abnormality in that eye. The afferent pupillary defect is a sensitive indicator of optic nerve dysfunction and, more specifically, visual field loss.[17] Retinal disease or amblyopia can also cause an afferent pupillary defect, but the disease process is usually severe and visual function is quite poor. Because the afferent pupillary defect is a relative measure of optic nerve function between eyes, bilateral symmetrical optic nerve involvement will result in a negative test.

Paradoxical Pupillary Constriction to Darkness

Another useful test is the "paradoxical pupillary constriction to darkness."[1,5,6] Figure 2-4 illustrates this phenomenon. As the room lights are turned off, the pupils, instead of dilating, will

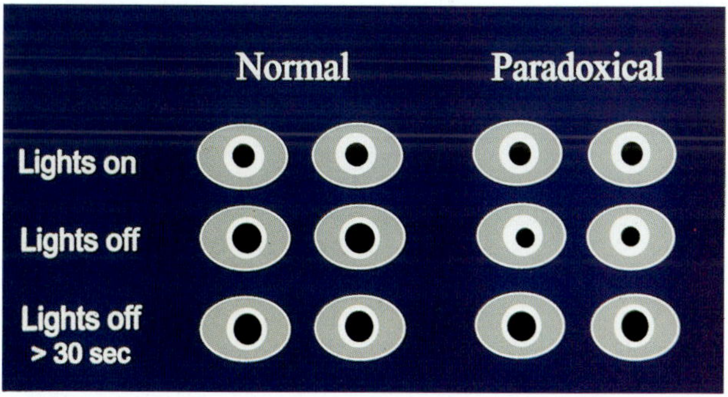

FIGURE 2-4. The paradoxical pupillary response to darkness is a momentary pupillary constriction immediately upon decreasing room illumination.

TABLE 2-3. Paradoxical Pupillary Phenomena.

Common causes
Congenital stationary night blindness
Congenital achromatopsia
Optic nerve hypoplasia
Rare causes
Leber's congenital amaurosis
Best's disease
Albinism
Retinitis pigmentosa

momentarily constrict. After 2 to 10s the pupils will undergo slow dilatation; this is best seen by providing some low-level side illumination as the lights are dimmed. This "paradoxical pupillary constriction to darkness" is indicative of optic nerve or retinal disease or both (Table 2-3).

Anisocoria

Occasionally the patient will present with one pupil larger than the other. The diagnostic dilemma is deciding whether the abnormality is the large pupil or the small pupil, or whether no abnormality exists at all. Usually, this can be accomplished with a few simple clinical observations (outlined in Table 2-4). It must be remembered that anisocoria is NOT a sign of severe unilateral retinal or optic nerve dysfunction. In an otherwise normal patient, a blind eye will not result in anisocoria.

TABLE 2-4. Anisocoria.

Diagnosis	*Pupil size*	*Response to light*	*Difference greater in:*	*Drug testing*
Essential anisocoria	1–2 mm difference	Normal	No change	None
Tonic pupil (Adie's)	Large	Absent	Light	Pilocarpine (0.1% constricts)
Horner's syndrome	Small	Normal	Dark	Cocaine 10% (poor dilation)
Pharmacological	Large	Absent	No change	Pilocarpine 2% (no constriction)
Oculomotor palsy	Large	Absent	No change	Pilocarpine (0.1% constricts)

Iris Defects

While examining the pupillary response, attention should also be directed toward the iris structure and color. An iris coloboma may indicate posterior segment abnormalities such as retinal or optic nerve colobomas. Iris transillumination defects are indicative of ocular albinism, which is associated with macular hypoplasia, decreased vision, and nystagmus. A complete absence of the iris (aniridia) is associated with nystagmus, cataracts, macular hypoplasia, and poor vision. Unequal pigmentation may be a sign of a congenital sympathetic paresis (congenital Horner's syndrome) with the paresis in the hypopigmented (lighter-colored) side.

MOTILITY

The major task in evaluating a child with a motility abnormality is trying to determine whether it is caused by a "common strabismus" or a potentially more serious acquired disorder. The acute nature of the presentation, which is often helpful in adults, can be confusing in children as many benign entities such as accommodative esotropia can "suddenly" appear. In addition, many congenital motility disturbances such as Brown's syndrome and Duane's syndrome can go unnoticed for quite some time. Careful observation for compensatory head positions, variability, or signs of aberrant regeneration may give a clue as to the acquired nature of the disorder. Examination of old photographs can be extremely useful in dating the onset of the strabismus. Because strabismus is often secondary to other ophthalmic abnormalities, a thorough eye exam including cycloplegic refraction (to rule out accommodative factors) is necessary. Because most neuro-ophthalmic motility disorders result from a weakness of one or more of the extraocular muscles, the motility evaluation hinges on whether the ocular rotations are normal. Although this can be difficult in children, various methods are available.

Begin by having the child look in the various fields of gaze. Colorful toys, noisy objects, or lights can be helpful in accomplishing this task. Occasionally, the child will resist looking in certain gaze positions, and other methods must be employed to assess a limitation. One of the most useful is the *"doll's head maneuver."* Because the child is often very apprehensive, he or she will remain fixated on the examiner instead of looking at the toy or light. In such circumstances, the examiner can rotate the child's head, thereby forcing the eyes into the desired position (Fig. 2-5). In doing so, any weakness can be determined just as effectively as having the child look into that gaze position.

A second maneuver using the same vestibular response can be employed with very young infants. It involves having the examiner rotate the infant in a circle (Fig. 2-6). This action stimulates the semicircular canals and forces the infant's eyes toward the direction of rotation.[7] Its main utility is in horizontal motility defects. This action also causes a jerk nystagmus to occur upon cessation, with the fast component to the opposite direction. Thus, when rotating an infant to the examiner's right, the child will exhibit a deviation to its left (examiner's right) with a right jerk nystagmus. This approach is extremely helpful in identifying sixth nerve palsies.

Occasionally, a child presents with an esotropia and, because of strong visual cross-fixation, attempts at assessing abduction are futile. In such circumstances, a trial of alternately patching the eyes in the clinic or at home may demonstrate the patient's normal ocular rotation. The Bielschowsky head tilt

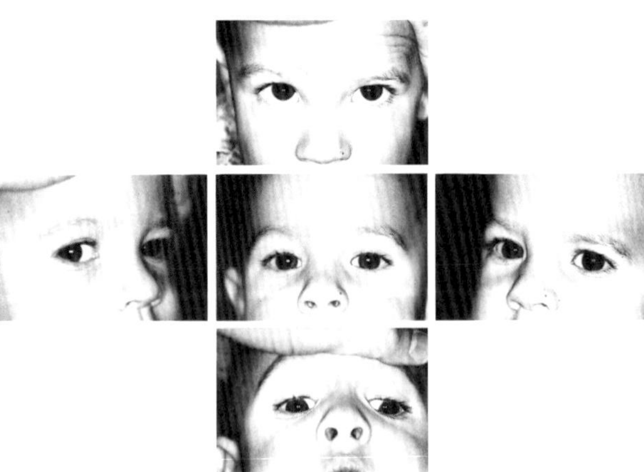

FIGURE 2-5. Doll's head maneuver to access ocular motility. The head is rotated by the examiner bringing the eyes into the various gaze positions. Note the marked exotropia on downgaze.

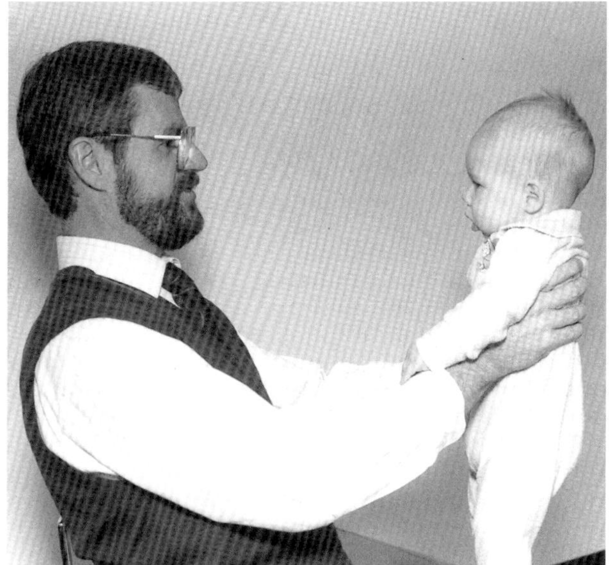

FIGURE 2-6. Testing ocular motility using the vestibular-ocular reflex. The child is rotated in a circle, which stimulates the semicircular canals, causing the eyes to deviate in the direction of rotation.

test, although not usually quantifiable in young children, can be used to detect an isolated cyclovertical muscle paresis. A vertical deviation seen while tilting the child's head to the side should raise the suspicion that a paralytic condition exists and further investigation is warranted.

Last, one can use the optokinetic drum or tape to assess ocular motor function. By rotating the drum to the patient's left, a pursuit movement to the left followed by a fast eye movement to the right (saccade) is elicited. Optokinetic testing is useful for monocular motility disorders because it helps demonstrate slower incomplete saccadic movements in paralytic extraocular conditions that are neurogenic, myoneural, or myopathic.[7] In addition, it can help to demonstrate weaknesses of gaze function and the absence of saccades in the presence of pursuit movements (congenital motor apraxia).

NYSTAGMUS

The child with nystagmus often presents a difficult diagnostic challenge. The clinician's primary responsibility is to determine whether the nystagmus is a sign of a significant central nervous system abnormality that requires immediate intervention. Fortunately, the great majority of children with nystagmus have ophthalmic etiology that can be diagnosed with simple office examination techniques.[11] In fact, more than 90% of children with nystagmus have some identifiable disorder of the anterior visual pathway. Although nystagmus can be confusing at first, a systematic and thorough evaluation will often elicit its etiology, suggest the appropriate additional laboratory tests, and provide valuable information to the parents concerning the child's future visual development and prognosis. There are several specific, recognizable, localizing types of nystagmus that direct the clinician to the appropriate diagnosis and evaluation (Table 2-5).

Describing Nystagmus

When describing a nystagmus, record as much information about the movement as possible. The nystagmus should be described by the type of movement, the frequency (the number of oscillations per unit of time), the amplitude (the distance traveled during the movement), and the direction, which may be horizontal, vertical, rotary, oblique, or circular (Fig. 2-7). A complete description often aids in the diagnosis and the follow-up of the patient's subsequent course.[4] Observing the nystagmus for an extended period of time is helpful in trying to determine its characteristics; this is particularly important in identifying periodic alternating nystagmus, a jerk nystagmus that changes directions every 60 to 90 s. Allowing the child to walk and move

TABLE 2-5. Localizing Types of Nystagmus.

Nystagmus	*Location/etiology*
Latent	Congenital
Manifest latent	Congenital
Spasmus nutans	Chiasm/suprachiasmal
Periodic alternating	Brainstem/cerebellum
See-saw	Midbrain/suprachiasmal
Retraction	Dorsal midbrain
Downbeat	Cerebellum/cervicomedullary junction
Opsoclonus	Neuroblastoma

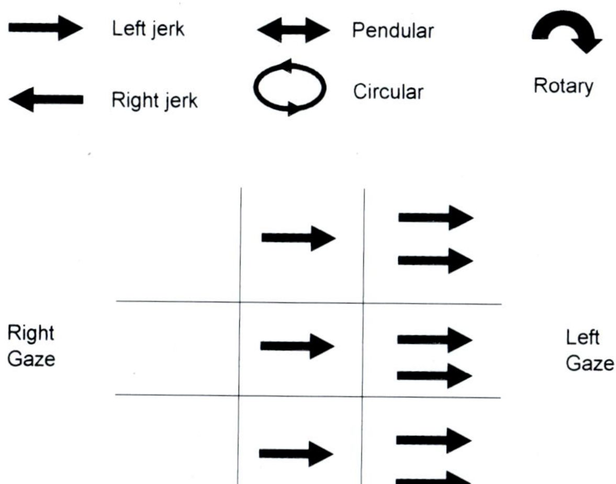

FIGURE 2-7. A schemata for recording nystagmus patterns, illustrating a left jerk nystagmus that worsens on leftgaze and improves on rightgaze. *Double* or *triple arrows* in any one block indicate increased movement in that gaze position. A combination of symbols can be used to fully record the movement pattern.

about the examination room will facilitate recognizing such factors as head positions, which may become more pronounced when the child is trying to move through the environment as opposed to sitting on the parent's lap.

Head Positions

Observations about head position or head movement can be very informative. Spasmus nutans, a benign form of acquired nystagmus, often has an associated head bob or torticollis. A patient with congenital motor nystagmus often develops a head turn to dampen the nystagmus. Although the presence of a preferred head position is not particularly helpful in deciding about etiology, it has some bearing on visual function and the type of nystagmus. Patients with a jerk nystagmus more often tend to develop head positions than patients with pendular nystagmus; this is because of *Alexander's law of nystagmus*, which states that a jerk nystagmus becomes worse when gazing in the direction of the fast component.[4] Thus, a left jerk nystagmus becomes

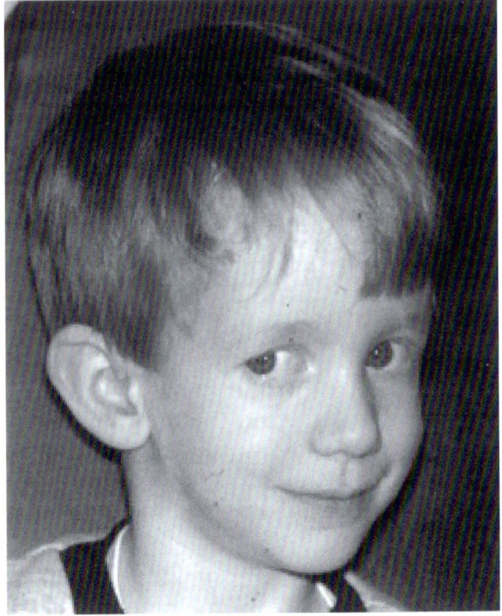

FIGURE 2-8. Example of head turn used in a patient with a left jerk nystagmus with a null point in rightgaze (Alexander's law).

much worse in leftgaze and improves dramatically on rightgaze. Therefore, a patient with a left jerk nystagmus will have a left face turn and a right gaze preference (Fig. 2-8). Old photographs can be helpful in documenting head positions.

CONFRONTATION VISUAL FIELDS

Visual field testing in children is limited to detecting altitudinal and hemianopic defects (bitemporal, homonymous). In children as young as 6 months of age, visual field testing can be accomplished by observing reflex eye movements to a visual stimulus. The technique is performed by having the examiner first attract the child's attention, and then a toy or some other interesting target is moved in quietly from the periphery. If the child makes an eye movement to fixate on the target, this is evidence that the peripheral field is intact (Fig. 2-9). This technique is quite useful in detecting homonymous and bitemporal hemianopias. It is less useful in altitudinal defects. In children as young as 2 years, "finger mimicking" visual fields can be

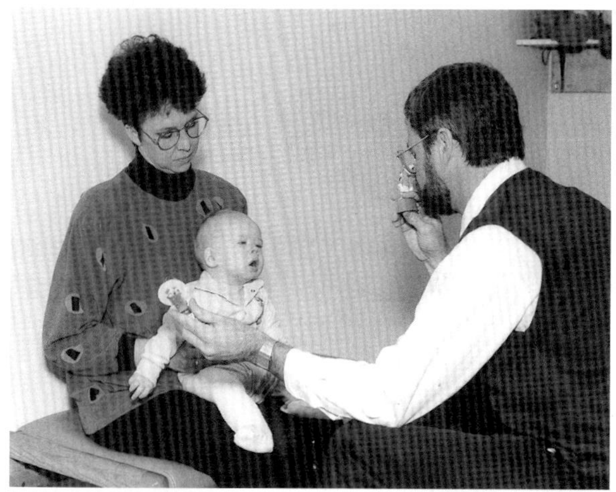

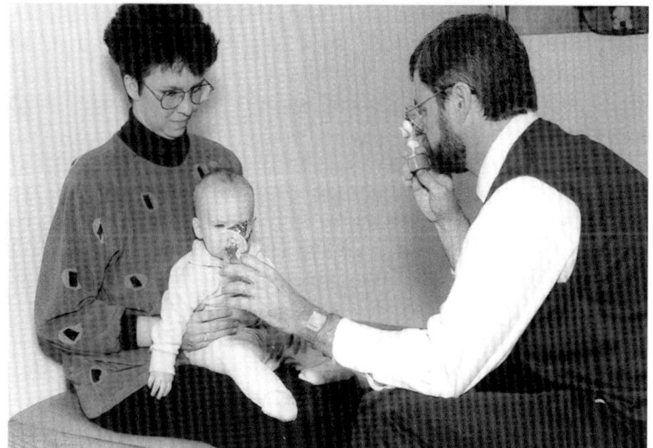

FIGURE 2-9. Testing visual fields in a young child. Begin by attracting the child's attention straight ahead (*top*). Then move an object in from the side. A head movement to the side of the target (*bottom*) indicates intact peripheral field.

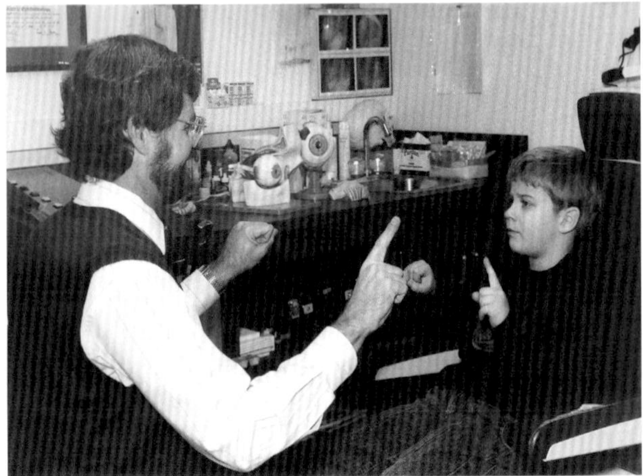

FIGURE 2-10. Finger mimicking visual fields. The child is asked to show the same number of fingers as the examiner. These should be displayed quickly to avoid fixation artifact.

obtained. Using this technique the child is asked to copy what the examiner is doing. Having the child display one, five, or no fingers by "mimicking" the examiner is a fairly reliable way to assess visual fields (Fig. 2-10). The numbers two, three, and four should be avoided as they are somewhat confusing at times. The fingers should be flashed quickly to avoid erroneous results obtained by the child fixating on the hand instead of the examiner.

Fixation is often difficult to control and is the major problem with this technique. A useful maneuver when attempting to evaluate the temporal visual field is to place the child's eye in full abduction; this prevents further eye movement laterally and minimizes a fixation artifact. This move cannot be done nasally as the nose blocks visual field assessment. Binocular visual field defects should be assessed first as the child may not cooperate for monocular testing because of the necessary eye occlusion. Finger "counting" visual fields can be performed in children over 3 years of age. The technique is similar to finger mimicking; however, the child "counts" the number of fingers presented. Simultaneous presentation in both hemifields is now possible, and subtler field defects can be detected. As before, the fingers should be flashed quickly and the numbers kept to one, five, or none. Altitudinal field defects are easier to test in this age group, and very reliable information can be obtained by this technique.

Goldman and automated perimetry can be performed on the child aged 6 to 7. Often children are playing sophisticated video games at home, and the test can be explained using such terms. Testing, however, should be kept simple because patience and fatigue are factors. Fixation is still a problem at this age, and constant surveillance is necessary to obtain a reliable field. When using the Goldman perimeter, two isopters are all that are necessary to detect most neuro-ophthalmic visual defects in children (V_4e, II_4e).[16] Automated perimetry is more difficult because the control programs are written to detect subtle field defects in adults and take more time than most children will tolerate. Before using more sophisticated tests, the examiner should begin with a simple confrontation technique to assess reliability. Visual field constriction is a common artifact because the child is hesitant to "make a mistake." This tendency tends to decrease with age.

COLOR VISION

Color, like beauty, is in the eye of the beholder. It is no more measurable by physical means than is the sensation of pain or the feeling of joy. The sensation of color can, however, be closely linked to physical attributes of the visual stimulus and to anatomic and physiologic properties of the afferent visual system.[8] The human process of color photoreception can be explained by the trichromatic theory. Early investigators hypothesized that there were three classes of cones in the human retina. Later experiments have confirmed the presence of exactly three types of color pigments in cone photoreceptors. These pigments have spectral sensitivity curves that peak at 450nm (blue cones), 540nm (green cones), and 580nm (red cones), and individuals with congenital color deficiencies have an absence of one or more pigments.[3]

The terms "protan" (red) and "deutan" (green) originate from the Greek words for "first" and "second" and denote the two most common kinds of red-green confusion, whereas blue-yellow confusions characterize the "tritan" (third) type of defect.[8] Congenital dyschromatopsias are mostly of the red-green type, binocular and stable throughout life. Color defects in patients with acquired dyschromatopsias frequently mimic

TABLE 2-6. Associated Color Vision Defects.

	Red-green	*Blue-yellow*
Optic nerve diseases		
Optic neuritis	X	
Toxic	X	
Leber's atrophy	X	
Compressive	X	
Traumatic	X	
Dominant atrophy		X
Chronic disc edema		X
Ischemic		X
Retinal diseases		
Retinal detachment (macula on)		X
Toxic		X
Peripheral chorioretinal dystrophies		X
Diabetic retinopathy		X
Retinoschisis		X
Cystoid macular edema		X
Cone dystrophy	X	
Juvenile macular degeneration	X	

Modified from Harper W. Acquired dyschromatopsias. Surv Ophthalmol 1987;32:10–32, with permission.

the abnormal patterns seen in those patients with congenital defects. It has been noted by Kollner and others that patients with diseases of the macula tended to have blue-yellow defects while those with diseases of the optic nerve tended to have red-green defects. Unfortunately, not all acquired defects behave in this manner, and significant exceptions exist. Table 2-6 lists the most common disease entities and their relative color defects.

The most accurate way to measure color vision is with the use of spectral light sources (Nagel anomaloscope). Because such testing is very difficult and time consuming, alternative methods based on pigmented surface colors were developed.[2] Tests that use this method are the pseudoisochromatic plates, the Farnsworth–Munsell 100 hue test, and Farnsworth D-15 test. By far the easiest test to use in children is the pseudoisochromatic plates. The plates consist of dots arranged in a particular pattern that can be read quite easily by the normal individual. The plates were designed to detect congenital dyschromatopsias but are inadequate for classification. The patterns are designed to show large letters, figures, or numbers, which are easily recognized even by children. Although the child may not know the letter or number illustrated, they can be asked to trace the figure with their finger. More sophisticated testing and classification can be performed with the Farnsworth–

Munsell 100 hue test or the Farnsworth D-15 test[2]; these involve arranging colored caps between pairs of reference caps that are placed at each end of a long narrow rectangular box. Characteristic patterns of confusion are seen in individuals with congenital and acquired color vision defects. This test requires a fair amount of cognitive ability, and children usually must be 6 or 7 years of age before such testing is possible.

FUNDUSCOPIC EXAM

The funduscopic exam is crucial in the evaluation of children with neuro-ophthalmic disorders, because most cases of visual loss or nystagmus are caused by an optic nerve or macular disorder that can usually be diagnosed with indirect ophthalmoscopy (Table 2-7). The test can be done by having the child cradled in the parent's lap, with the child's feet tucked under the parent's elbows, and the head supported by the parent's closed knees. If possible, to facilitate cooperation, keep the infant slightly hungry and feed the bottle during the fundus exam. If the child does provide some resistance, an assistant can be used to stabilize the head. The use of a lid speculum may be necessary, but every effort should be made to avoid it. Parents do not like the lid speculum and may become quite annoyed with the physician's "barbaric" techniques. Attempts at reassuring the parents that this is not uncomfortable, when the child is screaming loudly, usually are unsuccessful.

The older infant and young child can be persuaded into cooperating for the indirect ophthalmoscopy exam by making some

TABLE 2-7. Possible Etiology of Decreased Vision.

Age	*Monocular*	*Binocular*
Infant	Optic nerve hypoplasia Optic glioma	Optic nerve hypoplasia Chiasmal glioma Retinal dysplasia (Leber's congenital amaurosis) Albinism Delayed visual maturation
Child	Strabismus Neuroretinitis Optic neuritis	Hereditary optic atrophy Stargart's disease Pseudotumor cerebri
Teenager	Optic neuritis	Optic neuritis Macular dystrophies Leber's optic neuropathy

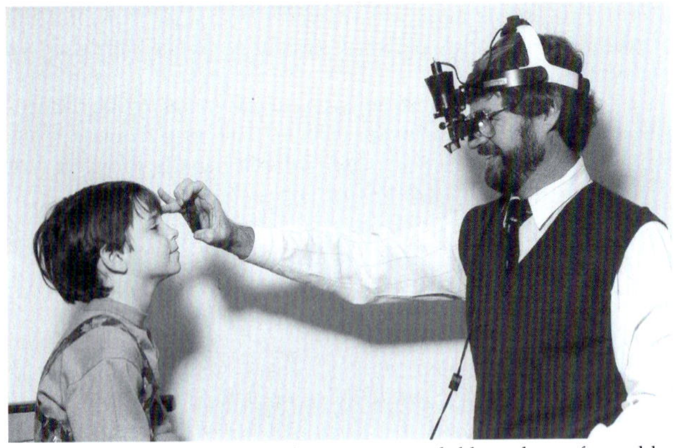

FIGURE 2-11. Indirect ophthalmoscopy in a child can be performed by using a 20 diopter lens. Control and stability can be obtained by resting the fingers on the child's forehead.

compromises in the quality of the exam. The first is to use as low illumination as possible. Although this does decrease the quality of the image, it is much better to get a "grade B" look of the fundus rather than a "grade A" view of the closed lids or inferior sclera. Second, avoid manipulating the lids as this usually causes the child to squeeze and results in the Bell's phenomena. By using a 20 diopter indirect lens and resting the fingers lightly on the child's forehead for support, the examiner can get an excellent view of optic nerve and macula (Fig. 2-11). Last, quick views should be obtained of each eye before prolonged retinal or optic nerve examination is attempted as all too often the child rapidly becomes uncooperative. A quick view of each eye is better than none at all. The peripheral fundus is rarely of neuro-ophthalmic significance but can be examined with a 28 diopter indirect lens if necessary.

GENERAL NEUROLOGICAL EVALUATION

The ocular findings must be evaluated in the context of the patient's overall neurological condition to reach a valid conclusion. In searching for associated neurological abnormalities, questions should be asked about such entities as seizures, ataxia, decreased hearing, and spasticity. In young infants, much can be learned by assessing general neurodevelopment as this will give some indication of neurological impairment. The best milestones to check are those which mothers tend to remember clearly (smiling, sitting, standing, walking, first words, feeding self, and bladder control), and the experienced mother should be asked to make comparisons with her other children. Discrepancies may have diagnostic value, because delay in a single area nearly always indicates a localized rather than a generalized defect.[15] Table 2-8 is a summary of some of the more common neurological milestones and their time of occurrence.

A detailed neurological examination in a child is beyond the expertise of most ophthalmologists, but a few areas are of particular concern. Helpful neuro-ophthalmic localizing information can be learned by assessing the trigeminal nerve (facial sensation), facial nerve (muscles of facial expression), and the auditory nerve (hearing). As an example, an abduction deficit plus ipsilateral facial weakness is most likely caused by a lesion in the brainstem (pons). An abduction weakness plus ipsilateral hearing loss and facial pain is most likely the result of inflammation of the petrous bone (Gradenigo's syndrome). Testing motor function and sensation in the upper and lower extremities, although less helpful from an ophthalmic standpoint, should also be attempted. Such information can be useful in guiding further neurological and neuroradiologic investigation. Only by considering the ocular abnormality within the context of the entire neurological system can appropriate therapy be recommended.

TABLE 2-8. Developmental Milestones in Infants and Children.

Age	*Motor activity*	*Social activity*
6 weeks	Lifts head while prone	Smiles
3 months	Holds objects in hands	Cooing noises
6–8 months	Sits, rolls over	Vocalizes displeasure Feeds self
9–12 months	Crawls, stands with support Walks holding on	Waves bye-bye Plays patty-cake Two to four words
12–15 months	Cruises, walks by self, throws objects Scribbles with crayon Builds tower with blocks	Requests by pointing Understands name of several objects Assists in dressing
18–24 months	Bends over and picks up objects Toilet trained Runs	Uses spoon Two to three sentences Knows some body parts

Data from Gesell and Amatruda. Developmental diagnosis. New York: Harper & Row, 1974; Illingworth. The development of the infant and young child: normal and abnormal. New York: Churchill Livingstone, 1980; Farmer TW (ed) Pediatric neurology. Philadelphia: Harper & Row, 1983, with permission.

References

1. Barricks M, Flynn J, Kushner B. Paradoxical pupillary responses in congenital stationary night blindness. Arch Ophthalmol 1977;95: 1800–1805.
2. Birch J. A practical guide for color-vision examination: report of the standardization committee of the international research group on color vision deficiencies. Ophthalmic Physiol Opt 1985;5:265–285.
3. Brown P, Wald G. Visual pigments in single rods and cones of the human retina. Science 1964;144:45–52.
4. Buckley E. Evaluation of the child with nystagmus. Semin Ophthalmol 1990;5:131–137.
5. Flynn J, Kazarian E, Barricks M. Paradoxical pupil in congenital achromatopsia. Int Ophthalmol 1981;3:91–96.
6. Frank J, Kushner B, France T. Paradoxic pupillary phenomena: a review of patients with pupillary constriction to darkness. Arch Ophthalmol 1988;106:1564–1566.
7. Glaser J. Neuro-ophthalmologic exam: general considerations and special techniques. In: Glaser J (ed) Neuro-ophthalmology. Philadelphia: Lippincott, 1990.
8. Hart W. Acquired dyschromatopsias. Surv Ophthalmol 1987;32:10–31.
9. Hemholtz H. Physiologic optics. New York: Optica Society of America, 1924.
10. Kestenbaum A. Clinical methods of neuro-ophthalmology examination. New York: Grune & Stratton, 1961.
11. Lambert S, Taylor D, Kriss A. The infant with nystagmus, normal appearing fundi, but abnormal ERG. Surv Ophthalmol 1989;34:173–185.
12. Levatin P. Pupillary escape in disease of the retina and optic nerve. Arch Ophthalmol 1959;62:768–770.
13. Linske A. Visual acuity in the newborn, with notes on some subjective methods to determine visual acuity. Doc Ophthalmol 1973;34: 259–265.
14. von Noorden K, Burian H. Visual acuity in normal and amblyopic patients under reduced illumination. Arch Ophthalmol 1959;65:533–540.
15. Paine R, Oppe T. Neurologic examination of children. Philadelphia: Lippincott, 1966.
16. Quinn G, Fea A, Minguini N. Visual fields in 4 to 10 year old children using Goldman and double arc perimetry. J Pediatr Ophthalmol Strabismus 1991;28:314–319.
17. Thompson H, Montague P, Cox T, Corbett J. The relationship between visual acuity, pupillary defect and visual field loss. Am J Ophthalmol 1982;93:681–688.

The Pediatric Low-Vision Patient

Anne Frances Walonker

The American Academy of Pediatrics states that 75% of learning during the early years is processed through vision; because vision is a learning sense, children with visual impairment may not learn to perform many tasks as quickly as those with normal vision. Children with subnormal vision often look and act like any other child in the classroom and on the playground making it difficult to distinguish them from normally sighted children. Children with low vision may wear thick glasses or even dark glasses, but they will run and jump as fearlessly as their playmates.

Never having known any other vision, these children are often unaware that their vision is less than that of other children, and the majority adapt quite well to their environment. Only a few children with low vision need special schools or a protected environment. The majority of these low-vision children function much better in a standard school system with the help of a resource teacher for some part of the school week. As much as is possible, these children need to be mainstreamed. They need to be expected to perform the same tasks and to assume the same responsibilities as normally sighted children of the same age.

INCIDENCE

According to the Centers for Disease Control (CDC), nearly 1 in 1000 children in the United States has some degree of low vision or is legally blind.[1] Not being able to see can alter how a child understands and functions in the world. Impaired vision can affect a child's emotional, neurological, and physical development by potentially limiting the range of experiences and the kinds of information to which a child is exposed.

CLINICAL FEATURES

Decreased vision in a child can be caused by many different processes, each one requiring a different method of treatment: either medical, surgical, or optical. If normal vision cannot be restored, then the use of both optical and nonoptical aids to enhance the remaining vision is necessary.

Whatever the cause of the decreased vision, early intervention is of the utmost importance for the child to adapt to the environment and to continue the learning processes without interruption. The clinical features that could alert a parent to signs of a visual problem in their child include, but are not limited to, nystagmus, strabismus, random eye movements, leukocoria, and corneal opacity.

CLINICAL ASSESSMENT

Clinical assessment of a child with a suspected visual impairment always consists of a very detailed clinical evaluation by a pediatric ophthalmologist, with ancillary testing such as electrophysiology and ultrasonography when appropriate.

The measurement of visual function should be done with targets appropriately sized for both the age of the child and the level of vision suspected, moving the child closer to the testing targets both for near and for distance. The visual requirements for each child should also be assessed because the various therapeutic modalities are age and task appropriate.

The importance of early diagnosis of the child's visual disability cannot be overstated. The earlier the disability is diagnosed, the earlier treatment intervention can begin. Early treatment may produce a better outcome by allowing a stepwise approach to planning the use of aids, both visual and nonvisual, for the short and long term. For those children with an inherited process, early diagnosis makes it possible to provide expedient and appropriate counseling for the families involved. Innumerable low-vision aids of various types are available for enhancing both distance and near vision. The type of device that is appropriate will change as the child becomes older and their visual requirements change and increase. The low-vision devices that are useful for children bear no relationship to those used by most adults.

Because reading is the child's access to learning, a visual aid that makes this task possible is one of the most important devices for these children. The phakic school-age child has an enormous range of accommodation. These children find that reading can be a simple matter of bringing the print close enough to their faces to magnify the image. A fixed-stand low-power magnifier (Fig. 3-1) to enhance these images is probably the most useful low-vision aid for these young children. When the magnifier is placed directly on the page, its fixed focus keeps the

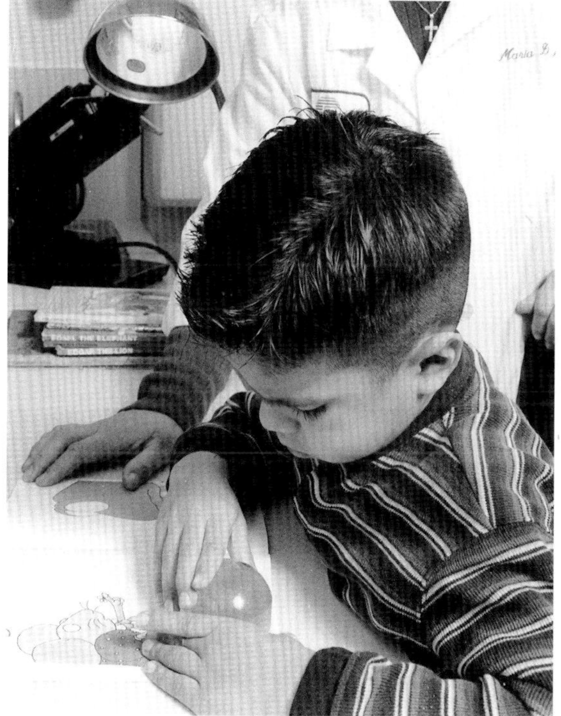

FIGURE 3-1. Low-power stand magnifier.

print clear at all times and lets the child run the device along the page. Even very young children learn to manipulate these devices, and they have been found more useful than many of the more technically sophisticated and costly aids available today.

The aphakic child has different needs. However, glasses or contact lenses with reading additions and the same fixed-focus stand magnifiers can be of great help to these children. The other aid that is exciting to young children with decreased vision is a monocular telescope (Fig. 3-2). It takes a little longer to master this device, but, once the child learns to use it, it opens up a whole new world. The small size of these telescopes makes

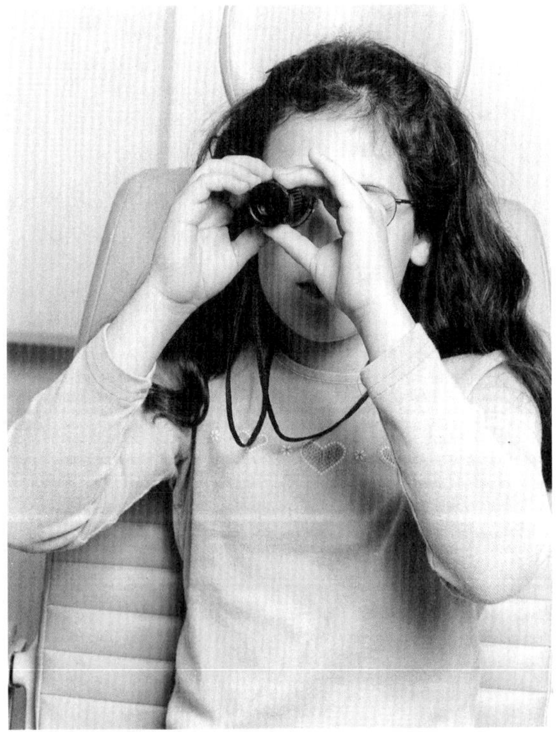

FIGURE 3-2. Monocular telescope.

them highly portable. A child can use this device anywhere and can share it with normally sighted friends, thus erasing the stigma associated with the use of a low-vision aid.

The social and academic success of a child with a visual disability depends largely on the expectations of the family and the understanding of the teachers and the school administrators; the focus should not be on the limitations that the visual disability creates but on the heights that these children can achieve. Teachers, classroom aides, and playground supervisors should be encouraged to treat these children no differently than they treat the others in the class. However, staff need to remain aware of the children's special needs and address these needs appropriately. Where these children are seated in the classroom, the distance between them and the blackboard, the size of the letters on the board, the color of the chalk used, and the angle of the glare from the windows are all as important as any optical or nonoptical visual aid being used.

Furnishing the family and the teachers with a detailed report of the size of print that the child can see for both near and distance work is most helpful. When there are problems with contrast on homework assignments (some copies are so poor that enlarging the print makes them impossible to read), a different type of copy for these children is important. For some children, a closed-circuit television (Fig. 3-3) facilitates reading when increased magnification is required, as the magnifying glass of increased power decreases the field of view. These devices are expensive, but an older child will find them very useful. Most schools with resource centers make them available, as do public libraries.

With increased awareness of and attention to those things that make schoolwork easier to handle, most children will adapt well to their less-than-normal vision, which will do more for their self-confidence than any expensive magnifier or complicated reading machine can possibly do. However, as the child becomes older and reading demands increase, these more sophisticated instruments will become appropriate and should be added to the armamentarium. Newer instruments include closed-circuit television cameras that can be used with computers and portable handheld devices that scan curved surfaces and have large-print readouts on the handles. There are many headborne devices, used for both distance and near reading, that are appropriate for adults who need them to maintain a career. These newer devices are not really necessary in the elementary

That's right!
What's right?
Meehoo!
That's what I want to know!
What's what you want to know?
Me who?
Yes, exactly!
Exactly what?
Yes, I have an Exactlywatt

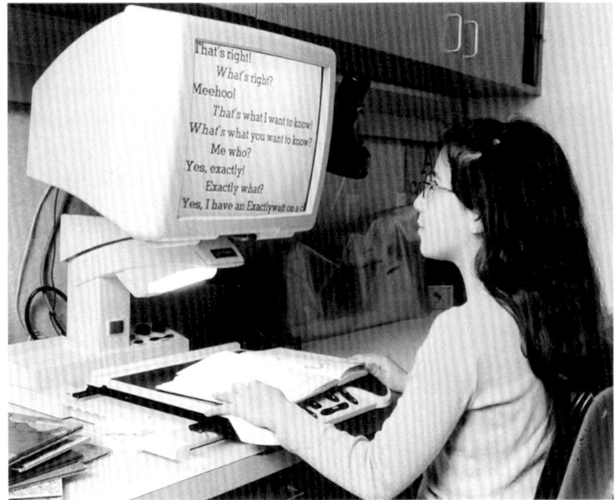

FIGURE 3-3. Closed-circuit television.

and high school classroom, but they may be more useful to college students who sit in large classrooms and who may find it necessary to copy notes from distant blackboards or screens.

There are some points to remember when evaluating a child for visual aids:

- Amblyopia can occur in the presence of another visual abnormality and should be treated vigorously. The better the vision, the less magnifying power needed.
- It is acceptable for moderate to high myopes to remove their glasses for near work.
- The accommodative range will decrease as these children get older, and a change in vision does not necessarily mean a worsening of a previously stable condition.
- There is no limit to the amount of reading aid that can be prescribed so long as this aid improves near vision.
- Only those visual aids that are needed for the currently performed tasks should be prescribed. For the young child, this will probably mean a stand magnifier for near tasks and a telescope for distance tasks.

RESOURCES

Bibliography from Pediatric Ophthalmology Consumer Resources

Madelyn Hall
Good Samaritan Hospital and Medical Center
1040 N.W. 22nd Avenue
Portland, OR 97219

"Vision and Vision Impairment" (a bibliography of books for children)
Pediatric Projects Incorporated
P.O. Box 1880
Santa Monica, CA 90406

"Selected readings for parents of preschool handicapped children"
National Library Service for the Blind and Physically Handicapped
Library of Congress
1291 Taylor Street NW
Washington DC 20542
1-800-424-8567

Additional Resources

National Association for the Visually Handicapped (NAVH)
305 East 24th Street
New York, NY 10010

American Foundation for the Blind
Customer Service Division
15 West 16th Street
New York, NY 10010

Reference

1. Centers for Disease Control. NECH Publ no 99-0444. National Center for Environmental Health, Centers for Disease Control. Washington, DC: 1999.

Breaking the News: The Role of the Physician

Nancy Chernus-Mansfield

Janet and Marc thought their life was as close to perfection as any family's life could be. Married for 8 years, they had one daughter, Missy, age 5, and Brian, age 3 months, their long-awaited son. At Brian's 3-month routine well-baby checkup, the pediatrician remarked that Brian might have strabismus because his eyes appeared to turn in and weren't "working together," as Janet later described it. The pediatrician was very reassuring, however, and told Marc and Janet that he would like the baby to be examined by a pediatric ophthalmologist "just to be on the safe side." Marc had recently started a new and more responsible job so it was decided that Janet would take Brian for the eye examination herself, to minimize the amount of time Marc was away from the office.

Thursday, July 14, began like many others for Janet. She got Missy off to kindergarten, kissed Marc goodbye, and packed up for the day's outing, an eye doctor's appointment. Preparing a 3-month-old to meet a new doctor was a challenge for Janet. She wanted Brian not only to look his best but to be his most alert and charming self.

When Janet arrived for the appointment, everything seemed easy enough. She filled out the routine medical information and was brought into the examining room. The doctor came in, introduced himself, and asked Janet some questions about Brian's development and about the pregnancy. As Brian was being examined, Janet began to feel twinges of anxiety. Brian was screaming. For the doctor to get a good look at his eyes, he explained to Janet that he would have to put a speculum in Brian's eyes to keep them open and in position. Unprepared for the papoose board they placed him on, or for the torturous-looking instrument the doctor used, Janet was becoming extremely upset. Finally the examination was complete, or so Janet thought. The doctor said he couldn't give a diagnosis, however, without some additional tests. Janet didn't understand. Why would crossed eyes require additional tests? The doctor would not comment. He told Janet he wanted more information and would arrange for her to go across the street to a facility that could do the tests. Quickly, Janet called her neighbor to make arrangements for Missy to be picked up from kindergarten. Although she was feeling upset by the morning's examination, Janet thought it best not to call and alarm Marc because she thought the doctor was probably just being thorough.

Janet took Brian across the street to the laboratory where they did electrophysiological tests. Fortunately, Brian had fallen asleep and the flashing lights and electrodes did not seem to bother him. The person who did the tests did not give Janet any information. He told her to return to her physician's office.

When Janet entered the doctor's office this time, she was feeling very apprehensive. She was ushered into the doctor's office, instead of an examining room. After about 15 long minutes, the doctor appeared. He sat down behind his desk, took out Brian's chart, and began to speak. From what Janet can remember, he said something like this: "The test confirmed what I have suspected. Your baby has a condition known as Leber's congenital amaurosis. This condition affects the optic nerves and, from my experience, I believe he is totally blind. There is no treatment. I am sorry. I wish you and your family the best of luck."

Janet can't remember what happened after that. She has no memory of her drive home, of picking up Missy, or of calling Marc. What she does remember is feeling that her life, Brian's life, Marc's life, and Missy's life were over. Nothing would ever be the same again.

Thursdays were busy days for Jack Smith, M.D. He had private patients in the morning and clinic patients all afternoon. At 38, he had achieved his dream of becoming a successful pediatric ophthalmologist. He had always had an interest in ophthalmology but, after his pediatric rotation, he decided that pediatric ophthalmology was a truly exciting field. Jack felt lucky that his wife of 12 years was always supportive of him and that all three of his children, Jack Jr., 10, Jennifer, 8, and Jason, 6, seemed happy and were proud of their dad. He enjoyed the challenge of his work in his private office as well as his research and teaching at the medical school. He had developed a particular interest in treating strabismus and had become the leading specialist in his area.

After arriving at his office, Jack surveyed his schedule and buzzed Karen, his "right arm," to send in the first patient. As he entered the examining room he saw Janet, an attractive thirtyish woman, gazing lovingly at her infant. Jack suspected that the baby had strabismus. The call from the pediatrician was brief, and indicated nothing out of the ordinary. Jack introduced himself and began the examination. Almost immediately he could feel a knot beginning in his stomach as he noted the presence of a nystagmus. By the time the baby was papoosed and the speculum was in place, he was really concerned. He thought, "Maybe it won't be as bad as I think it is; wait for the ERG." He would feel his discomfort build as he told Janet he wanted some additional tests. "No need to alarm her at this point," he thought. So he sent Janet across the street and proceeded to see the many other children waiting for their examinations.

At 11:45 A.M., the call came from the electrophysiology lab. Jack's suspicions were confirmed: Leber's—a totally blind baby. In 45 minutes he would be face-to-face with Janet. This was the only part of his practice he dreaded—giving bad news. What should he tell her? He wished he knew. "Does anyone?" he wondered. "I will just give her the facts. There's no way to sugarcoat this," he thought. Nothing had prepared him to break people's hearts.

Jack doesn't remember the details of Janet's reaction. He knew, of course, that she was extremely upset. Primarily, though, he felt overwhelming helplessness. None of his hard-won expertise could fix this baby; no patching, no surgery, no nothing. All Jack could do was hope that this family had the strength to cope with the diagnosis. The thought came, "If it was one of my kids, what would I do?" He dismissed that thought quickly. It was too painful. "I'm getting morbid; probably most of the kids do great, and their parents can handle their problems." At least Jack wanted to think so. He loved being a pediatric ophthalmologist because he could really help kids. It was so satisfying to see a child who had amblyopia, for example, and to know that with patching the child's vision would be assured. He didn't really know that much about what happened to the few blind children he had encountered. They seemed okay, but, Jack thought, to be fully honest, they were the patients with whom he spent the least time. There was, after all, nothing he could do for them.

Yet that day he couldn't shake the feeling of discomfort as he continued to see patients. His mind kept returning to Janet and the pain on her face. What would life be like for her and for her family? Janet seemed shocked when she heard the diagnosis, but she was very quiet. She hadn't said very much or even asked any questions other than, "Are you sure there is nothing that can be done?" He had said "No." Maybe, he thought in retrospect, just saying "no" was too brusque. He hated to admit there was nothing more he could do and that he was unable to offer further hope. Maybe he should have said more. Is there something else he could have done for her? He just didn't know.

PARENTAL REACTIONS TO THE DIAGNOSIS OF BLINDNESS

The impact of blindness on all family members is tremendous. Before the birth of any baby, we all have dreams and expectations about what the future holds. Expecting a child is a special time for most parents. Mothers and fathers love their baby long before it is born. They love the baby because they project onto their child all their dreams, fantasies, and expectations. For many parents, their hopes are realized when a healthy child is born. But for a moment try to imagine all these expectations and dreams destroyed by hearing the doctor say, "Your baby is blind." Parents are devastated. They experience a blow that is totally shattering. As Pearl Buck said when learning her daughter was mentally retarded, "All the joy of my life was gone."

Author Renee Nastoff, the parent of a child with a disability, eloquently described her pain when she wrote, "I fight the unseen enemy. I have reason for revenge but nothing against which to vent my outrage. My child is held hostage by a cruel twist of fate. Only a parent can comprehend the frustration of fighting an attacker that can't possibly be hurt. It is in the air all around me every moment of my life, overshadowing all decisions about my child, crushing and destroying the simple parental right to dream—about Little League, college, marriage, grandchildren. I can feel the enemy now, its fingers tightening at my throat, forcing what I thought were controlled tears. Sometimes it loosens its painful clasp, but never does it desert its hold on my life. I can't kill this stranger, and I can't break away. Yet it tries to force the very spirit of life from me. It will remain with me forever."

A parent experiences one of life's most devastating losses when a child is born with a disability. What the parent has lost is the anticipated perfect child—that very-much-loved-and-dreamed-of child to whom they have already become attached. Surprisingly, the degree of the baby's impairment is not always the crucial factor in determining the parent's reactions. The most important determinant is the parent's dreams for that child. Loss is the hardest thing that we, as human beings, experience. It is not an uncommon event that affects only certain people, nor is loss merely defined as death of a loved one. It actually touches each of us many times and in many ways in our lifetime. Loss shatters the dreams that are the most basic to a person's existence. Major losses with which we are all familiar include divorce, death, or illness. However, less profound losses can include the loss of physical attractiveness, career recognition, money, etc. The significance of the loss varies for each person and depends on how meaningful that particular loss is to the individual's identity. Loss is a common human experience cutting across all socioeconomic lines. The loss of the expected perfect baby is a major trauma in a family's life. The kinds of feelings that parents have in response to their child's visual impairment may be confusing to them. Feelings of shock, helplessness, fear, denial, depression, sadness, anger, guilt, disappointment, and uncertainty are natural and occur with intensity. Many parents have called this time a "mourning period" because the feeling of sadness is so acute. As one mother said: "I felt like my perfect baby had died and I had a different baby—a blind one." Another parent said, "I was so confused. What I expected to be the happiest time of my life turned out to be the saddest."

Grieving is a normal and spontaneous reaction to loss, but in our culture this normal reaction is often regarded as abnormal. Society may view people who are grieving appropriately as though they are behaving inappropriately. Grieving is the process that enables human beings to deal with loss. Yet parents report that the expression of their grief often cuts them off from the very support they need. As one father said, "I haven't cried since I was 12, but now whenever anyone asks about my son, I start to cry. I know that I make people uncomfortable and they often try to avoid me." This father's expression of his feelings is a healthy response that will eventually enable him to cope with his grief. It is part of the process of detaching from the child he wished for and forming an attachment to his actual child.

Another important and universal reaction parents express is an overwhelming need to understand the reason for their child's impairment. Parents say:

"The question 'why' is always in the back of my mind. Am I to blame?"

"When I was pregnant, I moved the furniture."

"There were various medications I was taking for my asthma. I often wonder, 'Was the medicine the cause of my baby's handicap?' "

"When I was pregnant with John, I couldn't quit work. We had no insurance, and I sometimes think maybe I could have taken it easier and should not have worried about the money. When I'm alone I start blaming myself."

It is natural for parents to look for reasons to explain their child's blindness. When a painful event occurs, it is human nature to feel that perhaps we could bear the pain better if we would understand why it happened, if we could make sense of something so senseless. When people feel lost, they want a road map, and answers seem to provide the needed map. For some people, medical explanations are helpful; for others, religious beliefs provide comfort; but for the vast majority of parents, there are no satisfying answers that relieve the pain or diminish the feeling that "life is not fair." Most of us have a deep sense of justice and fairness, and it is terribly hard to think that something this tragic can happen without a reason. Some fortunate families who are religious believe that, although they don't understand why, God has a purpose and this helps them cope with their child's disability. Many parents never find a reasonable explanation. People find it hard to think that a catastrophic disability happens randomly or that the world could be so chaotic that who or what a person is, or does, is of no consequence. Most of us grow up believing that justice prevails, that bad things happen to bad people and good things happen to good people. Reconciling this view with one's own life is very difficult for all of us. A physician once said, in helping a family deal with this issue: "Often people think that, because they took drugs in high school or had a teenage abortion, they may be responsible for the child's disability. I reassure my patients that all of us can find fault with ourselves in reviewing our lives. However, I tell parents that their previous behaviors have nothing to do with their child's disability. It is simply a random event, and they were unlucky. I find that my patients are very relieved when I reassure them about these issues."

Most parents do begin to cope quickly and in tandem with grieving. Although parents love their disabled child and make the necessary adjustments, their lives are never the same. The pain comes and goes forever.

BREAKING THE NEWS: THE ROLE OF THE PHYSICIAN

Physicians are often unaware the their role has a direct effect on the family's adaptation process. The way the physician presents the diagnosis to the family is crucial. For the rest of their lives, parents will remember not just what they were told, but the way in which it was communicated by the physician.

The following ingredients are necessary in a successful doctor–patient or doctor–parent interaction: consideration, truth, clarity, awareness, compassion, trust, accessibility, and professional kindness.

Consideration

Always sit down when talking to a family. Sit down in a private place, with no spectators. Do not appear rushed, even though you may have a waiting room full of patients. Look directly at the parents, make eye contact, and do not write or dictate into a recorder as you are talking. Try not to be interrupted when giving bad news; the family needs your undivided attention. During the diagnostic process, don't think out loud. This causes unnecessary anxiety. Don't talk with other medical personnel in front of the family; this can be accomplished before or after you have finished explaining the diagnosis. Above all, treat people as you would like to be treated in a like situation.

Truth

It is understandably difficult for the physician to give bad news. It is best to be direct, but not blunt. As one physician said, "There are many ways to say the same thing: truth doesn't mean brutality. Your face can stop a clock—when I'm with you, time stands still." Although both statements convey the same cognitive information, the emotional impact is significantly different.

Clarity

Give information using plain language. When parents are anxious, it interferes with understanding. Often physicians use medical jargon to protect themselves in this time of stress. Physicians must give the information clearly and directly. Sometimes in their discomfort, doctors unconsciously resort to excessive discussion or speculation about the disease or use too much intellectual discourse. This is not helpful to the family.

Awareness

Be aware of how the family is feeling. Acknowledge your own feelings as well. Recognize how you feel as a doctor giving a diagnosis for which there is no cure. Remember that the family is frightened and in more pain than you are and think about how the news is affecting them. Often physicians talk about disease or body parts to depersonalize the information and to depersonalize the enormity of the task of giving a difficult diagnosis.

Compassion

Allow yourself to feel compassion for your patient, for their parents, and for yourself. Compassion will not distort the professional relationship. Rather, your concern and discomfort about the diagnosis can be helpful to a family. Even if you are ill at ease or uncomfortable, the human connection your feelings can create may help the family to cope. Your expression, body language, and tone of voice are important. Your words will be etched forever in the memory of the family.

Trust

Parents must trust you not only as a physician who is medically competent, but as someone that they can count on to help them in this critical period. They must trust you to be honest at all times. Parents must also be able to trust that you recognize their pain and sorrow and will not abandon them.

Accessibility

Because of the emotional impact of the diagnosis, parents need to be able to talk with you more than once. Often it is helpful to leave the room for a period of time after the initial diagnosis has been delivered. Anxiety often blocks the ability to absorb information, and the family may need to have the diagnosis explained more than once. This response is normal and has nothing to do with their intelligence. Allow them some private time and then return 10 to 15 minutes later to review the information. Let the family know that you are available if they would like to schedule another appointment to talk about the diagnosis again or to answer any questions.

Professional Kindness

Professional kindness is the key to giving bad news. It encompasses all the ingredients previously discussed. It enables physicians to communicate with their patients in a helpful and meaningful way. It helps parents to come to terms with the diagnosis. Professional kindness is a tool, a means of helping people in a kind and humane way. Professional kindness lets parents know you care and are concerned about their welfare and the welfare of their child. Professional kindness will not tax the personal resources of a physician. Rather, it provides a concrete set of behaviors that can be relied upon even in the most serious situation.

SUMMARY

- Professional kindness works. Parents, and physicians themselves benefit.
- Treating families with professional kindness affects those families for the rest of their lives. Families who experience the lack of kindness are negatively affected forever, whereas those who experienced their doctor's concern feel cared about, which strengthens their ability to cope.
- Points to remember:
  a. Sit down.
  b. Make eye contact.
  c. Say you are sorry to have to give bad news.
  d. Give the diagnosis in a private setting.
  e. Explain the diagnosis simply and clearly.
  f. Do not take calls or allow interruptions while telling the news.

g. Allow the parents to cry or to express shock, grief, anger, or any other emotion they feel.
h. If you are too busy to spend sufficient time, arrange for another appointment so that parents can have adequate time to ask questions.
i. Do not try to ameliorate grief by saying such things as "It could be worse."
j. Try to give appropriate referrals. It helps both the family and the physician to be able to do something.
k. If possible, do not request payment from a family in shock. A staff member can contact the family at a later date.
l. Teach your staff about all these points. Insist on professional kindness in your office.

Acknowledgment. I thank Marilyn Horn, L.C.S.W., for all her hard work with the original subject matter.

APPENDIX

Parents need referrals. Contacting resources is something concrete parents can do for their child, and for many individuals, taking action also relieves anxiety. Resources are different in each state. We have prepared a list that gives you a place to start. Parents can use this list to find out what other resources may exist in their community.

Cancer

American Cancer Society
46 First St. NE
Atlanta, GA 30308
800/ACS-2345
404/320-3333

Candlelighters Childhood Cancer Foundation
1312 18th St. NW, Suite 300
Washington, DC 20036
800/366-2223
202/659-5136
(See also Visual Impairments for Retinoblastoma resources)

Cerebral Palsy

Canadian Cerebral Palsy Association
800 Wellington St., Suite 612
Ottawa, Ontario
Canada K1R 6K7
800/267-6572 (in Canada)
613/235-2144

United Cerebral Palsy Association
7 Penn Plaza, Suite 804
New York, NY 10001
800/USA-1UCP
212/268-6655

CHARGE Syndrome

CHARGE Accounts
c/o Quota Club
2004 Parkade Blvd.
Columbia, MO 65202
314/442-7604

Chronic Illness

N.O.R.D.
National Organization for Rare Disorders
P.O. Box 8923
New Fairfield, CT 06812
http://www.rarediseases.org

Magic Foundation
(Optic Nerve Hypoplasia)
1327 N. Harlem Ave.
Oak Park, IL 60302
709/383-0808
http://www.magicfoundation.org

Parents of Chronically Ill Children
1527 Maryland St.
Springfield, IL 62702
217/522-6810

Deaf/Blind

John Tracy Clinic
806 West Adams Blvd
Los Angeles, CA 90007
800/522-4582

Hydrocephalus

Hydrocephalus Association
2040 Polk St., Box 342
San Francisco, CA 94109
415/776-4713

Hydrocephalus Support Group
c/o Kathy McGowan
6059 Mission Rd., #106
San Diego, CA 92108
619/282-1070

National Hydrocephalus Foundation
22427 S. River Rd.
Joliet, IL 60436
815/467-6548

Lawrence Moon Bardet Biedl Syndrome

Lawrence Moon Bardet Biedl Syndrome Network
18 Strawberry Hill
Windsor, CT 06095
203/688-7880

Marfan Syndrome

National Marfan Foundation
382 Main St.
Port Washington, NY 10050
516/883-8712

Mental Retardation

Association for Retarded Citizens of the U.S.
500 E. Border St., Suite 300
Arlington, TX 76010
817/261-6003

Neurofibromatosis

National Neurofibromatosis Foundation
141 Fifth Ave., Suite 7-S
New York, NY 10010
800/323-7938
212/460-8980

Visual Impairments

American Foundation for the Blind
15 West 16th St.
New York, NY 10011
800/AF-BLIND (232-5463)
212/620-2043

American Printing House for the Blind
1839 Frankfort Ave.
P.O. Box 6085
Louisville, KY 40206-0085
502/895-2405

Association for Macular Diseases
210 East 64th St.
New York, NY 10021
212/655-3007

The Institute for Families of Blind Children
P.O. Box 54700
Mailstop #111
Los Angeles, CA 90054-0700
323/669-4649

National Association for the Visually Impaired
P.O. Box 317
Watertown, MA 02272-0317
800/562-6265
Fax: 617/972-7444
(Some areas have a state organization as well; NAPVI can direct the parent)

National Organization for Albinism and Hypopigmentation (NOAH)
155 Locust St., Suite 1816
Philadelphia, PA 19102
800/473-2310
215/545-2322

Parents and Cataract Kids (PACK)
c/o Geraldine Miller
P.O. Box 73
Southeastern, PA 19399
215/352-0719

Retinoblastoma International
4650 Sunset Blvd., M.S. 88
Los Angeles, CA 90027
323/669-2299
www.retinoblastoma.net

New England Retinoblastoma Support Group
603 Fourth Range Road
Pembroke, NH 03275

General Resources

The Family Resource Coalition
230 N. Michigan Avenue
Suite 1625, Dept. W
Chicago, IL 60601
(Identification of parent support groups all over the country)

Reaching Out: A Directory of National Organizations Related to Maternal and Child Health
38th and R Streets, NW
Washington, DC 20057
202/625-8400

Team of Advocates for Special Kids
100 W. Cerritos Ave.
Anaheim, CA 92805
714/533-8275

Other National Toll-Free Numbers:

American Council of the Blind 800/424-8666
Better Hearing Institute 800/424-8576
Epilepsy Information Line 800/332-1000
Cystic Fibrosis Foundation 800/344-4823
Downs Syndrome 800/221-4602
Easter Seal Society 800/221-6827
Health Information Clearinghouse 800/336-4797
Spina Bifida 800/621-3141

Fragile X Foundation 800/835-2246
American Kidney Fund 800/835-8018
National Information Center for Orphan Drugs and Rare Disease 800/336-4797
Sickle Cell Association 800/421-8453
Retinitis Pigmentosa (RP) Association International 800/344-4877
Local School Districts or State Departments of Special Education

Search on the Internet for most current information.

Ocular Motility Disorders

Mitra Maybodi, Richard W. Hertle, and Brian N. Bachynski

Normal individuals and most patients with common concomitant childhood strabismus have full ocular rotations (versions and ductions). This chapter is devoted to some of the more frequently encountered childhood disorders of the central and peripheral nervous systems, neuromuscular junction, and extraocular muscles that appear clinically to have incomitant ocular misalignments.

Analysis of ocular alignment, versions, ductions, forced ductions, and generated force allows the examiner to sort the causes of these limited eye movements into three general categories: (1) neuromuscular dysfunction, (2) restriction of the globe by orbital tissues, and (3) combined neuromuscular dysfunction and restriction (Fig. 5-1). Diagnosis in children is especially challenging because it is rarely possible to clinically test the force generated by extraocular muscle action. A general anesthetic is routinely required to perform forced ductions. It may therefore be necessary to base diagnostic and therapeutic decisions on incomplete clinical information, and the clinician must rely on familiarity with the epidemiologic and clinical characteristics of each disorder.

DISORDERS OF THE CENTRAL AND PERIPHERAL NERVOUS SYSTEMS

Eye movement disorders arising from disturbance of the normal neurophysiology may be classified as supra-nuclear, internuclear, or infranuclear.

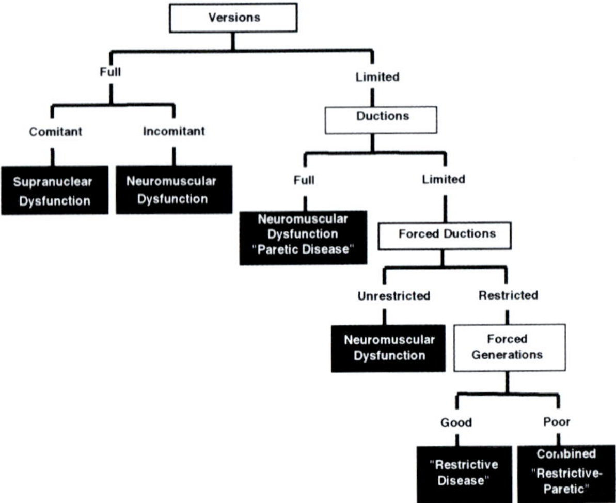

FIGURE 5-1. Clinical evaluation of range of eye movements. Versions and cover test measurements allow the examiner to decide whether the eye movements are normal (no limitation) or limited. Forced duction testing is used to differentiate a restriction (positive resistance to movement of the globe) from a "paresis" (no resistance to movement of the globe).

Supranuclear Eye Movements

Cranial nerves III, IV, and VI serve together with the extraocular muscles as a final mechanism that executes all eye movements. Supranuclear pathways initiate, control, and coordinate various types of eye movements. Several types of eye movements are briefly mentioned here (Table 5-1), but a detailed and lucid synthesis of current concepts of the neural control of eye movements can be found in many other sources.[288]

Physiology and Clinical Assessment

The *vestibular apparatus* drives reflex eye movements, which allow us to keep images of the world steady on the retinas as we move our heads during various activities. The eyes move in the opposite direction to the movement of the head so that they remain in a steady position in space. The semicircular canals are the end organs that provide the innervation to the vestibular nuclei, which in turn drive cranial nerves III, IV, and VI to compensate for rotations of the head. In contrast, the otoliths respond to linear accelerations of the head and to gravity when the head is tilted. You can easily test the effectiveness of input from the semicircular canals by testing the vestibulo-ocular reflex (VOR). First, hold your head still and observe an object such as your index finger as you move it side to side at about 1 to 3 cycles/s. The image is a blur. However, if you hold your finger steady and rotate your head from side to side at the same frequency, you are able to maintain a clear image.

Several forms of *saccades,* fast eye movements, can be clinically observed. *Voluntary* saccades may be *predictive,* in anticipation of a target appearing in a specific location; *command-generated,* in response to a command such as "look to the right"; *memory-guided*; or *antisaccades,* in which a reflexive saccade to an abruptly appearing peripheral target is suppressed and, instead, a voluntary saccade is generated in the equidistant but opposite direction. *Involuntary* saccades consist of *the fast phase of nystagmus* due to vestibular and optokinetic stimuli; *spontaneous saccades,* providing repetitive scanning of the environment, although also occurring in the dark and in severely visually impaired children; and *reflex saccades,* occurring involuntarily in response to new visual, auditory, olfactory, or tactile cues, suppressable by antisaccades.[83]

TABLE 5-1. Types of Eye Movements.

Type of eye movement	*Function*	*Stimulus*	*Clinical tests*
Vestibular	Maintain steady fixation during head rotation	Head rotation	Fixate on object while moving head; calorics
Saccades	Rapid refixation to eccentric stimuli	Eccentric retinal image	Voluntary movement between two objects; fast phases of OKN or vestibular nystagmus
Smooth pursuit	Keep moving object on fovea	Retinal image slip	Voluntarily follow a moving target; OKN slow phases
Vergence	Disconjugate, slow movement to maintain binocular vision	Binasal or bitemporal disparity; retinal blur	Fusional amplitudes; near point of convergence

OKN, optokinetic nystagmus.

The pathway of saccades originates in the visual cortex and projects through the anterior limb of the internal capsule, through the diencephalon. It then divides into dorsal and ventral pathways, the dorsal limb going to the superior colliculi, and the ventral limb (which contains the ocular motor pathways for horizontal and vertical eye movements) to the pons and midbrain. The superior colliculus acts as an important relay for some of these projections (Fig. 5-2).

The neurons responsible for generating the burst, or discharge, for saccades are classified as excitatory burst neurons (EBN); inhibitory burst neurons (IBN) function to silence activ-

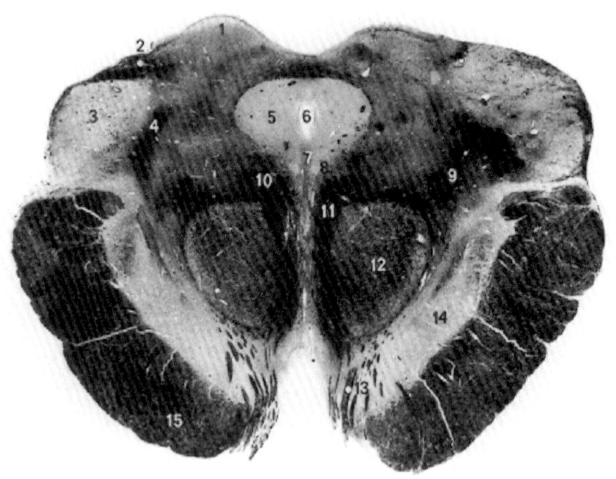

FIGURE 5-2. The superior colliculi are a pair of ovoid masses composed of alternating layers of gray and white matter; they are centers for visual reflexes and ocular movements, and their connections to other structures in the brain and spinal cord are varied and complex. Some of these other structures include the retina, visual and nonvisual cerebral cortex, inferior colliculus, paramedian pontine reticular formation, thalamus, basal ganglia, and spinal cord ventral gray horn. The fibers of the medial longitudinal fasciculus form a fringe on its ventrolateral side: *1*, superior (cranial) colliculus; *2*, brachium of superior (cranial) colliculus; *3*, medial geniculate nucleus; *4*, brachium of inferior (caudal) colliculus; *5*, central gray substance; *6*, cerebral aqueduct; *7*, visceral nucleus of oculomotor nerve (Edinger–Westphal nucleus); *8*, nucleus of oculomotor nerve; *9*, medial lemniscus; *10*, central tegmental tract; *11*, medial longitudinal fasciculus; *12*, red nucleus; *13*, fibers of oculomotor nerve; *14*, substantia nigra; *15*, basis pedunculi.

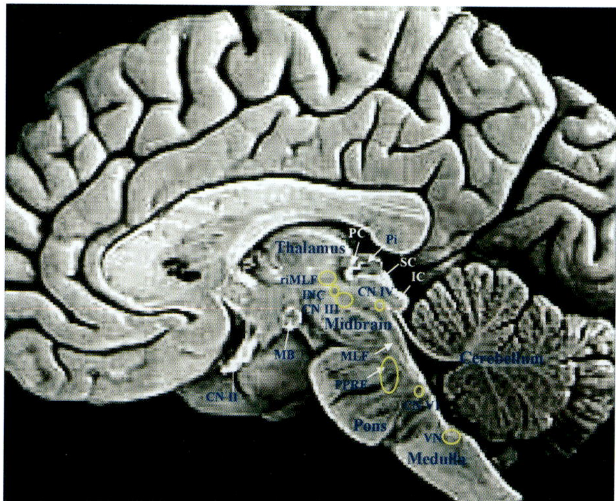

FIGURE 5-3. Brainstem structures controlling eye movements. Parasagittal section of the cerebrum and brainstem shows areas of the ocular motor nuclei and brainstem structures involved with internuclear and supranuclear pathways. *PC*, posterior commissure; *SC*, superior colliculus; *IC*, inferior colliculus; *Pi*, pineal; *riMLF*, rostral interstitial nucleus of the medial longitudinal fasciculus; *INC*, interstitial nucleus of Cajal; *CN III, IV, VI*, cranial nerve III, IV, VI; *MLF*, medial longitudinal fasciculus; *PPRF*, paramedian pontine reticular formation; *VN*, vestibular nuclei.

ity in the antagonist muscle during the saccade. In the brainstem, the rostral interstitial nucleus of the medial longitudinal fasciculus (riMLF) and the pontine paramedian reticular formation (PPRF) provide the saccadic velocity commands, by generating the "pulse of innervation" immediately before the eye movement, to cranial nerves III, IV, and VI. Horizontal saccades are generated by EBN in the PPRF, which is found just ventral and lateral to the MLF in the pons (Figs. 5-3, 5-4, 5-5), and by IBN in the nucleus paragigantocellularis dorsalis just caudal to the abducens nucleus in the dorsomedial portion of the rostral medulla. Vertical and torsional components of saccades are generated by EBN and IBN in the riMLF, located in the midbrain.

Following a saccade, a "step of innervation" occurs during which a higher level of tonic innervation to ocular motoneurons keeps the eye in its new position, against orbital elastic forces

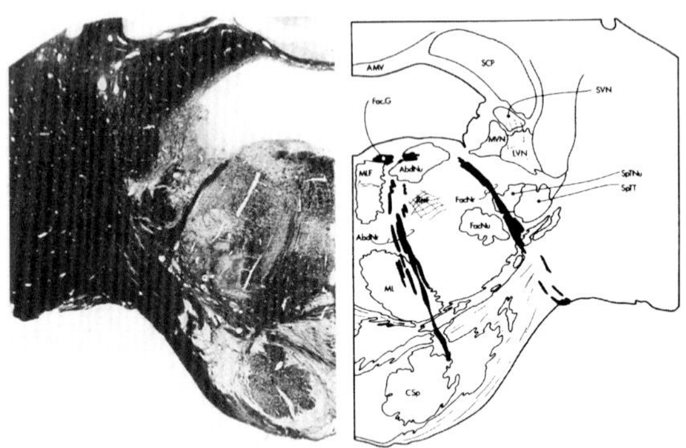

FIGURE 5-4. Transverse section of caudal pons. *AbdNu*, abducens nucleus; *AbdNr*, abducens nerve; *AMV*, anterior medullary velum; *CSp*, corticospinal tract; *FacG*, internal genu of facial nerve; *FacNr*, facial nerve; *FacNu*, facial nucleus; *LVN*, lateral vestibular nucleus; *ML*, medial lemniscus; *MLF*, medial longitudinal fasciculus; *MVN*, medial vestibular nucleus; *RetF*, paramedian pontine reticular formation; *SCP*, superior cerebellar peduncle; *SpTNu*, spinal trigeminal nucleus; *SpTT*, spinal trigeminal tract; *SVN*, superior vestibular nucleus. (Adapted from Haines DE. Neuroanatomy: an atlas of structures, sections, and systems. Baltimore: Urban & Schwarzenberg, 1983, with permission.)

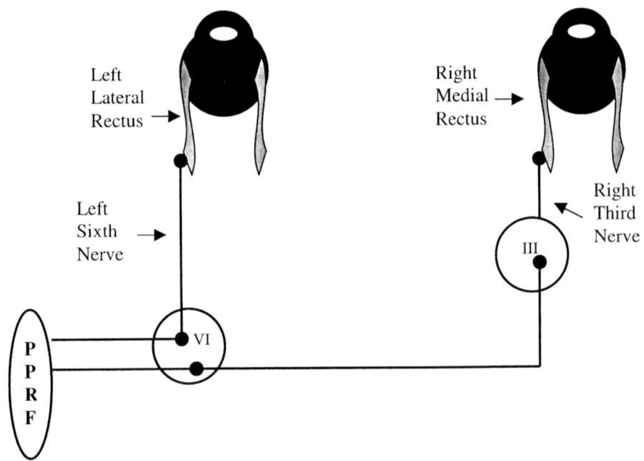

FIGURE 5-5. Schematic of brainstem pathways coordinating horizontal saccades. The PPRF, after receiving input from the ipsilateral cortical centers and superior colliculus, stimulates two sets of neurons in the abducens nucleus: (1) those that send axons to innervate the ipsilateral lateral rectus and (2) those whose axons join the MLF and subsequently activate the medial rectus subnuclei of the contralateral third nerve. *PPRF*, paramedian pontine reticular formation; *VI*, sixth cranial nerve nucleus; *III*, third cranial nerve nucleus.

that would restore the eye to an anatomically "neutral" position. For horizontal saccades, the step of innervation comes from the neural integrator (see following), primarily from the nucleus prepositus–medial vestibular nucleus complex. The eye is held steady at the end of vertical and torsional saccades by the step of innervation provided from the interstitial nucleus of Cajal in the midbrain.[288]

In addition to burst neurons, omnipause neurons, located in the nucleus raphe interpositus in the midline of the pons, between the rootlets of the abducens nerves, are essential for normal saccadic activity. Continuous discharge from omnipause neurons inhibits burst neurons, and this discharge only ceases immediately before and during saccades.[288]

Other burst neurons termed long-lead burst neurons (LLBN) have also been identified that discharge 40ms before saccades, whereas the previously mentioned burst cells discharge 12ms before saccades. Some LLBN lie in the midbrain, receiving projections from the superior colliculus and projecting to the pontine EBN, medullary IBN, and omnipause neurons. Other LLBN lie in the nucleus reticularis tegmenti pontis (NRTP), projecting mainly to the cerebellum but also to the PPRF. It appears that LLBN receiving input from the superior colliculus may play a crucial role in transforming spatially coded to temporally coded commands, whereas other LLBN may synchronize the onset and end of saccades.[288]

If an abnormality of saccadic eye movements is suspected, the quick phases of vestibular and optokinetic nystagmus (OKN) can be easily evaluated in infants and young children. To produce and observe vestibular nystagmus, hold the infant at arm's length, maintain eye contact, and spin first in one direction and then in the other. An OKN response can be elicited in the usual manner by passing a repetitive stimulus, such as stripes or an OKN drum, in front of the baby first in one direction and then in another. In addition, reflex saccades are induced in many young patients when toys or other interesting stimuli are introduced into the visual field. Older children are asked to fixate alternately upon two targets so that the examiner can closely observe the saccades for promptness of initiation, speed, and accuracy.

Smooth pursuit permits us to maintain a steady image of a moving object on our foveas and thereby to track moving targets with clear vision. The pathways for smooth pursuit have not been fully elucidated, but it appears that frontal and extrastriate visual cortex transmits information about the motion of both the target and the eyes to the dorsolateral pontine nuclei (DLPN). This complex signal travels from the DLPN to the cerebellum (paraflocculus, flocculus, and dorsal vermis), and from the cerebellum via the vestibular and fastigial nuclei to its final destination, the ocular motor nerve nuclei III, IV, and VI. Unilateral lesions in the cortex and cerebellum affect smooth pursuit toward the side of the lesion.

Vergences are eye movements that turn the eyes in opposite directions so that images of objects will fall on corresponding retinal points. Two major stimuli are known to elicit vergences: (1) retinal disparity, which leads to fusional vergences, and (2) retinal blur, which evokes accommodative vergences. Convergence of the eyes, accommodation of the lens, and constriction of the pupils occur simultaneously when there is a shift in fixation from distance to near; together, these actions constitute the *near triad*.

The neural substrate for vergence lies in the mesencephalic reticular formation, dorsolateral to the oculomotor nucleus. Neurons in this region discharge in relation to vergence angle (vergence tonic cells), to vergence velocity (vergence burst cells), or to both vergence angle and velocity (vergence burst-tonic cells). Although most of these neurons also discharge with accommodation, experiments have shown that some do remain predominantly related to vergence.[32] Like versional movements, a velocity-to-position integration of vergence signals is necessary. The nucleus reticularis tegmenti pontis (NRTP) has been shown to be important in the neural integration, that is, velocity-to-position integration, of vergence signals. The cells in NRTP that mediate the near response appear to be separate from the cells which mediate the far response. Lesions of NRTP cause inability to hold a steady vergence angle. NRTP has reciprocal connection with the cerebellum (nucleus interpositus) and receives descending projections from several cortical and subcortical structures.[32,288]

The *cerebellum* plays an important role in eye movements. Together with several brainstem structures, including the nucleus prepositus and the medial vestibular nucleus, it appears to convert velocity signals to position signals for all conjugate eye movements through mathematical integration. Because of this, all the structures involved in this process are often referred to as the *neural integrator*. The role of the neural integrator in horizontal saccades was mentioned earlier.

To test the neural integrator clinically, observe fixation, fixation in eccentric gaze, saccades, pursuit, and OKN and also test for rebound nystagmus and VOR cancellation. To examine for rebound nystagmus, first ask the patient to fixate on a target from the primary position, then to refixate on an eccentric target for 30 s, and finally to return to the original primary position target. A patient with rebound nystagmus will show transient nystagmus with the slow phases toward the previous gaze position. To evaluate a child's VOR cancellation, it is easiest to place your hand on top of the patient's head to control both the head and a fixation target that will extend in front of the child's visual axis. You may use a Prince rule with a picture attached. Ask the child to fixate on the target as you passively rotate both the head and the target side to side. If the child is unable to cancel the VOR, you will observe nystagmus instead of the steady fixation expected in normal subjects.

Patients with faulty neural integration may show gaze-evoked nystagmus, impaired smooth pursuit, inability to cancel the vestibulo-ocular reflex during fixation, saccadic dysmetria, defective OKN response, or rebound nystagmus. Most frequently, gaze-evoked nystagmus is seen in conjunction with use of anticonvulsants or sedatives. However, because 60% to 70% of brain tumors in children are subtentorial, acquired eye movement abnormalities suggesting defective neural integration, whether isolated or associated with other neurological deficits, alert the examiner to investigate for a serious central nervous system abnormality.[39,110,132] Structural anomalies affecting the brainstem and cerebellum, for example, the Arnold–Chiari malformation, as well as metabolic, vascular, and neurodegenerative disorders, may also produce abnormalities of the neural integrator.

Reflex eye movements such as the vestibulo-ocular reflex and Bell's phenomenon are easy to elicit clinically and are very useful for gross localization of neural lesions. When both saccades and smooth pursuit in a certain direction are limited, the examiner tries to stimulate eye movements in that same direction with a doll's head (oculocephalic) maneuver, spin test, or forced lid closure. If any of the reflex eye movements are intact, the appropriate cranial nerve(s) and extraocular muscles(s) are clearly functioning, and the defect is necessarily supranuclear.

and the head begins to rotate toward the object of interest. Next, the head continues to rotate past the intended target, allowing the tonically deviated eyes, which are now in an extreme contraversive position, to come into alignment with the target. Finally, as the eyes maintain fixation, the head rotates slowly back so that the eyes are in primary position. This apparent use of the VOR to refixate continues for several years, but with increasing age, patients demonstrate less prominent head thrusting and may even be able to generate some saccades although these are abnormal.[97,542]

In some infants, generalized hypotonia may be associated. This hypotonia seems to be more pronounced in boys and improves with increasing age. These babies later demonstrate the motor delay, incoordination, and clumsiness that have been noted in the literature.[153,395]

Clinical Assessment The parents of children are asked about any associated developmental abnormality. A complete ophthalmic examination is performed to rule out any strabismus or amblyopia, as strabismus has been reported in 22% of these patients in one series.[195] Vision, electroretinogram (ERG), and visual evoked potential (VEP) are normal in the congenital saccade initiation failure patients.[164,451] Any coexistent abnormal vision, nystagmus, or abnormal ERG or VEP suggests associated disease.[451] Neurological abnormalities or dysmorphic features are further investigated by the appropriate subspecialists. A brain MRI is necessary for any suspected neurological disorder, to look for any midline malformation, particularly around the fourth ventricle and cerebellar vermis.[83]

Systemic Associations Significant structural abnormalities of the central nervous system (CNS) may be associated, such as lipoma[477] or brainstem tumor.[540] Joubert's syndrome is associated with cerebellar hypoplasia and agenesis of the corpus callosum.[282] A neuroradiologic correlation has been made in children with saccade initiation failure, in which 61% of 62 children had abnormal scans, primarily the brainstem and cerebellar vermis; however, significant abnormalities in the cerebral cortex and basal ganglia were also found.[450]

Gaucher's disease,[185,197] ataxia telangiectasia[7,473] and its variants, and Niemann–Pick variants[100] may also present with the inability to generate saccades as well as blinking and head thrusting before refixation. Unlike congenital saccade initiation failure, these disorders generally involve vertical as well as horizontal saccades and, of course, eventually manifest systemic signs.

Early-onset vertical saccade initiation failure has been observed in children with lesions at the mesencephalic–diencephalic junction, presumably infarcts resulting from perinatal hypoxia.[135,219]

Inheritance Occasional familial occurrence,[196,345,387,398,501] increased frequency in males, and occurrence in monozygotic twins[67] suggest a genetic process in some cases. Association with nephronophthisis has been described in two patients, each of whom exhibited deletions on chromosome 2q13.[55]

Treatment No treatment is available for congenital saccade initiation failure, but associated strabismus is treated accordingly.

Prognosis The visual and clinical prognosis of those patients with the congenital type is good. Many can adapt over time to allow gaze shifts with less head thrusting and can even generate some saccades, albeit still abnormal.[97,542]

Induced Convergence Retraction/Parinaud or Dorsal Midbrain Syndrome

Lesions of the posterior commissure in the dorsal rostral midbrain (see Fig. 5-2) may result from many disease processes and can affect a variety of supranuclear mechanisms, including those that control vertical gaze, eyelids, vergence, fixation, and pupils. Other terms such as *pretectal syndrome, Koerber–Salus–Elschnig syndrome, Sylvian aqueduct syndrome, posterior commissural syndrome,* and *collicular plate syndrome* all refer to this condition.

Incidence A report of 206 patients with pretectal syndrome in one neurologist's practice at a general hospital in southern California indicated the incidence to be 2.3% of all patients examined by this neurologist in an 18-year period.[255] Of these 206 patients, 71 exhibited induced convergence retraction.

Etiology and Systemic Associations The pretectum was confirmed as the critical structure that is affected in this disorder, investigated clinicopathologically in humans[91] and experimentally in monkeys.[371,372] Also, isolated interruption of the

TABLE 5-3. Causes of Childhood Dorsal Midbrain Syndrome.

Classification by cause	*Specific etiologies*
Tumor	Pineal germinoma, teratoma and glioma; pineoblastoma; others[386]
Hydrocephalus	Aqueductal stenosis with secondary dilation of third ventricle and aqueduct, or with secondary suprapineal recess compressing posterior commissure,[89,366] commonly caused by cysticercosis in endemic areas
Metabolic disease	Gaucher[100,492]; Tay–Sach; Niemann–Pick[154]; kernicterus[214]; Wilson's disease[265]; others
Midbrain/thalamic damage	Hemorrhage; infarction
Drugs	Barbiturates[138]; carbamazepine; neuroleptics
Miscellaneous	Benign transient vertical eye disturbance in infancy; trauma; neurosurgery[445]; hypoxia; encephalitis; tuberculoma; aneurysm[102]; multiple sclerosis

posterior commissure in humans produces the entire syndrome of upward gaze palsy, pupillary light–near dissociation, lid retraction, induced convergence retraction, skew deviation, and upbeat nystagmus.[251] Among the many underlying causes of this condition are hydrocephalus, stroke, and pinealomas. Table 5-3 lists other reported etiologies and systemic associations.

Clinical Features and Assessment The constellation of deficits are (1) vertical gaze palsy, (2) light–near dissociation of the pupils, (3) eyelid retraction (Collier's sign), (4) disturbance of vergence, (5) fixation instability, and (6) skew deviation.

Limitation of upward saccades is the most reliable sign of the convergence retraction. Upward pursuit, Bell's phenomenon, and the fast phases of vestibular and optokinetic nystagmus may also be affected either at presentation or with progression of the underlying process. It is rare for upgaze to be unaffected. Pathological lid retraction and lid lag are also common (Collier's sign).

When the patient attempts upward saccades, a striking phenomenon, convergence and globe retraction, frequently occurs; this is not true nystagmus, despite the common description of this clinical finding as convergence-retraction nystagmus, because there is no true slow phase. This action is best elicited with down-moving OKN targets because each fast phase is replaced by a convergence-retraction movement. Cocontraction of the extraocular muscles has been documented during this convergence-retraction jerk.[161]

Unlike the pathways from upward saccades, the pathways for downward saccades do not appear to pass through the posterior commissure (Figs. 5-3, 5-6). Perhaps because of this, disturbances of downgaze are not as predictable or uniform. Usually down-going saccades and pursuit are present, but they may be slow. Sometimes, especially in infants and children, there is a tonic downward deviation of the eyes that has been designated the "*setting sun*" sign, and down-beating nystagmus may also be observed. The "setting sun" sign may also be seen in children with hydrocephalus.

Convergence spasm may occur during horizontal saccades and produce a "pseudoabducens palsy" because the abducting eye moves more slowly than the adducting eye.[113] This phenomenon can cause reading difficulties early in the course of dorsal midbrain syndrome because it provides an obstacle to refixation toward the beginning of a new line of text. Indeed, older children may present with numerous pairs of corrective

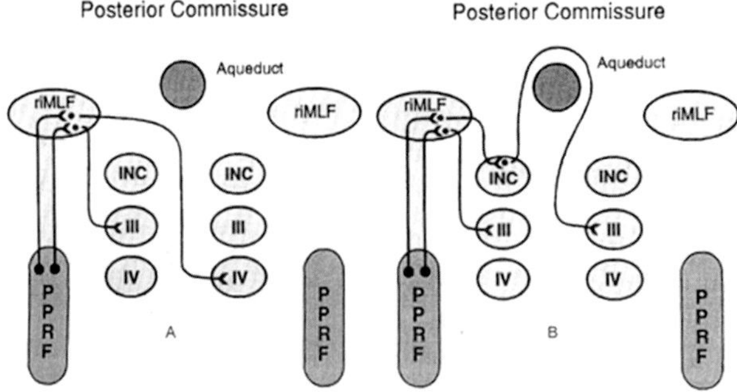

FIGURE 5-6A,B. Schematic of brainstem pathways coordinating downward **(A)** and upward **(B)** saccades. **(A)** Downward saccades. The PPRF activates neurons in the riMLF that send fibers caudally to synapse upon the inferior rectus subnucleus of the ipsilateral third nerve and the contralateral superior oblique nucleus. Not shown in this diagram, fibers from the contralateral PPRF carry corresponding signals simultaneously. **(B)** Upward saccades. The PPRF activates neurons in the riMLF that send fibers through the posterior commisure to the superior rectus subnucleus of the contralateral third nerve and fibers to the inferior oblique subnucleus of the ipsilateral third nerve. Not shown in this diagram, fibers from the contralateral PPRF carry corresponding signals simultaneously. *riMLF*, rostral interstitial nucleus of the medial longitudinal fasciculus; *INC*, interstitial nucleus of Cajal; *III*, third cranial nerve nucleus; *IV*, fourth cranial nerve nucleus; *PPRF*, paramedian pontine reticular formation.

spectacles that have been prescribed due to their "vague" complaints about reading and other near work. In other patients complaining of difficulties with near vision, convergence may be paralyzed. "Tectal" pupils are usually large and react more poorly to light than to near, and anisocoria is not uncommon.

All children with convergence retraction deserve thorough, prompt neurological and neuroradiologic evaluation because timely intervention may be decisive. The natural history of this disorder is dependent on the underlying etiology.

Treatment The underlying medical cause requires investigation and primary treatment. Once the condition is stable for a period of time, from 3 to 12 months, surgery has been performed with some success. In addition to treating the coexistent diplopia from skew deviation or horizontal strabismus, which may be surgically corrected, the anomalous head posture from defective vertical gaze may also be treated by inferior rectus recession or vertical transposition of horizontal recti during simultaneous horizontal strabismus correction.[74] Faden operation (posterior fixation suture, or retroequatorial myopexy) on both medial recti to control convergence spasms and bilateral superior rectus resection to alleviate the anomalous head posture have also been reported.[465]

Prognosis The medical prognosis is dependent upon the underlying etiology. In the aforementioned review of 206 patients, only 20 patients died: 11 of tumors, 7 after strokes, and 1 with transtentorial hernation with tuberculous abscess. The good prognosis in this series may have been skewed by the preponderance of patients with cysticercal hydrocephalus.[255]

The prognosis of strabismus surgery in all eviating anomalous head posture and diplopia was good in all three patients in one study after a minimum of 6 months follow-up.[74] In another report, head posture and ocular motility improved beyond expectation and remained satisfactory after a minimum of 1 year follow-up.[465]

Transient Vertical Gaze Disturbances in Infancy Vertical gaze abnormalities may be benign and transient in infants. Four babies with episodic conjugate upgaze that became less frequent over time have been described.[6,113] During these episodes, normal horizontal and vertical vestibulo-ocular responses could be observed.

Tonic downgaze has been observed in 5 of 242 consecutively examined healthy newborn infants[215] as well as in other infants.[113,285] Again, the eyes can easily be driven above the primary position with the vestibulo-ocular reflex. Also, the eyes show normal upward movements during sleep. In contrast, infants with hydrocephalus who manifest the "setting sun" sign do not elevate the eyes during sleep or with an oculocephalic maneuver.

Premature infants with intraventricular hemorrhage may also develop tonic downgaze, usually in association with a large-angle esotropia.[480] These infants do not elevate the eyes with vestibular stimulation. Upgaze often returns during the first 2 years of life, but the esotropia does not resolve when upgaze returns.

Double Elevator Palsy/Monocular Elevation Deficiency

Monocular deficiency of elevation, that is, an apparent weakness of both the superior rectus and inferior oblique muscles, has been termed *double elevator palsy* or *monocular elevation deficiency*. This deficit may be caused by mechanical restriction of the globe or neural dysfunction at the supranuclear, nuclear, or infranuclear level. Congenital double elevator palsy of supranuclear origin is confirmed on clinical examination if the affected eye elevates during Bell's phenomenon or doll's head maneuver.[44,52]

Spasm of the Near Reflex

Spasm of the near reflex, also referred to as *convergence spasm*, is characterized by intermittent spasm of convergence, of miosis, and of accommodation.[95] Symptoms include headache, photophobia, eyestrain, blurred vision, and diplopia. Patients may appear to have bilateral sixth nerve palsies, but careful observation will reveal miosis and high myopia (8–10 D) on dry retinoscopy, accompanying the failure of abduction.[172] This key clinical clue prevents misdiagnosis and misdirected testing.[172,182,252,430]

Most commonly, spasm of the near reflex is psychogenic, and treatment may include simple reassurance, psychiatric counseling, or cycloplegia with bifocals. However, a number of cases of spasm of the near reflex associated with organic disease have been reported.[487] In a series of seven patients, two had posterior fossa abnormalities (cerebellar tumor, Arnold–Chiari malformation), two had pituitary tumors, one had a vestibulopathy, and two had antecedent trauma.[112] None of these patients appeared to have a personality disorder, and none complained of significant disability. Nevertheless, no clear causal relationship or unified neuroanatomic localization has been established. It is prudent to keep in mind that just as any patient with organic disease may also have a functional disorder, disturbances that are clearly functional do not exclude coexisting organic disease.

Internuclear Opththalmoplegia

In the absence of peripheral lesions such as myasthenia gravis, *failure of adduction combined with nystagmus of the contralateral abducting eye* is termed *internuclear ophthalmoplegia* (INO) and localizes the lesion to the medial longitudinal fasciculus (MLF) unequivocally.

Etiology

The abducens nucleus consists of two populations of neurons that coordinate horizontal eye movements (see Fig. 5-5). Fibers from one group form the sixth nerve itself and innervate the ipsilateral lateral rectus muscle; fibers from the second group join the contralateral MLF and project to the subnucleus of the third nerve, which supplies the contralateral medial rectus muscle. In this way, the neurons of the sixth nerve nucleus yoke the lateral rectus with the contralateral medial rectus.

Clinical Features

Clearly, lesions of the abducens nucleus will cause an ipsilateral conjugate gaze palsy. Lesions of the MLF between the midpons and oculomotor nucleus, in turn, disconnect the ipsilateral medial rectus subnucleus from the contralateral sixth nerve nucleus and cause diminished adduction of the ipsilateral eye on attempted versions (see Fig. 5-3). The signs of INO may be accompanied by an ipsilateral hypertropia or skew deviation.

Clinical Assessment

A subtle adduction deficit is best appreciated when repetitive saccades are attempted; the adducting eye will demonstrate a slow, gliding, hypometric movement in conjunction with overshoot of the abducting eye. Usually, the ipsilateral eye can be adducted with convergence, but convergence will also be impaired if the MLF lesion is rostral enough to involve the medial rectus subnucleus.

Systemic Associations

Similar to dorsal midbrain syndrome, INO is an anatomic rather than etiological diagnosis. A host of structural, metabolic, immunological, inflammatory, degenerative, and other processes can interfere with the function of the MLF and nearby structures. In young adults, multiple sclerosis is by far the most common cause of INO.[342] Multiple sclerosis also underlies most cases of bilateral INO. Although patients with bilateral INO generally remain orthotropic in primary position, they sometimes exhibit an exotropia in the *wall-eyed bilateral internuclear ophthalmoplegia (WEBINO)* syndrome.[311] Additional causes of INO include Arnold–Chiari malformation,[23,99,118,533] hydrocephalus,[352] meningoencephalitis,[64,226] brainstem or fourth ventricular tumors,[99,439,482,496] head trauma,[49,84,254] metabolic disorders, drug intoxications, paraneoplastic effect, carcinomatous meningitis, and others. Peripheral processes, particularly myasthenia gravis and Miller Fisher syndrome, may closely mimic INO and should be considered in any patient with INO-like eye movements.

Treatment and Prognosis

The first goal is to treat the underlying etiology. For example, steroid therapy is necessary in multiple sclerosis, and blood pressure management is required for a hypertensive stroke. After this initial consideration, if the disorder persists and remains stable for at least 6 months, the accompanying exotropia may be corrected by surgery. In a series of three patients treated surgically for diplopia caused by bilateral INO (from brainstem vascular disease) with exotropia of 55 to 70 prism diopters, favorable results were achieved by bilateral medial rectus resections and bilateral lateral rectus recessions (with one lateral rectus on an adjustable suture in each of the three).[74] After a minimum of 6 months postoperative follow-up, all three patients achieved excellent cosmesis. In one of the three patients, binocularity was restored in the primary position, in the second diplopia was eliminated in primary and downgaze, and in the third diplopia was completely eliminated.

Ocular Motor Cranial Nerve Palsies

The processes that produce ocular motor nerve palsies in infants and children, as many neurological diseases in this age group, are commonly diffuse.

General Clinical Considerations

Muscle paralysis is diagnosed by the inability of the eye to move in the direction of action of the particular muscle voluntarily and reflexively, tested by the doll's head maneuver, spin test (looking for vestibular nystagmus), or forced lid closure (looking for Bell's phenomenon). Paresis of a muscle may be detected on testing of versions, at which time version in a particular direction may be limited but ductions may appear full. If the muscle is totally paralyzed, the ductions will be limited as well; in this case, if it is possible to perform a forced duction test, the test would reveal no restriction in the direction of action of a paretic muscle. However, after long-standing muscle paresis, the muscle may become tightened, and forced duction testing in the direction opposite to that of the muscle action would reveal restriction.

A subtle paresis is best appreciated when repetitive saccades are attempted; the eye will demonstrate a slow, gliding, hypometric movement in the direction of action of the particular muscle(s), in conjunction with overshoot of the other eye in that direction. The *primary deviation*, or the measured strabismus when fixing with the normal eye, is smaller than the *secondary deviation*, which is the strabismus measured when fixing with the restricted or paretic eye.

Significant factors in evaluating a child with ocular motor cranial palsies include (1) age of the child, (2) history of previous cranial nerve palsies or relevant systemic disease, (3) recent history of febrile illness, immunization, trauma, or exposure to toxins, (4) accompanying neurological symptoms or signs, and (5) the course under careful, regular observation.

Any child exhibiting an ocular motor nerve palsy accompanied by other neurological signs deserves a consultation with a neurologist and a thorough, timely workup. It is incumbent upon the ophthalmologist to detect and treat any amblyopia that may occur. Also, prevention of amblyopia, by alternate patching, for example, can be considered in severely amblyogenic conditions such as third nerve palsies.

The following discussion sets out an approach to the recognition and initial management of *isolated* third, fourth, and sixth nerve palsies and reviews some common childhood causes of combined ocular motor nerve palsies.

SIXTH NERVE PALSIES

ETIOLOGY AND SYSTEMIC ASSOCIATIONS

Acquired sixth nerve palsies, whether isolated or not, are usually caused by tumors (especially glioma and medulloblastoma) and trauma (47%–62%).[3,24,191,269,287,405] A significant number of cases are also due to inflammatory causes such as meningitis (including from Lyme disease), Gradenigo's syndrome,[117] cerebellitis, and postviral sixth nerve palsy. The clinician is also faced with numerous other possible etiologies (Table 5-4).

CLINICAL FEATURES AND ASSESSMENT

As previously mentioned, a lesion affecting the sixth nerve nucleus produces an ipsilateral horizontal gaze palsy. Injury to the nerve at any other location along its course results in absent or poor abduction of the ipsilateral eye (Fig. 5-7).

Of course, poor abduction is not specific to sixth nerve palsies and may also be caused by disorders of the neuromuscular junction (e.g., myasthenia gravis), restrictions (e.g., medial orbital wall fractures with tissue entrapment), and inflammation (e.g., orbital myositis). The examiner considers and excludes these possibilities before establishing the diagnosis of sixth nerve palsy. If a congenital anomaly of innervation, such as Duane's syndrome, is clearly identified as the cause of abduction deficit, no further investigation of the eye movement abnormality is necessary.

Acute comitant esotropia can also follow head trauma (usually minor), febrile illness, migraine, or occlusion of an eye or may not be related to any obvious inciting cause.[75,170,385,460] This condition is distinguishable on examination from a bilateral sixth nerve palsy. However, although an acute comitant esodeviation without accompanying signs is usually benign, it may in some cases be the harbinger of an intracranial tumor such as cerebellar astrocytoma or pontine glioma[29,526] or other pathology such as a Chiari 1 malformation.[517] Absence of symptoms or signs such as headaches, papilledema, or nystagmus may not rule out the possibility of an intracranial pathology. Therefore, a thorough ophthalmic examination is performed. MRI is

TABLE 5-4. Etiology of Infranuclear Sixth Nerve Palsy.

Location/signs	*Etiologies*
Fascicle Ipsilateral VIIth nerve palsy, facial analgesia, loss of taste from anterior two thirds of tongue; peripheral deafness; Horner's syndrome, contralateral hemiparesis	Tumor; demyelination; hemorrhage; infarction
Subarachnoid space Papilledema; other cranial nerve palsies	Meningitis; meningeal carcinomatosis; trauma; increased intracranial pressure causing downward pressure on brainstem; after lumbar puncture, shunt for hydrocephalus, spinal anesthesia, or halopelvic cervical traction; clivus tumor; cerebellopontine angle tumor; berry aneurysm; abducens neurinoma
Petrous apex Ipsilateral seventh nerve palsy; pain in eye or face; otitis media, leakage of blood or cerebrospinal fluid from ear; mastoid ecchymosis; papilledema	Mastoiditis; thrombosis of inferior petrosal sinus; trauma with transverse fracture of temporal bone; persistent trigeminal artery, aneurysm, or arteriovenous malformation
Cavernous sinus/superior orbital fissure Ipsilateral Horner's syndrome; ipsilateral IIIrd, IVth, Vth cranial nerve involvement; proptosis; disc edema; orbital pain; conjunctival injection	Cavernous sinus thrombosis; carotid-cavernous fistula; tumor; internal carotid aneurysm
Orbit Ipsilateral IIIrd, IVth, Vth cranial nerve involvement; proptosis; disc edema; orbital pain; conjunctival injection	Tumor; pseudotumor
Uncertain	Transient abducens palsy of newborn; after febrile illness or immunization; migraine; toxic; idiopathic

indicated if the esotropia is unresponsive to correction of refractive error, there is no history of flu-like illness, or no improvement is seen over the course of 1 to 4 weeks.

Natural History and Clinical Workup

Newborns may demonstrate a transient sixth nerve palsy that is frequently unilateral and occasionally accompanied by a temporary ipsilateral seventh nerve palsy.[53,267,291,400] Simple observa-

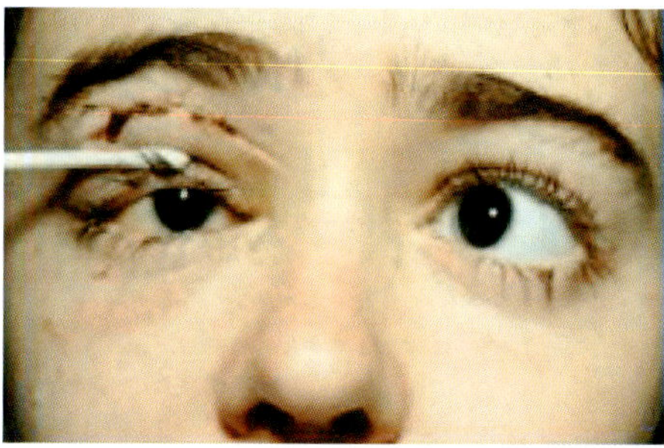

FIGURE 5-7. Right sixth cranial nerve palsy. These photos show the limitation of abduction on attempted right gaze typical of a sixth cranial nerve palsy. Forced duction testing of this patient's right eye showed no restriction to abduction.

tion is generally sufficient because resolution typically occurs within 4 to 10 weeks.

Older infants and children may develop transient isolated sixth nerve palsies 1 to 3 weeks after nonspecific febrile or respiratory illnesses,[267,405] after a specific viral illness such as varicella,[350] after immunization,[522] before mononucleosis,[273] or without any obvious precipitating factor.[435] Some of these palsies may recur, and the recurrences have no serious implications.[2,60,65,399,474,476] Again, aggressive investigation is not warranted, but two simple studies are advised: (1) a complete blood count with differential, which may show lymphocytosis as evidence of a recent viral infection, and (2) examination of the ears for otitis media. The parents are warned to observe for any new signs or symptoms. Careful reexamination at regular intervals is essential; deterioration or improvement in lateral rectus function provide important evidence for or against a progressive mass lesion. Most children in this group recover abducens function within 10 weeks, although a prolonged (9 months) palsy may rarely occur.[267]

Persistence, without improvement, or deterioration of an isolated sixth nerve palsy in a child beyond about 3 months requires an intensive neurological, neuroradiologic, and otolaryngologic evaluation. In adults, a substantial number of isolated sixth nerve palsies that last beyond 6 months are caused by potentially treatable, often slow-growing, tumors.[111,159,426] In a Mayo Clinic series of 133 children with acquired sixth nerve paresis, 15 presented with an isolated sixth nerve palsy due to tumor.[405] Of these, 12 developed additional neurological signs within a few weeks, whereas 3 patients took 2 to 3 months to develop additional signs. An additional problem is that a physician may not always be able to confirm that the sixth nerve palsy in a child is isolated. Therefore, if close follow-up to resolution of the palsy or paresis is not possible, neuroimaging is recommended.[24]

Treatment

Amblyopia prevention is always key in children younger than 7 to 9 years of age. Providing full hyperopic correction also relieves the demand for accommodation and thus decreases the chance of worsening esotropia.

Treatment options include botulinus toxin injection and surgery. One approach is to inject botulinus toxin into the antagonist medial rectus muscle to prevent tightening of the unopposed medial rectus,[442,444] sometimes allowing binocular vision in primary position, while the palsy is resolving.[218] Reducing medial rectus contracture with botulinus toxin injection may also improve a surgical result.[302]

Prognosis

Spontaneous recovery of abduction in childhood sixth nerve palsy or paresis is much less common than in adults. The rate of residual strabismus was found to be 66% in one study of any sixth nerve palsy or paresis in patients 7 years of age and younger, likely a result of permanent structural deficits without complete recovery in the setting of tumor and hydrocephalus-shunt malfunction as the most frequent etiologies. The rate of amblyopia in this study was 20%, thus highlighting the need for parent education and close follow-up.

The highest rates of spontaneous recovery have been reported in idiopathic (67%[24]), infectious (50%[24]), inflammatory (90%[191]), and traumatic (33%–50%[24,191]) cases.

Fourth Nerve Palsy

Etiology and Systemic Associations

Of the many causes of trochlear palsy in childhood (Table 5-5), "congenital" and traumatic are by far the most common.[191,209] The cause of most congenital trochlear palsies remains unknown, but aplasia of the trochlear nucleus has been reported to accompany the absence of other cranial nerve nuclei.[10,317,464] The superior oblique tendon or muscle is often the primary

TABLE 5-5. Etiology of Fourth Nerve Palsy.

Location/signs	*Etiologies*
Nucleus and fascicle Contralateral Horner's syndrome	Trauma; tumor; demyelination; after neurosurgery; nuclear aplasia; arteriovenous malformation; hemorrhage; infarction
Subarachnoid space Papilledema; other cranial nerve palsies	Trauma; tumor; increased intracranial pressure; after lumbar puncture or shunt for hydrocephalus; spinal anesthesia; meningitis; mastoiditis
Cavernous sinus/superior orbital fissure Ipsilateral Horner's syndrome, ipsilateral IIIrd, Vth, VIth nerve involvement; proptosis; disc edema; orbital pain	Tumor; internal carotid aneurysm; Tolosa–Hunt syndrome
Orbit Ipsilateral IIIrd, VIth nerve involvement; proptosis; enophthalmos; disc edema; orbital pain; conjunctival/episcleral injection	Tumor; trauma; inflammation
Uncertain location	Congenital; idiopathic

problem. Laxity of this tendon has been described on forced duction testing[381] and correlates well with the presence of attenuated superior oblique muscles on orbital MRI.[432] Therefore, congenital cases may be more correctly termed congenital superior oblique palsy/underaction instead of fourth nerve palsy. Absence of the superior oblique muscle altogether is also in the differential of an apparent congenital superior oblique palsy.[87]

The trochlear nerves are particularly vulnerable to closed head trauma when there may be contrecoup of the tectum of the midbrain against the edge of the tentorium.[292] In this way, the nucleus or fascicle may be injured within the substance of the midbrain, or the nerve itself may be contused as it exits the brainstem dorsally and passes laterally around the midbrain (see Fig. 5-3). The proximity of the two trochlear nerves to each other at the site of their crossing in the anterior medullary velum (roof of the Sylvian aqueduct; see Fig. 5-4) explains the high incidence of bilateral involvement after coup-contrecoup, closed head trauma.[286]

Clinical Features and Assessment

Vertical deviations may also result from other processes, such as abnormal neuromuscular transmission, restriction, inflammation, skew deviation, dissociated vertical divergence, small nonparalytic vertical deviations associated with horizontal strabismus, and paresis of other cyclovertical muscles. The clinical assessment of a vertical deviation is carefully executed to exclude these various possibilities.

It is important to ask about previous extraocular muscle surgery or orbital trauma and to obtain any history that suggests myasthenia gravis or skew deviation. The examiner notes any anomalous head position (Figs. 5-8, 5-9), versions, ductions, cover test measurements in cardinal fields of gaze, any secondary deviation, forced (Bielschowsky) head tilt test measurements, presence or absence of both subjective and objective torsion, and presence or absence of dissociated vertical deviation. Forced ductions, Tensilon testing, and other supplemental tests are performed as appropriate.

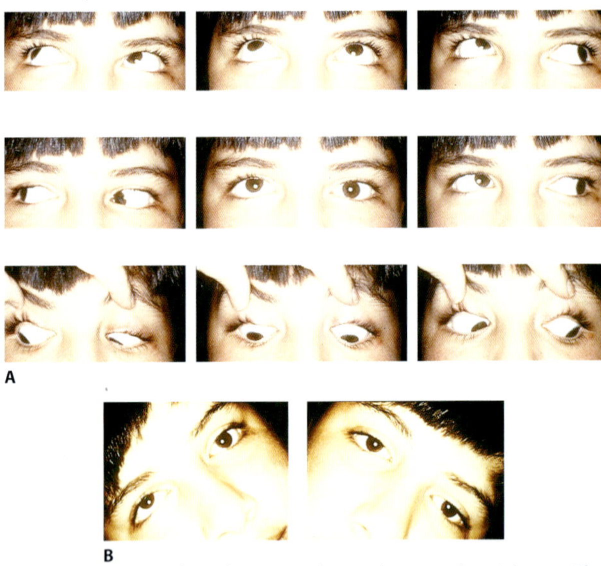

FIGURE 5-8. (**A**) Unilateral congenital cranial nerve palsy, right eye. The photograpph demonstrates a right hypertropia that increases in left gaze. There is slight underaction of the right superior oblique nad significant overaction of the right inferior oblique muscle. (**B**) The photograph of head tilt test, with right hypertropia increasing on tilt right and diminishing on tilt left. Positive head tilt with the right hyper increasing in left gaze indicates a right superior oblique palsy.

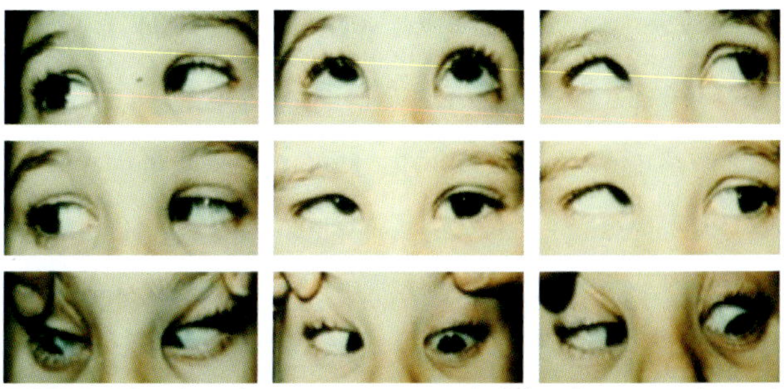

FIGURE 5-9. Bilateral asymmetric congenital fourth nerve palsy and esotropia. Note that the right superior oblique palsy is more severe than the left, and there is a right hypertropia in primary position. There is significant superior oblique underaction, right side more than left side. A significant V-pattern is present. There is a right hypertropia in right gaze and a left hypertropia in left gaze.

Several other comments regarding the clinical evaluation are crucial.

1. The familiar "Parks–Bielschowsky three-step" test helps to combine information from cover test measurements and the Bielschowsky head tilt phenomenon.[59,370] This test is only useful when there is a *palsy* of a *single* cyclovertical muscle and can therefore only be applied after the careful assessment just described.[281] A fourth nerve palsy would reveal hypertropia, worsening on horizontal gaze in the direction contralateral to the hypertropic eye, and worsening on head tilt ipsilateral to the hypertropic eye. Infants with congenital superior oblique palsies present with a head tilt, whereas older children and adults with decompensated congenital palsies complain of vertical and/or torsional diplopia.[323]

To diagnose a congenital superior oblique palsy, old photographs are helpful, often revealing a long-standing head tilt. Also, vertical fusional amplitudes frequently exceed the normal range of 3 to 4 prism diopters. The presence of a suppression scotoma when assessing diplopia or the presence of fusion also aids in establishing the chronicity of the condition as suppression is usually a childhood adaptation mechanism. Moreover, the presence of facial asymmetry may be associated with a long-standing head tilt from early childhood.[176,202,338,528] The presence of facial asymmetry may not be a specific sign for congenital superior oblique palsy, however, because patients with acquired superior oblique palsy and heterotopic rectus muscles exhibited similar features of facial asymmetry.[502] The causal relationship of the head tilt due to an abnormal superior oblique is not established.[373] Hemifacial changes are often associated with plagiocephaly as a craniofacial anomaly, and craniofacial anomalies are commonly associated with anomalous extraocular muscles.[124]

2. The examiner also checks for bilateral and asymmetrical superior oblique palsies, because the larger paresis may "mask" the smaller until unilateral surgery is performed.[274,280] Bilateral involvement should particularly be suspected after closed head injury. Findings that suggest bilaterality include alternation of hypertropia with fixation, gaze, or head tilt: excyclotorsion of 10° or more: and V-pattern esotropia.[286]

3. Excyclodeviations usually occur with trochlear palsies, may accompany restrictions and myasthenia gravis, and are less commonly seen with skew deviations.[494] The triad of skew deviation, head tilt, and *incyclo*torsion of the hypertropic eye is termed the *ocular tilt reaction*, an entity that can mimic fourth nerve palsy on the traditional three-step test.[128] Therefore, examination for torsion, by double-maddox rod or simple fundoscopy, is essential in distinguishing a fourth nerve palsy from ocular tilt reaction.

Inheritance

Rarely, congenital superior oblique palsy may be familial.[28,198] The mode of inheritance in the described families has not been determined.

Natural History

Long-standing congenital superior oblique palsy may decompensate in adulthood for a variety of reasons, including trauma, with the presenting symptom of vertical diplopia. As for traumatic cases, most cases of unilateral injury do resolve (see following). Also, after long-standing fourth nerve palsy, a "spread of concomitance" may be observed where the deviation in rightgaze and leftgaze are nearly equal, although the differential deviation in right versus left head tilt persists. This spread of concomitance has been attributed to a "contraction" of the ipsilateral superior rectus muscle.[26]

Treatment

Most surgeons wait 6 to 12 months before deciding on strabismus surgery for traumatic cases, to await spontaneous resolution of the deviation or stability in measurements. For congenital cases presenting with head tilt in infancy, surgery may be performed as soon as possible to correct the head posture and thus to aid in normal development of the neck muscles and the alignment of cervical vertebrae. It is unknown, however, whether early strabismus surgery can prevent or reverse facial asymmetry. For the large head tilts in infancy, a superior oblique tuck may treat the head tilt quickly; the benefit of normalizing head posture with this procedure may outweigh the resultant iatrogenic Brown's syndrome.

For long-standing fourth nerve or superior oblique palsy, a variety of options exist. One approach is to operate on one muscle for vertical deviations of up to 15 prism diopters and to consider two-muscle surgery in deviations above 15 prism diopters. The first choice of procedure is often ipsilateral inferior oblique muscle weakening. The second procedure often performed when the deviation is greater than 15 prism diopters is either ipsilateral superior rectus recession,[26] when the vertical deviation is worse in upgaze, or contralateral inferior rectus recession, when the deviation is worse in downgaze.[202]

A fast and easy approach to deciding which muscle to weaken first is to perform a "modified Parks three-step test"[205] to determine which muscle is *overacting* and then to weaken that muscle first. This modified three-step test is performed in the same manner as the traditional one, except for the first step, in which the *overacting* vertical muscles are circled in each eye (instead of the traditional method of circling the presumed weak vertical muscles).

In the case of bilateral palsy, bilateral inferior rectus recession and Harada–Ito procedures are recommended, both able to treat excyclotorsional diplopia.

Prognosis

When a child presents with a postinfectious, isolated trochlear palsy that cannot be explained as congenital, traumatic, restrictive, myasthenic, or neoplastic, the prognosis is good and observation alone is sufficient.

Overall prognosis for recovery of isolated fourth nerve palsies in adults and children was reported to be 53.5% combined (1000 total patients from 2 months to 91 years of age, 90% of whom were over 19 years and 75% of whom were over 35 years of age).[424] Unilateral traumatic fourth nerve palsies in a series of 24 pediatric and adult patients (ages 7–78 years; mean, 35.4 years),

46% of whom sustained minor head trauma, resulted in 75% resolution.[483] Another series reported 65% resolution in unilateral but 25% in bilateral cases of traumatic fourth nerve palsy.[479]

Third Nerve Palsy

Etiology and Systemic Associations

In childhood, a third nerve palsy typically keeps company with other neurological findings, which aid in localization and diagnosis (Table 5-6), but isolated palsies do occur and are generally congenital, traumatic, infectious, or migrainous.[191,225,257,326,339,440] An acquired, isolated oculomotor nerve palsy in a child may also result from tumor, preceding viral illness, bacterial meningitis (most commonly pneumococcal, *Haemophilus influenzae* type b, or *Neisseria meningitidis*), or immunization.[76,77,86,191,225,257,309,326,339,347,430,440,446] Rarely, children may demonstrate gradually progressive paresis because of a slowly growing tumor[1] or a truly cryptogenic oculomotor palsy. Posterior communicating aneurysms, although extremely rare in children, should be considered as well.[313] Microvascular infarction due to atheroscler-

TABLE 5-6. Etiology of Infranuclear Third Nerve Palsy.

Location/signs	***Etiologies***
Fascicle Ipsilateral cerebellar ataxia; contralateral rubral tremor; contralateral hemiparesis; vertical gaze palsy	Demyelination; hemorrhage; infarction (rare in childhood)
Subarachnoid space Papilledema; other cranial nerve palsies	Meningitis; trauma or surgery; tumor; increased intracranial pressure; uncal herniation
Cavernous sinus/superior orbital fissure Ipsilateral Horner's syndrome; ipsilateral IVth, Vth, VIth nerve involvement; proptosis; disc edema; orbital pain; conjunctival/episcleral injection	Cavernous sinus thrombosis; tumor; internal carotid artery aneurysm; carotid–cavernous fistula; Tolosa–Hunt syndrome; pituitary apoplexy; sphenoid sinusitis, mucocele; mucormycosis
Orbit Ipsilateral IVth, Vth, VIth nerve involvement; proptosis; enophthalmos; disc edema; orbital pain; conjunctival/episcleral injection	Trauma; tumor; inflammation
Uncertain location	After febrile illness or immunization; migraine; idiopathic

sis, hypertension, or diabetes mellitus, a common cause of isolated third nerve palsy in adults, is extremely rare in children.

Clinical–Anatomic Correlation

The anatomic organization of the third nerve nucleus, like that of the sixth nerve nucleus, provides constraints that help differentiate the rare nuclear third nerve palsy from an infranuclear third nerve palsy. Because the superior rectus subnucleus supplies the contralateral superior rectus muscle, and the central caudal nucleus innervates both levator muscles, damage to a single oculomotor nerve nucleus gives rise to contralateral superior rectus weakness and bilateral ptosis. Also, because of the arrangement of the three medial rectus subnuclei and the visceral nuclei within the oculomotor nucleus, a nuclear third nerve palsy is not likely to produce isolated medial rectus involvement or unilateral pupillary involvement. In addition, other midbrain signs such as vertical gaze abnormalities are often associated with lesions of the oculomotor nucleus (see Fig. 5-6).

Because the oculomotor nerve innervates the levator palpebrae superioris, the sphincter of the pupil and ciliary body, as well as four extraocular muscles (the medial rectus, superior rectus, inferior rectus, and inferior oblique), it is easy to identify a complete infranuclear third nerve palsy by the presence of ptosis; a fixed, dilated pupil; and a "down-and-out" eye position resulting from the unopposed lateral rectus and superior oblique muscles (Fig. 5-10). However, third nerve palsies can be "partial"; any individual sign or combination of signs may be present and, if present, may be complete or incomplete. Numerous patterns can therefore arise.

Clinical Features and Assessment/Natural History

Oculomotor nerve palsies, like abducens and trochlear nerve palsies, should be distinguished from myasthenia and mechanical restrictions. Clinically observable involvement of the pupil or signs of *oculomotor synkinesis* (aberrant regeneration) establish involvement of the third nerve, assuming pharmacological and traumatic mydriasis can be excluded.

The manner through which neural impulses become misdirected is not always clear.[455] Misrouting of regenerating motor axons is firmly documented[152,392,456] and corroborates the frequent clinical observation of the appearance of synkinesis at about 8 to

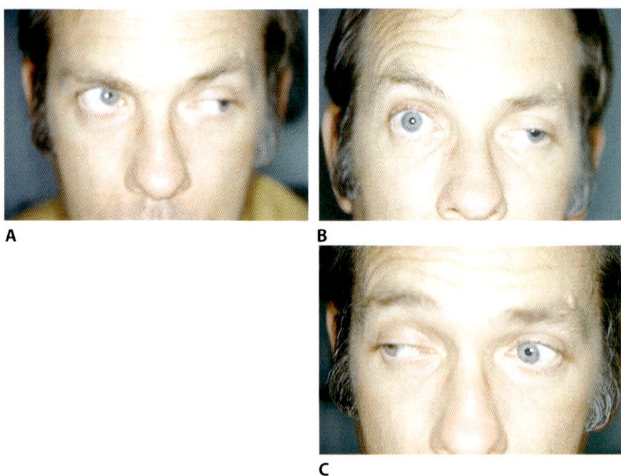

FIGURE 5-10. Patient with traumatic left third nerve palsy. The top photograph shows the classic appearance of a left third nerve palsy with ptosis and the eye in a down and out position. The left photograph shows full abduction, left eye. The bottom right photograph shows left eye with limited adduction. Note, there is lid retraction and miosis, left eye, on attempted adduction indicating aberrant innervation of the levator muscle and pupillary sphincter with part of the medial rectus nerve.

12 weeks after an acute palsy.[277] However, aberrant regeneration cannot comfortably account for transient oculomotor synkinesis[239,289,454] or spontaneous "primary" oculomotor synkinesis.[66,105,289,436,493] Ephaptic transmission, conduction of a nerve impulse across a point of lateral contact, and synaptic reorganization of the oculomotor nucleus are two proposed theories of synkinesis.[289,455] The presence of oculomotor synkinesis has not been reported with demyelination, but it does not otherwise narrow the differential diagnosis of third nerve palsy in the pediatric age group.

Congenital third nerve palsy is usually incomplete and unilateral and is frequently associated with oculomotor synkinesis and "miosis" of the pupil in the affected eye.[191,326,504] Although many children with congenital oculomotor nerve palsies have no associated neurological findings, some do,[41] and a thorough neurological evaluation of these infants is suggested. If there are additional neurological signs or bilateral third nerve palsies, MRI may also provide useful information.[175]

Rarely, paresis and spasm of the extraocular and intraocular muscles innervated by the third nerve may alternate, typically every few minutes, to produce *oculomotor palsy with cyclic spasms*.[295] With few exceptions, these cycles accompany congenital, rather than acquired, oculomotor palsies and continue throughout life. In some instances, several months to several years may elapse between the discovery of the paresis and the onset of the cyclic spasms. Investigation is not necessary unless the third nerve palsy is acquired or there is progressive neurological dysfunction. The pathogenesis of this phenomenon remains obscure.[272]

Ophthalmoplegic migraine generally begins in childhood[40] but may even be seen in infancy.[13,534] It is an uncommon disorder despite the fact that 2.5% of children experience a migraine attack by age 7 and 5% by age 15.[43] Symptoms of migraine in children include nausea, vomiting, abdominal pain, and relief after sleep in 90%.[419] The headaches, which may be accompanied by an aura, are often unilateral and throbbing in quality. Family history is positive in 70% to 90%. With ophthalmoplegic migraine, the patient characteristically experiences pain in and about the involved eye, nausea, and vomiting; often the third nerve palsy ensues as the pain resolves. Full recovery of third nerve function within 1 to 2 months is typical, but resolution may be incomplete and oculomotor sykinesis has been reported.[355] Multiple attacks may occur, and years may pass between episodes.[133] Most patients with ophthalmoplegic migraine have normal angiograms, but one 31-year-old with recurrent episodes of ophthalmoplegic migraine, which had begun at age 5, and partial third nerve palsy since age 7, demonstrated a small perimensencephalic vascular anomaly.[224]

Aneurysms have been reported to cause isolated third nerve palsies during the first and the second decades of life[71,135,157,158,313,383] and carry a high risk of mortality or significant morbidity if left undetected and untreated. On the other hand, aneurysms appear to be rare in children.[158,495] Angiography with general anesthesia can be risky in the childhood age group, and the gap between the sensitivity of angiography and MRI for detecting aneurysms continues to narrow. The clinician assesses all these variables along with the history and physical examination to decide on the appropriate workup for each patient. For example, in the child under age 10 with a family history of migraine who presents with nausea, vomiting, and headache, followed by third nerve palsy as these symptoms resolve, that is, with typical ophthalmoplegic migraine, angiography may not be necessary.[166] However, when a third nerve palsy acquired in childhood cannot be explained on the basis of the clinical examination or noninvasive neuroimaging, the cerebrospinal fluid should be evaluated and angiography considered.

Treatment

After diagnosis and treatment of the underlying disorder, observation of any recovery of oculomotor nerve function is necessary before surgical intervention. When partial or full recovery occurs, it often does so within 3 to 6 months but it may take 1 year or more. Surgical treatment includes strabismus surgery and ptosis correction. The latter is approached with caution in an eye that lacks a functional Bell's phenomenon because of the risk of exposure keratopathy.

Prognosis

Two recent series have found fair to poor visual and sensorimotor outcome in oculomotor nerve palsy/paralysis of children with comparable mix of congenital, traumatic, and neoplastic cases.[339,440] The best ophthalmologic outcome with measurable stereopsis was in the resolved cases (3 of 20; 15%) in the first study, and in 4 of 31 patients with partial third nerve palsy in the second study, 2 of whom had spontaneous resolution. In the first series, amblyopia therapy was most effective with congenital causes, but treatment results were poor with other causes; young children with posttraumatic and postneoplastic oculomotor nerve injuries demonstrated the worst ophthalmologic outcomes.

Combined Ocular Motor Nerve Palsies

As the oculomotor, trochlear, and abducens nerves are in relatively close physical proximity from brainstem to orbit, it is not surprising that many diseases occurring at numerous locations can affect these nerves simultaneously.

Clinical Assessment

The evaluation begins by establishing that the eye movement abnormality is due to cranial nerve disease rather than supranuclear lesions, disorders of the neuromuscular junction, restrictive or inflammatory myopathies, or chronic progressive "neuromyopathies," for example, Kearns–Sayre syndrome. In the presence of a third nerve palsy, the fourth nerve function is tested by observing for intorsion of the affected eye in downgaze. If multiple ocular motor nerve palsies are indeed present, a thorough history and examination, neuroimaging of the rostral brainstem, cavernous sinuses, and orbits, and examination of the cerebrospinal fluid (CSF) are typically necessary to distinguish between the myriad possible localizations and etiologies. Prompt diagnosis is particularly important for children with infections or pituitary apoplexy; the latter is often accompanied by severe headache, ophthalmoplegia caused by rapid expansion into the cavernous sinus, and rapid mental status deterioration.

ETIOLOGIES

Processes in the brainstem (tumor, encephalitis), subarachnoid space (meningitis, trauma, tumor), and of uncertain localization (postinfectious polyneuropathy) tend to *produce bilateral combined ocular motor nerve palsies* whereas processes in the cavernous sinus/superior orbital fissure (tumor, pituitary apoplexy, cavernous sinus thrombosis, carotid-cavernous fistula) and orbit (trauma, tumor, mucormycosis) usually cause *unilateral combined ocular motor nerve palsies*.

The ophthalmologist needs to be familiar with certain *generalized neuropathies* that may initially present with *acute ophthalmoplegia*. In a series of 60 patients with acute bilateral ophthalmoplegia, *Guillain–Barre* and *Miller Fisher syndromes* accounted for the diagnosis in 15 of 28 patients under age 45.[253] The bulbar variant of *Guillain–Barre syndrome (acute postinfectious polyneuritis)* frequently presents as a rapidly progressive, painless ophthalmoplegia. Early in the course, involvement of eye movements may be incomplete and mimic either unilateral or bilateral oculomotor nerve palsies, but complete ophthalmoplegia with or without involvement of the pupils and accommodation typically evolves within several days. Partial ptosis usually accompanies severe limitation of eye movements,[413] but levator function may be entirely normal or completely absent. Some degree of cranial nerve involvement occurs in about 50% of children with Guillain–Barre syndrome,[413] and in the setting of rapidly progressing bilateral ophthalmoplegia, dysfunction of other cranial nerves, particularly bilateral facial nerve involvement, strongly supports the diagnosis of acute postinfectious polyneuritis.

A variety of infections have been reported to precede Guillain–Barre syndrome in 50% to 70% of children; these include gastroenteritis, tonsillitis, measles, mumps, varicella, pertussis, hepatitis, Epstein–Barr virus, *Campylobacter jejuni*, coxsackie virus, and nonspecific upper respiratory infections. Two of these, varicella[103,521] and acute Epstein–Barr virus infection,[184] precede or accompany the onset of Guillain–Barre syndrome with noteworthy frequency in children and young adults. Paresthesias, often painful, commonly appear early in the course, and signs of meningeal irritation may also appear early in children. Although a rise in CSF protein levels without pleocytosis is the rule, it generally does not occur for several days to weeks after the onset of symptoms and, in a small percentage of patients, is not observed at all. The patient should be referred to a neurologist for management in a hospital setting with materials for tracheostomy and mechanical ventilation readily available.

Ophthalmoplegia (external and sometimes internal), ataxia, and areflexia constitute *Miller Fisher syndrome*,[155] and diplopia is usually the first symptom. At least 20 children (under age 18 years) with Miller Fisher syndrome have been reported.[50] A preceding febrile or "viral" illness may be reported with many of the same infectious agents previously listed.

Although the eye movements often suggest unilateral or asymmetrical bilateral abducens pareses, many patterns have been reported including horizontal gaze palsy, upgaze palsy,[249] pupil-sparing oculomotor nerve palsy, and pseudointernuclear ophthalmoplegia.[30,125,478,520] All these eye movement patterns generally progress to severe bilateral ophthalmoplegia within 2 or 3 days. Ptosis and pupillary involvement may occur but are often absent.[78] Limb and gait ataxia typically appear 3 or 4 days after the ophthalmoparesis but are, at times, concurrent with it. Areflexia is almost invariably present by the end of a week.[141] An association with demyelinating optic neuropathy has also been reported.[368,488]

Miller Fisher syndrome is considered to be a variant of Guillain–Barre syndrome. However, there is some controversy as to the site of the lesion in Miller Fisher syndrome,[8,315,414,415,488] whereas Guillain–Barre is clearly a peripheral neuropathy. Clinical observations suggesting the possibility of CNS involvement in Miller Fisher syndrome have included apparently supranuclear eye movement abnormalities[314,459] and clouding of consciousness.[8,50] In some cases, evoked potentials[232] and MRI[416] have been normal; in others, CT images[121,541] and MRI[136,163] have displayed clear abnormalities in the brainstem as well as in the cerebral white matter and cerebellum. In yet another group, absent F waves and H reflexes on peripheral nerve testing and markedly abnormal electroencephalograms suggested both peripheral and central involvement.[50] Two neuropathological studies demonstrated normal CNS in both,[119,378] and another showed inflammatory infiltration of peripheral and cranial nerve roots[25]; however, central chromatolysis in the nuclei of the third, fourth, fifth, and twelfth nerves and of the anterior horn cells has also been reported.[186] Additionally, anticerebellar antibody has been found to be reactive to a significantly greater number of bands on Western blotting of serum from Miller Fisher patients (6 of 7) compared to that of Guillain–Barre (3 of 6) or healthy controls (4 of 10).[227]

As with acute postinfectious polyneuritis, if the CSF is examined late enough in the course, the protein concentration is elevated in most cases.[141] A useful diagnostic tool is the presence of antiganglioside antibodies in serum of patients with Guillain–Barre and Miller Fisher syndromes. Patients with Guillain–Barre syndrome subsequent to *Campylobacter jejuni* enteritis frequently have IgG antibody to GM_1 ganglioside. Miller Fisher syndrome is associated with IgG antibody to GQ1b and GT1a ganglioside in 90% of cases.[527,539] Moreover, acute ophthalmoparesis without ataxia has also been found to be associated with anti-GQ1b antibody, suggesting that this is a milder variant of Miller Fisher syndrome.[539] These antibody findings are evidence for the molecular mimicry theory of postinfectious autoimmune pathology.

Despite its dramatic and alarming presentation, Miller Fisher syndrome generally has a benign prognosis. Careful observation is, however, recommended because ophthalmoplegia occurred early in one case of childhood Guillain–Barre syndrome that progressed to respiratory failure.[179] Occasionally, "relapsing Miller Fisher syndrome" appears to occur,[434,506] which should not be confused with recurrent ocular motor palsies that may accompany a rare familial syndrome of recurrent Bell's palsy.[9] Treatment of Guillain–Barre and Miller Fisher syndromes may, in severe cases, require plasmapheresis or intravenously administered immunoglobulin.[241,538]

Acute hemorrhagic conjunctivitis caused by enterovirus 70 can be accompanied by dysfunction of any of the cranial or spinal motor nerves,[220,246,513] resulting in a polio-like paralysis (radiculomyelitis) in approximately 1 in 10,000 patients infected with this virus.[535] Cranial nerve involvement occurred in 50% of the patients in one series.[246] Solitary seventh or fifth nerve palsies were most common, followed in frequency by combined fifth and seventh nerve palsies. Prognosis correlates with severity and pattern of cranial nerve involvement; patients with mild weakness and involvement of cranial nerves VII, IX, and X tend to resolve fully, whereas those with severe weakness and involvement of cranial nerves III, IV, V, and VI often do not significantly improve. Optic atrophy may also occur. Treatment is only symptomatic.

Anomalies of Innervation

Some ocular motility disturbances, both congenital and acquired, arise when an inappropriate nerve or nerve branch innervates an extraocular muscle. Such "miswiring" immediately suspends the laws of extraocular motor physiology (e.g., Hering's and Sherrington's laws) and produces bizarre, intriguing eye movements. In certain cases, electromyographic (EMG) and pathological studies have confirmed the defective anatomy and physiology underlying the clinical presentation. Although miswiring can generate many types of abnormal eye movements, only the more common anomalous motility patterns are detailed here.

Sixth Nerve

Duane's Syndrome

Duane's syndrome is characterized by retraction of the globe and narrowing of the lid fissure on attempted adduction as well as limited eye movements. Three forms of abnormal motility have been classified[217]:

Type I: limited abduction with intact adduction (Fig. 5-11)
Type II: limited adduction with intact abduction
Type III: limited abduction and limited adduction

Incidence Duane's syndrome has been reported to account for 1% to 4% of all strabismus cases.[122]

Etiology Electromyographic data indicate that the medial and lateral recti contract simultaneously, that is, they "co-contract," and may thereby produce both the retraction of the globe into the orbit and the limitation of eye movement.[216,217,308] One can speculate as to how different distributions of inappropriate neural input from the oculomotor and abducens nerves to the lateral and medial recti could produce each of the three patterns of limited ocular motility seen in Duane's syndrome. This

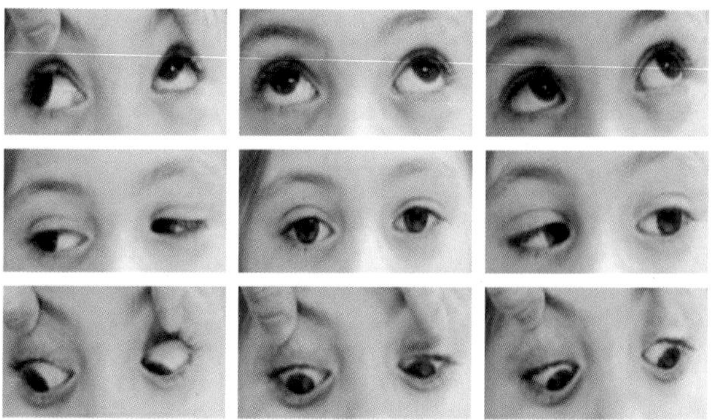

FIGURE 5-11. Duane's syndrome, left eye. This montage demonstrates the limitation of abduction (*middle, right photo*), palpebral lid fissure narrowing on adduction (*middle, left photo*), upshoot in adduction (*top, left photo*), and "Y" pattern (*middle, top photo*) seen with Duane's syndrome.

aberrant innervation is thought to be a result of congenitally deficient innervation of the VIth nucleus, leading to a fibrotic lateral rectus muscle (Fig. 5-12).

Neuropathological investigations of three patients with Duane's syndrome have all revealed aplasia or hypoplasia of the abducens nucleus and nerve, and in two of these cases, branches of the third nerve "substituted" for the defective sixth nerve by supplying some of its fibers to the lateral rectus. The first case was unilateral and demonstrated a hypoplastic lateral rectus muscle in addition to hypoplasia of the abducens nucleus and nerve.[310] In a second patient with bilateral type III Duane's syndrome, both abducens nuclei and nerves were absent; also, both lateral recti were found to be partially innervated by the inferior division of the oculomotor nerves and were histologically normal in innervated areas but fibrotic in areas not innervated.[213] The third patient had unilateral, left type I Duane's syndrome and showed, as did the previous case, absence of the sixth nerve, partial innervation of the lateral rectus by the inferior division of the oculomotor nerve, and fibrosis of the lateral rectus muscle in areas not innervated. However, although the left abducens nucleus was hypoplastic, containing less than half the number of neurons seen in the right nucleus, both medial longitudinal fasciculi were normal and the remaining cell bodies in the nucleus were interpreted to be internuclear neurons. This

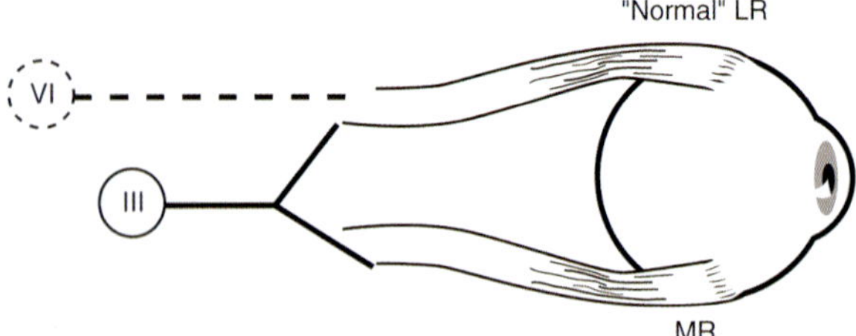

"Early" onset embryonic aberrant CN III innervation

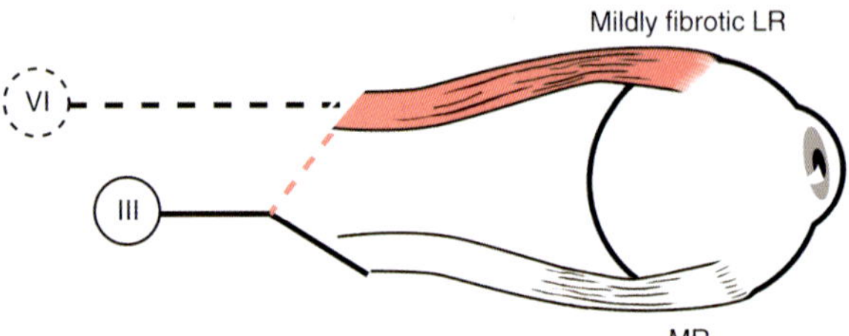

"Later" onset embryonic aberrant CN III innervation

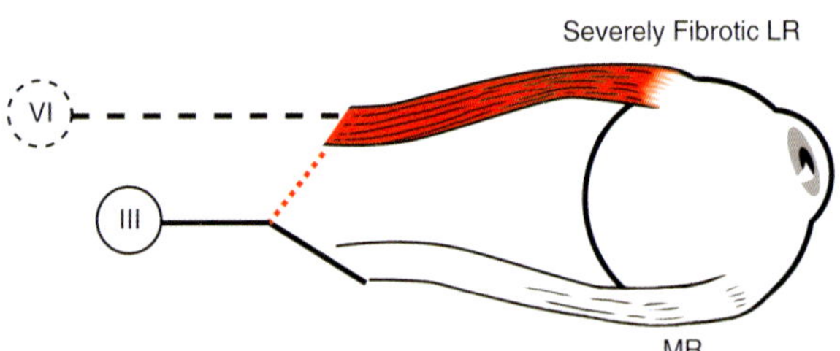

"Late" onset embryonic aberrant CN III innervation

finding corroborates the clinical observation that, in unilateral type I Duane's syndrome, adducting saccades in the unaffected eye are usually normal.[177,322,333] This finding also indicates an exquisitely specific neural deficit. Electrophysiological techniques such as auditory evoked potentials[237] and eye movement recordings[351,537] have suggested that there may be other associated brainstem dysfunction, but these studies have not produced conclusive evidence or have not been reproducible.[403,481]

"Upshoots" and/or "downshoots" on attempted adduction are common motility findings. Theoretically, the cause of the upshoots and downshoots may be mechanical, innervational, or a combination of the two. In most cases, the mechanics of the lateral rectus seem to be largely responsible because weakening or eradicating the action of a tight lateral rectus results in significant reduction or elimination of upshoots and downshoots. The "bridle-effect theory" postulates that vertical sideslip of a tight lateral rectus across the adducting globe produces these movements[234,510]; however, neuroimaging has not confirmed vertical displacement of the lateral rectus during upshoots and downshoots.[62,511] In certain individuals, an innervational anomaly may account for upshoots and downshoots. For example, one of the authors (B.N.B.) has observed that continued severe upshoot on adduction in a patient whose lateral rectus was detached from the globe and allowed to retract far

FIGURE 5-12. Proposed embryonal etiopathogenesis of Duane's syndrome as a congenitally deficient innervation syndrome. The developing cranial nerves have a "trophic" function on the developing mesenchyme of the future extraocular muscles. If there is late or no innervation to the developing mesenchyme, the muscle becomes dysplastic, fibrotic, and inelastic. If there is early aberrant innervation of the developing mesenchyme by cranial nerve III, the lateral rectus has a "normal" architecture but abnormal innervation, leading to limited abduction only (type I). The later during embryogenesis the innervation, the more dysplastic the lateral rectus, leading to limited adduction as well (type III). The balance between the quantitative amount of aberrant innervation and the degree of lateral rectus fibrosis creates relatively different patterns of abduction and adduction, leading to the different "types" of Duane's syndrome. Type II Duane's syndrome (not depicted) may be caused by more innervation from the third cranial nerve to the lateral rectus compared to the medial rectus. *Dotted lines* represent absent or hypoplastic innervation; *dashed lines* represent later onset of innervation; *thickness of lines* represents quantitative amounts of innervation. *LR*, lateral rectus; *MR*, medial rectus; *III*, oculomotor nucleus; *VI*, abducens nucleus.

into the orbit before suture adjustment. In addition, there is EMG evidence for cocontraction of appropriate cyclovertical muscles and the lateral rectus during upshoots and downshoots[217,322,443]; such co-contraction could play a substantial role in some cases.

Clinical Features and Natural History Most large series indicate that females represent about two-thirds of cases and that the left eye is affected in about two-thirds of unilateral cases. Approximately 75% are type I; type III accounts for most of the rest, and type II is quite rare. Types I and II may occasionally coexist in the 10% to 20% of cases that are bilateral. Many Duane's syndrome patients are orthotropic in primary position or with a small head turn and have excellent binocular function.[229,391,402] Although amblyopia can occur in the involved eye, the reported incidence of amblyopia as well as anisometropia varies widely.[448,491] Most Duane's syndrome patients ignore or are unaware of sensory disturbances,[300] but occasionally an older child presents with "acute" awareness of diplopia in the appropriate fields of gaze.

As mentioned, upshoots and downshoots on attempted adduction may occur and may be accompanied by A, V, or X patterns, giving the appearance of oblique muscle dysfunction.

Clinical Assessment Other diseases should be considered in the differential diagnosis. Rarely, acquired orbital disease may produce limitations of abduction and retraction, thereby mimicking Duane's syndrome. This effect has been observed with medial orbital wall fractures, fixation of muscle by orbital metastases, orbital myositis, and a variety of other conditions.[165,266,367,469]

Systemic Associations Although Duane's syndrome is usually an isolated finding, it may accompany any of a multitude of other congenital anomalies in 5% to 57% of cases (Table 5-7).[307,363,377]

Inheritance Familial cases are not uncommon, and an autosomal dominant mode of inheritance best fits most, but not all, of the reported pedigrees.[126] Duane's syndrome, sensorineural deafness, upper limb defects, facio-auriculo-vertebral anomalies, and genitourinary and cardiac malformations appear as isolated findings or in combination throughout certain families and may all, perhaps, be ascribed to a highly pleiotropic autosomal dominant gene that is frequently nonpenetrant.[198a,361] Studies of

TABLE 5-7. Congenital Anomalies Associated with Duane's Syndrome.

Structure	*Associated anomalies*
Ocular/external	Microphthalmos; coloboma; heterochromia iridis; flocculi iridis; congenital cataract[33,34,363] Ptosis; nevus of Ota; hypertelorism; prominent epicanthus[33,34,210,377,448] Epibulbar dermoid[307,363,377,379]
Neural	Optic nerve anomalies[34,120,248,261,307,377]; DeMorsier syndrome[5] Sensorineural deafness[261–264,307,448] Seventh nerve palsy[106,307,377,428] Marcus Gunn jaw winking[230,307] Gusto-lacrimal reflex[58,307,393] Fourth nerve palsy[307] Möbius syndrome[307]
Musculoskeletal	Craniofacial anomalies; skeletal anomalies; Klippel–Feil syndrome; Goldenhar's syndrome; Marfanoid hypermotility syndrome; cleft lip/palate; muscular dystrophy[34,35,106,212,261–264,307,361,363,377,379,393,421,448]
Miscellaneous	Cardiac anomalies[35,307,377] Genitourinary anomalies[106,377] Noonan syndrome Fetal alcohol syndrome[211] Congenital panhypopituitarism[107] Oculocutaneous albinism[208]

monozygotic twins have revealed both concordance and discordance in more than one family.[207,247]

Two recent reports of large families with autosomal dominant Duane's syndrome, one in the U.K. and the other in Mexico, have both found linkage to chromosome 2q31.[20,148] Other reports have found deletions in chromosome 8q in patients with Duane's syndrome associated with other abnormalities such as mental retardation and hydrocephalus.[79,505]

Treatment A patient with unacceptable primary position deviation, head position, globe retraction, upshoot, or downshoot may require surgery. All these factors as well as the relative contributions of mechanical and innervational factors are considered during surgical planning. As a general recommendation, resections of the horizontal recti of an affected eye is usually avoided because this may increase globe retraction. Otherwise, the surgical approach is individualized.[275] Depending on the situation, a wide variety of techniques may prove helpful, including transposition of the vertical recti with or without medial rectus recession,[169,331] Y-splitting of the lateral rectus,[410] adjustable sutures,[388] and posterior fixation sutures.[293,510]

Prognosis Recession of horizontal rectus muscle eliminates the face turn in 79% of cases and significantly reduces the face turn in most of the remaining patients.[276,388] Undercorrection of primary position esotropia may occur postoperatively as the amount of recession needs to be larger than indicated in the tradition tables for concomitant strabismus; rerecession is recommended for these cases if the initial recession was less than 8 mm or if forced duction testing still indicates restriction. The occasional overcorrections may be reversed by advancing the recessed muscle or recessing the antagonist horizontal rectus muscle if tight.[171,348,353]

Synergistic Divergence

Synergistic divergence is a striking motility pattern consisting of an adduction deficit with simultaneous bilateral abduction on attempted gaze into the field of action of the involved medial rectus.[109,514,525] As with Duane's syndrome, cocontraction of the lateral and medial recti has been demonstrated on EMG,[525] and it has therefore been suggested that synergistic divergence may be placed along the Duane's "spectrum" of congenital anomalous innervation. In this conceptual scheme, synergistic divergence is similar to type II Duane's syndrome, except that the larger part of the branch of the third nerve "intended" for the medial rectus is misdirected to the lateral rectus. The globe retraction characteristic of Duane's syndrome does not accompany synergistic divergence, presumably because there is so little innervation to the medial rectus. However, this hypothesis has not been verified by clinicopathological study, and saccadic velocity studies in two patients indicate that the abducens nerve may not necessarily be absent or severely hypoplastic.[188]

Synergistic divergence has been observed as early as 5 months of age,[108] may be bilateral,[187,188,486] and has been associated with other abnormalities including Marcus Gunn jaw-winking,[72,73,187] ipsilateral congenital Horner's syndrome,[238] arthrogryposis multiplex congenita,[109] congenital fibrosis syndrome, and oculocutaneous albinism.[72,73]

Surgical crippling of the ipsilateral lateral rectus has been combined with a variety of other procedures such as medial rectus resection and superior oblique tenotomy and inferior oblique myectomy[330] to eliminate the simultaneous abduction as well as to correct the exotropia in primary position.[188]

Other types of anomalous innervation that may involve the sixth nerve include congenital or acquired synkinesis of the levator and lateral rectus during abduction,[242,343] acquired trigemino-abducens synkinesis with abduction accompanying jaw movements,[312,349,453] congenital twitch abduction on attempted upgaze,[271] or lateral gaze synkinesis on downward saccades.[503]

Third Nerve

Oculomotor Synkinesis

Oculomotor synkinesis (aberrant regeneration of the third nerve) commonly accompanies third nerve palsies, usually those of congenital or traumatic origin, but also those caused by aneurysm, migraine, or tumor. This condition is discussed in detail in the section on third nerve palsies. Although oculomotor synkinesis is, perhaps, the most familiar form of anomalous innervation involving the oculomotor nerve, other patterns do occur.

Vertical Retraction Syndrome

Vertical retraction syndrome is exceedingly rare with only several case reports in the literature.[258,376,389,433,518] Typically, elevation or depression of the globe is limited, and when attempted, it is associated with narrowing of the lid fissure and retraction. There may be an associated horizontal deviation that is greater with gaze in the direction of the limited vertical eye movements. Forced ductions are positive, although this does not preclude a central mechanism.

EMG study of one patient revealed lateral rectus muscle contraction on upgaze and downgaze. Eye movement recordings of this and two other patients in the same study showed a twitch abduction of the occluded eye on upward saccades, followed by a postsaccadic drift back and a slower abduction in downgaze; this phenomenon was seen in each nonfixing of all three patients, suggesting a synergistic innervation between the abducens nerve and the upper and lower divisions of the oculomotor nerve.

EMG in one atypical case of vertical retraction syndrome showed cocontraction of the vertical recti in upgaze, downgaze, and adduction, and electro-oculography was also consistent with an anomalous innervational pattern.[389] The clinical findings included exotropia; poor elevation and adduction; retraction of the globe on upgaze, downgaze, and adduction; and downshoot on adduction.

Marcus Gunn Jaw-Winking

Marcus Gunn jaw-winking is not usually accompanied by abnormal eye movements but is included here as another instance of anomalous innervation. This congenital trigemino-oculomotor synkinesis links innervation of jaw and eyelid levator muscles and is characterized by congenital ptosis, usually unilateral, with elevation of the ptotic lid when the jaw is moved. This ipsilateral associated ptosis accounts for 5% to 10% of all congenital ptosis.[57,193]

Etiology Because normal subjects demonstrate EMG cocontraction of the muscles supplied by the oculomotor nerve and certain muscles of mastication supplied by the trigeminal nerve,[427] Marcus Gunn jaw-winking may represent an exaggeration of a physiological synkinesis that is normally present but clinically undetectable. The precise mechanism for failure of higher inhibition remains unclear. EMG evidence and histological study of the levator muscles suggest an underlying brainstem process because the levator muscles are involved bilaterally.[204,299,427]

Clinical Features There are two major categories of trigemino-oculomotor synkinesis. The first, and most common, consists of external pterygoid-levator synkinesis and is characterized by lid elevation when the jaw is projected forward, thrust to the opposite side, or opened widely. In the second form, internal pterygoid-levator synkinesis, lid elevation is triggered by clenching of the teeth. Rarely, a number of stimuli other than pterygoid contraction can cause eyelid elevation, and these include smiling, inspiration, sternocleidomastoid contraction, tongue protrusion, and voluntary nystagmus. Conversely, in an unusual case of trigemino-oculomotor sykinesis, pterygoid contraction was associated with contraction of the inferior rectus rather than the levator, thereby producing monocular bobbing eye movements rather than eyelid elevation.[356]

Marcus Gunn jaw-winking typically presents shortly after birth with rhythmic elevation of the affected upper lid during feeding. The ipsilateral associated ptosis may be of any degree of severity. A significant number of patients have amblyopia, anisometropia, strabismus, superior rectus palsy, or double elevator palsy.[57,193]

Natural History It is interesting to note that, in many cases, parents remark that the synkinesis seems less apparent as the child becomes older. As this observation is not supported by objective examination, it may occur because the child learns to control both lid position and excursion.

Systemic Associations Marcus Gunn jaw-winking can be bilateral; has been reported in association with other forms of anomalous innervation such as synergistic divergence, Duane's syndrome, and trigemino-abducens synkinesis; and is rarely familial or associated with heritable diseases such as Waardenburg syndrome, Rubinstein–Taybi syndrome (author's observation; M.M.), Hirschsprung megacolon, neuroblastoma, and neurofibromatosis type 1.[94,268,316]

Treatment Strabismus, amblyopia, and anisometropia are treated when necessary. Surgical management of the ptosis may be achieved by conventional levator resection in mild cases of jaw-winking. In moderate to severe cases, bilateral levator excision and bilateral frontalis suspension have been shown to provide satisfactory correction of both jaw-winking and ptosis. The frontalis suspensions may be achieved by using fascia lata, either autologous or homologous, or strips of the levator muscle after transsecting the muscle, but still attached distally via the aponeurosis to the tarsus.[45,259]

Seventh Nerve

The seventh nerve may also be involved in several anomalous innervational patterns that do not affect eye movements but may present to the ophthalmologist.

Intrafacial Synkinesis

Intrafacial synkinesis commonly appears after peripheral facial nerve palsies; branches of the regenerating seventh nerve are misrouted to inappropriate muscles. Frequently, for example, the orbicularis oculi contracts simultaneously with lower facial muscles, and there may be significant narrowing of the palpebral fissure with smiling. Other patterns can occur and, on occasion, are bothersome enough for a patient to require botulinus toxin injection or surgery.[22,390,411]

Marin–Amat Syndrome

This syndrome, also known as *inverse Marcus Gunn phenomenon*, is a rare disorder in which the upper eyelid *falls* when the mouth opens. This syndrome is observed after peripheral facial nerve palsies and has been suggested to be a result of aberrant reinnervation. However, EMG shows inhibition, rather than excitation, of the affected levator muscle during external pterygoid contraction,[296] and absence of orbicularis oculi activity may differentiate this condition from the typical forms of intrafacial synkinesis. Wide jaw opening causes synkinetic contraction of the orbicularis oculi and lid closure, possibly triggered by stretching of the facial muscles.[394]

DISORDERS AT THE NEUROMUSCULAR JUNCTION

Myasthenia Gravis in Infancy

Myasthenia gravis in the infant takes one of three clinical forms.

Transient Neonatal Myasthenia

Transient neonatal myasthenia is seen in approximately one of seven infants born to mothers with myasthenia gravis. All these babies develop a weak cry and difficulty sucking in the first several days of life, and about half become generally hypotonic. This condition, caused by antiacetylcholine receptor antibody (anti-AChR antibody) received by the baby from the mother's circulation,[292] responds promptly to anticholinesterase agents but will resolve in 1 to 12 weeks if untreated.[344,530] There is no relapse or long-term sequela.

Familial Infantile Myasthenia Gravis

Familial infantile myasthenia is rare, appears in children of mothers without myasthenia gravis, and presents in early infancy with ptosis, poor suck and cry, and secondary respiratory infections. Episodic crises of severe respiratory depression and apnea are precipitated by fever, excitement, or vomiting.[151,180,406] Other features include hypotonia, proximal muscle weakness, and easy fatigability, but the extraocular muscles are usually not involved. Inheritance of familial infantile myasthenia gravis has been reported to be autosomal recessive with localization to the telomeric region of chromosome 17, on 17p13.[90] A candidate gene under study for this disease in the 17p region is synaptobrevin-2, a synaptic vesicle protein; this protein probably participates in neurotransmitter release at a step between docking and fusion.[221] This disorder responds to anticholinesterase medications and tends to ameliorate with age.

Congenital Myasthenic Syndromes

A third type of myasthenia seen in infants is the group of congenital myasthenic syndromes, a heterogeneous group of disorders that may affect presynaptic or postsynaptic mechanisms. Various acetylcholine receptor subunit defects as well as genetic defects in endplate acetylcholinesterase have been related to different congenital myasthenic syndromes.[144]

The frequency of congenital myasthenic syndromes varies from 8% to 21% in reported series of childhood myasthenia gravis, reportedly higher where consanguineous marriages are frequent.[18,340] In the fetal period, decreased fetal movements have been reported, resulting in arthrogryposis multiplex congenital, congenital flexures, and contractures of multiple joints.[498] Affected patients are born to mothers without myasthenia and may demonstrate ptosis and ophthalmoparesis during infancy. Severe generalized weakness may also present in the postnatal period with frequent apneic episodes, recurrent aspiration, failure to thrive, and poor sucking. Other patients may present during the first or second year of life with ocular signs and only mild systemic signs. Although ptosis was reported to be present in all of seven patients in one series,[340] it was generally mild and not incapacitating.

These disorders persist throughout life and can be distinguished from acquired myasthenia gravis and from each other by combining clinical, electrophysiological, ultrastructural, and cytochemical investigations.[144–146] Tensilon testing can be positive, and a patient may respond to a trial of pyridostigmine. Presence of anti-AChR antibody excludes this disease.[340] Inheritance in one type termed *slow-channel congenital myasthenia gravis* has been attributed to mutations in the AChR subunit genes, and depending on which subunit is mutated, the disease is transmitted in an autosomal dominant or autosomal recessive fashion. Treatment in congenital myasthenic syndrome patients is generally supportive, and the use of acetylcholinesterase inhibitors is disease specific. Surgery for stable strabimsus in a child can yield a stable long-term result.[340]

Autoimmune Myasthenia Gravis

Incidence

Acquired myasthenia gravis affects overall about 1 in 20,000 per year to 0.4 in 1,000,000 per year.[519] Girls are affected two to six times as frequently as boys, and the incidence of the condition increases progressively through childhood until the end of the second decade of life. Afer the age of 50 years, males predominate; the mean age of onset in women is 28 years and in men 42 years.[519] Among the various childhood forms of myasthenia gravis, a recent series identified 25 (71%) of 35 children as having the autoimmune disease.[340]

Etiology

Acquired myasthenia gravis is an autoimmune disorder. The myasthenic patient has fewer available skeletal muscle acetylcholine receptors because of antibodies produced against these receptors[130] and also because of complement activation.[16] Neuromuscular transmission is thereby poised to fail. Normally, with repetitive stimulation of a motor nerve, the amount of acetylcholine released from that nerve diminishes. In the delicately balanced myasthenic, this decrease in neurotransmitter may well lead to a failure of muscular response. In this context, it is easy to understand why muscle fatigue is the clinical hallmark of myasthenia gravis and why the constant activity of the extraocular muscles, among other activities,[243,354] particularly predisposes them to demonstrate fatigue. The exact reasons for predilection for the extraocular muscles are under study, one explanation potentially lying in the differential expression of acetylcholine receptor subunits in extraocular versus skeletal muscle.[47,244,301]

A number of medications are known to produce myasthenia gravis in normal individuals or to exacerbate already existing disease. The list includes D-penicillamine, antibiotics, anticonvulsants, intravenous contrast dye, anticholinesterase agents, neuromuscular blocking agents, antiarrhythmic drugs, phenothiazines, beta-blockers, and quinine. For example, myasthenia produced by D-penicillamine is indistinguishable from primary acquired myasthenia clinically, immunologically, and electrophysiologically.[519]

Clinical Features

Several general clinical observations may be made concerning myasthenia gravis. Muscle weakness is not accompanied by other neurological signs; muscle function, which may fluctuate even within the course of an office visit, is improved by cholinergic medications; and extraocular, facial, and oropharyngeal muscles are most commonly involved. Beyond this, there are numerous variations of presentation, and no single sign is solely reliable.

Natural History

Of patients who present initially with purely ocular symptoms and signs, 50% to 80% subsequently develop generalized myasthenia within about 2 years.[519] In a large study of 1487 patients with myasthenia, 53% presented with ocular symptoms.[183,519] Of the entire group of myasthenic patients in this study, 15% continued to demonstrate purely ocular manifestations (with follow-up to 45 years; mean, 17 years). Of the 40% of patients in this study with strictly ocular involvement during the first month after onset of symptoms, 66% developed generalized disease. Of these who subsequently developed generalized disease, 78% did so within 1 year, and 94% within 3 years after onset of symptoms and signs.

In a series of 24 children in Toronto with acquired autoimmune myasthenia (age, 11 months to 16 years; median age, 4.7 years), 14 (58%) patients initially had ocular involvement only (median follow-up time, 2.6 years). Of these 14, 5 (36%) progressed to generalized myasthenia gravis in a mean time of 7.8 months (range, 1–23 months). Patients with ocular myasthenia presented at an average of 6.8 years; those with systemic disease presented on average at 7.1 years.[340]

Clinical Assessment

Variable diplopia or ptosis most often prompt an ophthalmologic evaluation. Patients with these symptoms are evaluated for signs and symptoms of generalized myasthenia such as facial weakness, dysphonia, arm or leg weakness, chewing weakness, and respiratory difficulties. In "ocular myasthenia," however, the findings are restricted to the levator and extraocular muscles. Because there is no stereotypical myasthenic eye movement, this diagnosis should be considered in any child with an unexplained, acquired ocular motility disturbance and clinically normal pupils, particularly when the deviation is variable, whether or not ptosis is present. Any pattern of abnormal motility is suspect, including an apparent gaze palsy, internuclear ophthalmoplegia,[167] isolated cranial nerve palsy,[423] one and one-half syndrome,[116,468] incomitant strabismus, accommodative and vergence insufficiency,[101] and gaze-evoked nystagmus.[250,288] Prolonged OKN may demonstrate slowing of the quick phases; large saccades may be hypometric; small saccades may be hypermetric; and characteristic "quiver movements," which consist of an initial small saccadic movement followed by a rapid drift backward, may be seen.[46,288]

In addition to the eye movements, lid function is assessed. Ptosis can be elicited or accentuated by fatiguing the levator palpebrae superioris with prolonged upgaze or repeated lid closure. Because Hering's law of equal innervation applies to the levator muscles as it does to the extraocular muscles, the contralateral lid may be retracted but falls to a normal position when the ptotic lid is lifted with a finger. Through the same mechanism, in bilateral ptosis, manual elevation of one lid increases the amount of ptosis on the other side by diminishing the amount of innervation necessary to fixate. Cogan's lid twitch sign can be elicited in some myasthenic patients by having the patient look down for 20s and then making an upward saccade to the primary position; the lid twitches upward one or more times and then slowly drops to its ptotic position. Finally, the orbicularis oculi muscles are often weak, and the patient may not be able to sustain lid closure.

Examination of the patient before and after the administration of anticholinesterase agents is, arguably, of more limited use in children than in adults. This method may be most helpful in children whose history and physical examination do not permit a clear diagnosis yet who have such significant deficits in lid elevation or ocular motility that a response is easily observed. A positive test consists of the direct observation of a weak muscle becoming stronger after the administration of intravenous edrophonium hydrochloride (Tensilon) or intramuscular neostigmine methylsulfate (Prostigmin). The initial dose is 2mg, given up to 10mg total. The onset of action for Tensilon is 30s, lasting up to 5min. This drug is contraindicated in patients who are elderly or have heart disease, and other workup should be performed before considering the Tensilon test. Intramuscular Prostigmin is longer acting than Tensilon and allows more time for measurement of changes, but its absorption rate and hence onset of action are quite variable; its onset of action is generally between 15 to 20 min and the peak response occurs about 30 to 40 min after administration. In children the dose is 0.02 mg/kg, always with a total of less than 1.5 mg; and in adults the dose is 1.5 mg, with atropine 0.6 mg, coadministered.[279] Choice of drug can be individualized according to the endpoints that are being assessed and to the ability of the child to cooperate.

To make a decisive observation, it is important, both before and after giving these drugs, to quantitate as accurately as possible the function of the affected muscle(s) through measurement of pertinent indicators such as lid height in primary position, levator function, saccadic velocities, ocular movement, ocular alignment, and orbicularis strength. After administering Tensilon, the examiner observes for tearing and lid fasciculations as evidence of cholinergic effect, and draws no conclusion if a paradoxic decrease in muscle function occurs, because this may happen in the presence or absence of myasthenia. Positive responses after either drug are fairly reliable evidence for myasthenia but can, on rare occasions, occur in nonmyasthenic patients. False-negative responses, however, are common and therefore do not exclude myasthenia gravis.

Alternatively, a rest test may be used by allowing the patient to rest with eyes closed for a period of 10 to 15 min.[337] An "ice test" has also been reported to improve ptosis[173,278,425] and motility[142] after applying an ice pack to the eyes for 2 to 5 min. However, subsequent report of four patients[337] revealed no difference among an ice test, a heat test, or a rest test, so long as the rest period was at least 10 to 15 min.

Further diagnostic testing may include anti-AChR antibody titer and electromyography. EMG is particularly useful in generalized myasthenia but is difficult to perform in a frightened, uncooperative child. The electromyographer looks for a characteristic decrement in the muscle action potentials with repetitive supramaximal nerve stimulation and for the "jitter phenomenon" on single muscle fiber studies, difficult responses to elicit and observe even in a cooperative patient. Anti-AChR antibody is most helpful in generalized myasthenia as it is reportedly present in 80% to 90% of those patients but only 50%

or fewer of ocular myasthenics.[149,463,519] According to other reports, specifically on juvenile myasthenia gravis patients, the frequency of postive AChR antibody was between 56% and 63%.[4,15,19]

Systemic Associations

Associated immune disorders to be considered in children include rheumatoid arthritis, juvenile-onset diabetes mellitus, asthma, and thyroid disease; neoplasia (breast cancer, uterine cancer, carcinoma of the colon, pinealoma) is also seen.[408] Thymoma rarely occurs in children although it is recognized to accompany 10% of myasthenia gravis.

Inheritance

Inheritance is usually sporadic. Approximately 1% to 4% of cases are familial without a clear Mendelian pattern. This familial predisposition may be due to predilection for autoimmunity in general.

Treatment

Once the ophthalmologist diagnoses or strongly suspects myasthenia, a neurologist generally directs further testing and treatment. The ophthalmologist's role remains important, however. In addition to monitoring the motility and lid dysfunction and providing symptomatic relief for these disorders, the ophthalmologist should be alert to the possibility of amblyopia. If not promptly detected and attended to, amblyopia can be extremely difficult to treat, particularly when there is sufficient ptosis to necessitate taping or a ptosis crutch for the lid during occlusion of the sound eye.

Current therapy aims to increase the amount of acetylcholine available through the use of anticholinesterase agents or to diminish the autoimmune reaction with corticosteroids, other immunosuppressive agents, such as azathioprine, cyclosporin A, and mycophenolate mofetil,[93,150] plasmapheresis, or thymectomy. Supervision of these treatments is clearly in the bailiwick of the neurologist. It is worth noting that anticholinesterase agents are not as effective in ameliorating ocular motility as they are for other manifestations of myasthenia[149] nor are they as effective as steroids[462] or other treatments directed against the autoimmune response.[431] However, because of the risks and complications, the use of steroids, immunosuppressives, plasmapheresis, and thymectomy in pure ocular myasthenia gravis remains controversial.[68,365,441] In a recent pilot study, cyclosporin A was found to be effective in a series of eight patients, resulting in complete remission in seven of the eight, with a mean follow-up of 14 months; the eighth patient was noncompliant.[80]

Strabismus surgery has been performed on patients with stable deviations of at least 5 months, using conventional strabismus surgical techniques.[115,360] The presence of systemic disease is an important consideration in deciding on the method of anesthesia, although general anesthesia is not an absolute contraindication when the disease is clinically controlled.

Prognosis

The prognosis for survival, improvement, and remission in a child with myasthenia gravis is better than that in an adult, according to most studies.[327,408,462] Rodriquez and coworkers[408] studied 149 children who were less than 17 years old at the onset of autoimmune myasthenia gravis and had a median follow-up of 17 years with minimum follow-up of 4 years. An estimated 80% of these patients were alive at age 40, about 90% of the survival expected in the general population. Improvement or remission was seen in 79% of the 85 patients who underwent thymectomy and 62% of the remaining 64 patients. In the smaller Toronto series, children required an average of 2 years on medication before entering remission.[340] Complete remission in adults has been reported as 40% to 70%, generally achieved after 1 to 3 years of treatment.[519]

In 9% of children in the Rodriquez series, the disease remained strictly ocular; this is comparable to the 14% found in a large adult series observed over a similar interval.[183] In the Toronto series, 38% of the 24 children remained strictly ocular, although the mean follow-up period was 3.5 years.[340] Children with ocular myasthenia gravis may also show prolonged remissions and respond well to steroid therapy on relapse.[412,437]

The result of strabismus surgery for myasthenia gravis has reportedly been favorable in two studies, after a follow-up of 4 months to 14 years (median, 12 months).[115,360] In these two studies combined, 2 of 10 patients required reoperations, and 1 of the 10 required prisms postoperatively.

Botulism

Numerous pharmacological agents and toxins may interfere with transmission at the neuromuscular junction. The neurotoxin produced by the bacterium *Clostridium botulinum* irreversibly impedes the intracellular mechanisms responsible for the release of acetylcholine from the presynaptic nerve terminals.[458]

Etiology

The different neurotoxins produced in botulism exhibit different clinical characteristics. Type E botulism is usually associated with eating seafood; pupillary abnormalities and ptosis may be seen as early signs. Gastrointestinal symptoms are more prevalent in type E and type B. The most severe form is type A, which carries the highest risk for ventilatory support and the highest mortality.

Clinical Features

Children may develop botulism from ingestion of contaminated food, wound infection, or intestinal infection in infants. Infants usually come to attention because of lethargy, weakness, feeding difficulty, a feeble cry, and constipation.[240] Older children report nausea, vomiting, blurred vision, dysphagia, and pooling of secretions in the mouth, followed by generalized weakness and diplopia. In both groups, ophthalmologic findings are common and may include any type or degree of external ophthalmoplegia, dilated pupils that react poorly to light, and ptosis.[485]

In one outbreak of 27 patients in the U.K., the complaints were of blurred vision in 78%, drooping lids in 56%, and double vision in 30%. In this report, 11 of 14 (79%) of reviewed records revealed sixth nerve palsy and 13 of 14 (93%) revealed accommodative paresis, both of which were early ophthalmic signs. The severity of ophthalmoparesis was a good indicator of the overall severity and progression of disease. When there was ventilatory failure, it occurred 12 h after third cranial nerve palsy.[457]

In another report, it was noted that sixth cranial nerve palsy may be the initial neurological manifestation of type B botulism.[485] In 8 of 11 (73%) of their patients diagnosed with third nerve palsy, respiratory insufficiency eventually ensued.

Quivering eye movements on attempted saccades have also been observed and analyzed on eye movement recordings, consisting of hypometric saccades with subnormal and stuttering velocities.[200]

Clinical Assessment

Because botulism may be difficult to distinguish clinically from Guillain–Barre syndrome,[241] pupillary findings, which are rare in Guillain–Barre, become particularly important. Botulism may also be mistaken for myasthenia gravis (again, the pupils are helpful; a Tensilon test may be falsely positive in mild forms of botulism[457]), sudden infant death syndrome, and hypothyroidism in infants. In infants, EMG is the primary means of diagnosis.[241]

Treatment

Treatment is essentially supportive. Antitoxin has been shown only to shorten the duration of illness in type E botulism, but is considered in patients with botulism as soon as the diagnosis is suspected as it can only act before the toxin is irreversibly bound to its receptor. Adverse reactions to the antitoxin have been reported in up to 20% of patients. Guanidine, a drug that enhances release of acetylcholine from the presynaptic nerve terminal, has only a slight effect on limb and ocular muscles and no effect on respiratory muscles.[457]

Prognosis

Recovery does not occur until new neuromuscular junctions are established, a process that may take weeks to months. The mortality from this condition in the United States has been reported as 7.5%; this figure is higher in developing countries.[457]

DISORDERS OF THE EXTRAOCULAR MUSCLES

Abnormal extraocular muscles may limit eye movements through decreased function or through restriction. The pattern of limitation may simulate neural and neuromuscular disorders

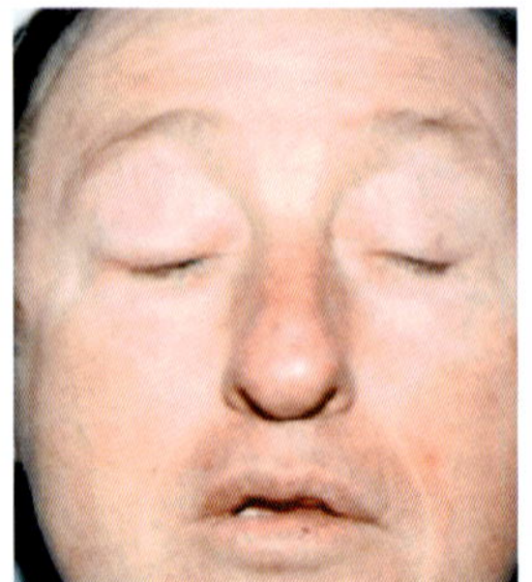
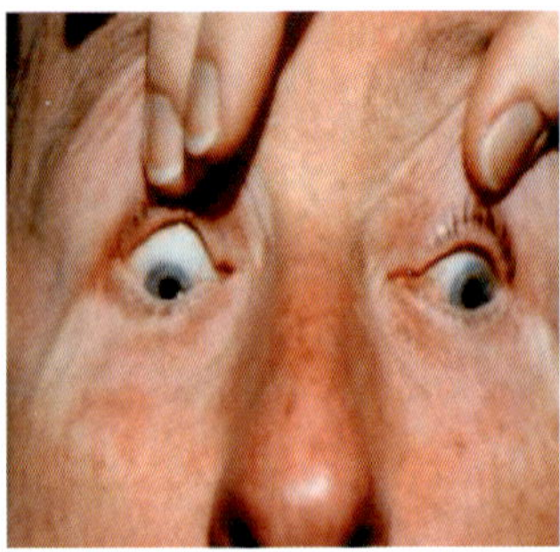

FIGURE 5-13. Fibrosis of the extraocular muscles. Severe ptosis (*right photo*) and eyes fixed in depression with minimal to no movement typical of severe fibrosis of the extraocular muscles.

so closely that force ductions, special imaging (echography, CT, MRI), or even surgical exploration may be necessary for differentiation.

These disorders may be either congenital or acquired. Congenital anomalies of the extraocular muscles include agenesis, duplication, abnormal origins and insertions, fascial anomalies, and fibrous bands.[297,500,508,509,529] *Congenital absence of one or more extraocular muscles* limits movement of the globe in the direction of action of the missing muscle(s) and may mimic a nerve palsy. Indeed, in one series of presumed congenital superior oblique palsies for which a superior oblique tuck was deemed necessary and attempted, 18% of the patients were found to have congenital absence of the superior oblique.[201] Agenesis and other forms of maldevelopment of the extraocular muscles have long been recognized and associated with craniofacial anomalies.[124,384]

At times, certain extraocular muscles mechanically restrict eye movements from birth, for example, in the *congenital fibrosis syndrome* (Fig. 5-13) or *congenital Brown's syndrome*. Acquired disorders such as *trauma, dysthyroid myopathy, acquired Brown's syndrome*, and *orbital myositis* may all cause weakness or restriction of extraocular muscles. Although investigation of these disorders requires careful attention to the history and systemic health of the child as well as local ocular and orbital signs, such advertence is frequently rewarded.

DISORDERS OF NERVE AND MUSCLE

Kearns–Sayre Syndrome (Chronic Progressive Ophthalmoplagia)

CLINICAL FEATURES AND NATURAL HISTORY

Ptosis and chronic progressive limitation of eye movements, usually without diplopia, are features of a variety of disorders. Among these, Kearns–Sayre syndrome (KSS) is singularly apt to come to attention in childhood, most often because of ocular signs. The triad of external ophthalmoplegia, heart block, and retinal pigmentary degeneration identified in the original description of KSS[256] remains the cornerstone of diagnosis, although a multitude of associated signs have since been recognized (Table 5-8).

The eye movements in KSS show gradually progressive limitation, which is usually symmetrical and affects all directions of gaze. Bell's phenomenon and eye movement responses to caloric stimulation or head rotation are also slowly lost. Anticholinesterase agents do not improve the range of eye movements. Pupils remain normal. The lids are typically ptotic and often close weakly because of involvement of the orbicularis

TABLE 5-8. Manifestations of Kearns–Sayre Syndrome.

System	*Findings*
Cardinal features	Chronic progressive external ophthalmoplegia; degenerative pigmentary retinopathy; cardiac conduction defects/sudden death; no family history
Musculoskeletal	Short stature; "ragged-red" fibers by light microscopy of muscle tissue; skeletal and dental anomalies
Neurological	Elevated CSF protein; deafness; vestibular dysfunction; cerebellar ataxia; "descending" myopathy of face and limbs; mild corticospinal tract signs; subnormal intelligence; demyelinating polyradiculopathy; slowed electroencephalogram; decreased ventilatory drive/sudden death; spongiform degeneration of cerebrum and brainstem
Endocrine	Diabetes mellitus; hypogonadism; hypoparathyroidism; growth hormone deficiency; adrenal dysfunction; hyperglycemic acidotic coma/death; elevated serum lactate and pyruvate
Other	Corneal edema; nephropathy

Source: Modified from Glaser JS, Bachynski BN. Infranuclear disorders of eye movement. In: Glaser JS (ed) Neuro-ophthalmology, 2nd edn. Philadelphia: Lippincott, 1990:402, with permission.[166]

oculi. Indeed, generalized facial weakness is frequent and contributes to a typical facial appearance.

Affected fundi demonstrate a diffuse pigmentary retinopathy that characteristically involves the posterior pole as well as the periphery and generally consists of a "salt-and-pepper" pattern of pigment clumping. Commonly both rod and cone function are reduced on electroretinography,[341] and although it has been noted that only 40% of patients have decreased visual acuity or night blindness,[54] photoreceptor function can diminish insidiously with time.

Systemic Associations

Cardiac conduction defects, a cardinal feature of KSS, can be heralded by an interval of enhanced conduction at the A-V node and may lead to death at any time.[88,404] Other systemic associations include small stature, ataxia, deafness, raised cerebrospinal fluid protein, diabetes, and hypoparathyroidism (see Table 5-8).

Clinical Assessment

On any patient suspected of KSS, an electrocardiogram is performed. Abnormal blood lactate and pyruvate levels may be found. On skeletal muscle biopsy, "ragged-red fibers" and abnormal mitochondria are expected. In diagnosing patients suspected of KSS but with an incomplete constellation of findings, analysis of muscle mtDNA to look for mitochondrial deletions may be more critical than mitochondrial morphological examination (see following).[178] The brain MRI of patients with KSS may show normal or atrophied brain, but the characteristic finding is a combination of high-signal foci in subcortical cerebral white matter, brainstem, globus pallidus, or thalamus.[92]

Etiology

A protracted and shifting debate over the etiology and nosology of KSS has continued for decades. Early on, *chronic progressive external ophthalmoplegia (CPEO)* was considered to be an isolated myopathy of the extraocular muscles, with occasional weakness of the extremities.[260] However, many subsequent reports described CPEO in conjunction with multisystem disease, with KSS itself serving as a good example. When spongiform degeneration of the brainstem and cerebrum, which is observed on neuropathological examination of patients with

KSS, was highlighted,[114] the neural structures governing eye movements became suspect. Next, myopathological findings pointed investigators in yet a different direction. In CPEO, light microscopy of muscle preparations processed with the modified Gomori trichrome stain frequently demonstrates "ragged-red" muscle fibers among normal extraocular muscle fibers, orbicularis oculi fibers, and, at times, other skeletal muscle fibers. With electron microscopy, these ragged-red fibers as well as other muscle fibers demonstrate markedly abnormal mitochondria. In KSS, such abnormal mitochondria were detected in a variety of other tissues as well, including sweat glands,[245] liver cells,[174] and cerebellar neurons.[438] Experimental infusion of a chemical that uncouples oxidative phosphorylation produced reversible ragged-red fibers.[318] This morphological evidence combined with biochemical abnormalities indicating mitochondrial dysfunction led to speculation about the role of mitochondrial DNA (mtDNA) in the pathogenesis of these disorders.

INHERITANCE

The majority of KSS and CPEO cases are sporadic. In one review, only a single family demonstrated more than one person manifesting the entire KSS.[420] When small pedigrees with multiple individuals exhibiting CPEO have been reported, transmission has generally been maternal and compatible with mitochondrial inheritance,[140,223,236] but paternal transmission of CPEO has also been observed, suggesting a defective autosomal nuclear gene in some cases.[139,140,467]

New techniques in molecular biology have triggered an explosion of studies of mtDNA in patients with KSS and CPEO.[178,334] A significant proportion of these patients show large-scale heteroplasmic deletions in mtDNA, and these deletions play a pivotal role in the pathogenesis of these disorders. *Heteroplasmy* denotes the presence of several different mtDNA in a cell, some of which may be pathogenic. KSS and CPEO patients have heteroplasmy in different proportions depending on the tissue studied[222]; large-scale deletions of mtDNA have been observed in muscle of 80% of KSS patients and 70% of those with CPEO.[178] Based on these observations, it has been suggested that CPEO and KSS are different severities along the same clinical spectrum.[131,178]

Another finding that may explain the overlap between the clinical presentations of KSS and CPEO is that patients with these two diseases have identical mtDNA deletions, but in KSS they are localized to the muscle and neural tissues, whereas in CPEO they are localized to muscle. Another disease called Pearson syndrome also has the identical deletions as in KSS and CPEO but is localized to the blood. In fact, patients with Pearson syndrome may develop KSS later in life.

On the other hand, mtDNA duplications have been observed in KSS but not in CPEO patients,[178] a difference that lends support to the idea that these are two distinct clinical entities, as suggested earlier.[54]

The severity of disease in patients with mitochondrial deletions apparently depends on a variety of factors: (1) the degree of heteroplasmy, or the distribution of normal and mutant mitochondria; (2) the nature of the mitochondrial mutation; (3) reduction in absolute amounts of normal mtDNA; and (4) a homoplasmic mutation that leads to a large deletion.[178]

Treatment and Prognosis

The prognosis for patients with KSS is fair, and treatment is largely symptomatic. Patients can frequently be managed with a cardiac pacemaker[382] to obviate conducting fibers that, on pathological study, are fibrotic and infiltrated by fat.[156,160] Despite cardiac pacing, patients may die suddenly of inadequate brainstem ventilatory response to hypoxia.[82,104]

Abrupt and fatal endocrine dysfunction may also be triggered by steroids,[38] and there can be hypersensitivity to agents used during induction of general anesthesia.[233] For many pediatric patients, however, it is the relentless progression of neurological deficits, especially weakness and ataxia, rather than the possibility of sudden demise, that proves to be particularly trying.

Preliminary reports suggest that administration of coenzyme Q10, a quinone found in the mitochondrial oxidative system (with reported doses of 60–120 mg daily for 3 months in one patient,[357] 50 mg 3 times a day for 3 months in two others[359]), may improve A-V block as well as normalize serum pyruvate and lactate levels[358]; improve neurological function without an effect on the ophthalmoplegia or the electrocardiogram[70]; and increase respiratory vital capacity when used with succinate.[452]

Surgery is generally not recommended for either ptosis or strabismus in these patients as it is a progressive disease. Surgical correction of ptosis would involve a high risk of exposure keratopathy, especially because the eye will lose its Bell's phenomenon during the course of the disease and corneal wetting would not occur. Diplopia from strabismus may be treated with prisms and, as a last resort, monocular occlusion.

Myotonic Dystrophy

Myotonic dystrophy, also known as dystrophia myotonica or Steinert's disease, is an autosomal dominant multisystem disorder with variable phenotype. Early investigators focused on muscle as the primary site of involvement; subsequent studies revealed that the nervous system[231] as well as a variety of other tissues are affected in addition to the muscles. At least two main types of myotonic dystrophy exist, termed DM1 and DM2. Two other described forms, called proximal myotonic myopathy (PROMM) and proximal myotonic dystrophy (PDM), are closely linked to the DM2 locus and may be caused by the same genetic defect with different phenotypic expression.

Incidence

Myotonic dystrophy is considered as one of the most frequent "dystrophies" in adulthood, with a prevalence of approximately 5 in 100,000 in white European populations.[401]

Etiology

The fascinating pathogenesis of DM1 has been described as a result of various mechanisms.[319] The most important factor is the expanded trinucleotide cytosine-thymidine-guanine (CTG) repeats in the 3′-untranslated region of the disease gene, dystrophia myotonica protein kinase (DMPK) gene, which leads to decreased DMPK messenger RNA (mRNA) expression and protein levels. However, DMPK knockout mice showed only mild muscle weakness and abnormal cardiac conduction. On further investigation, it was found that the expanded trinucleotide repeat in the mRNA is toxic to the muscle, because when transgenic mice were developed that express human skeletal actin—unrelated to the DMPK gene—with expanded CTG repeats in the 3′-untranslated region, the mice developed myotonia and myopathy.[304]

A significant correlation exists between age of onset and number of CTG repeats and a general correlation between the degree of CTG expansion and the severity of disease manifestations. Mildly affected patients have 50 to 150 repeats, classic DM1 patients have 100 to 1000, and congenital cases may have more than 2000.[319]

The exact pathological mechanism remains unclear, but a theory unifying the protean manifestations of the disease has been proposed, namely that the fundamental defect is a generalized abnormality of cell membranes.[418] Recent evidence supports the hypothesis that DMPK deficiency is associated with sodium channel abnormality in DM.[336]

Clinical Features and Natural History

Unlike KSS, ocular motility abnormalities in myotonic dystrophy are commonly subclinical and have been observed for the most part in adults. A number of authors have described progressive limitation of voluntary eye movements as well as markedly decreased maximum saccadic velocity and reduced smooth pursuit gain, but it is not clear whether these eye movement disorders result from a neurological or myopathic defect or both.[14,123,143,290,364,449,484,503] Clinical myotonia, that is, delayed muscular relaxation, most strikingly affects the limb muscles (e.g., persistent grip), but may on occasion involve the extraocular muscles[134]; immediately after sustaining gaze in a certain direction, the patient cannot promptly move the eyes in the opposite direction. Bell's phenomenon is particularly useful to elicit sustained upgaze in an infant or uncooperative child.

Although the manifestations of myotonic dystrophy usually become apparent in adolescents or young adults, detailed questioning often documents symptoms during the first decade of life, and the disease can, at times, affect infants and young children distinctly.[127] For the ophthalmologist, a characteristic facial appearance (facial diplegia, triangular-shaped mouth, and slack jaw) and weak orbicularis function typically without ptosis suggests the possibility of myotonic dystrophy in a young child. Bilateral facial weakness is the most characteristic feature of early-onset myotonic dystrophy and is frequently misdiagnosed as Möbius syndrome (see following section). With increasing age, the more familiar facial appearance of myotonic dystrophy (narrow, expressionless, "hatchet" face with hollowing of cheeks and temples) evolves because wasting of the facial muscles occurs, and ptosis becomes far more common.

PROMM, PDM, and DM2 are also autosomal dominant myotonic dystrophy without the CTG repeat expansion at the

DM1 locus. PROMM and PDM predominantly involve proximal muscles, and DM2 involves distal muscles. All three have been linked to chromosome 3q21.3 and may be various phenotypes of the same disease. These patients also develop posterior subcapsular cataracts with onset before 50 years of age. They do not exhibit ophthalmoplegia, however.[320]

CLINICAL ASSESSMENT

Bilateral iridescent and posterior cortical lens opacities are useful for establishing a clinical diagnosis[27]; they may be identified in young children but are often not seen until the teenage years. Clear electroretinographic abnormalities with normal-appearing fundi may be observed early on,[69] and a subgroup of patients demonstrate visual loss and observable pigmentary retinopathy later in the course of the disease. Additional ophthalmic signs are listed in Table 5-9.[37] A negative family history does not exclude the diagnosis because a parent with myotonic dystrophy may be affected so mildly as to be unaware of it.[374] Careful evaluation of the parents can therefore prove helpful.

Beside the slit lamp examination for cataracts, other primary diagnostic tests include DNA testing for an enlarged CTG repeat, examination for muscle and nonmuscle manifestations, and EMG for subclinical myotonia. Secondary tests include serum creatinine kinase, which is often mildly elevated in

TABLE 5-9. Ophthalmic Manifestations of Myotonic Dystrophy.

Structure	*Findings*
Eyelids	Ptosis; myotonic lag (due to delayed relaxation of levator); orbicularis weakness; myotonic closure (due to delayed relaxation of orbicularis)
Motility	Slow saccades with full ductions and versions; myotonia induced by Bell's reflex, convergence, or eccentric gaze; partial to complete ophthalmoplegia (usually symmetrical)
Globe	Cataracts (subcapsular polychromatophilic opacities; posterior cortical spokes; posterior subcapsular plaques; mature cataracts); short depigmented ciliary processes; hypotony; iris neovascular tufts (resulting in spontaneous hyphema); keratitis sicca; macular and peripheral retinal pigmentary degeneration; miotic, sluggishly reacting pupils
Miscellaneous	Decreased ERG responses; elevated dark-adaptation thresholds; generalized constriction of visual fields

Source: From Ref. 37, with permission.

diseased individuals, and muscle biopsy, which frequently shows an increase in central nuclei, fiber atrophy, and ringed fibers.

Inheritance

The interesting feature of this disease is that when it is passed on from one generation to the next in autosomal dominant fashion, the severity of disease increases. The phenomenon of progressive earlier onset and greater severity of disease is termed *anticipation*; this is particularly true for cases of female transmission, which can lead to the congenital cases of the disease. Increased severity in the subsequent generations is associated with increased expansion of the CTG repeats.[303]

DM1 gene has been mapped to chromosome 19q13.3. DM2, PROMM, and PDM have all been linked to chromosome 3q21.3, but the gene defect(s) has not yet been identified.[320]

Systemic Associations

In addition to facial diplegia, infants frequently demonstrate hypotonia, delayed motor and intellectual development, feeding difficulties, neonatal respiratory distress, and talipes.[192] In adults, diabetes, pituitary dysfunction, widespread involvement of the smooth muscle of the gastrointestinal tract, premature balding, and gonadal atrophy may all be seen.

Treatment and Prognosis

Comprehensive medical care of patients with myotonic dystrophy is essential. Prompt intervention may become necessary at any time because of associated, potentially life-threatening, cardiac conduction defects. Periodic EKGs are obtained to detect heart block, which may require a pacemaker. Drugs such as procainamide, quinine, and propranolol are avoided in patients with cardiac involvement. Endocrinological management is necessary for those patients who also have diabetes or pituitary dysfunction.

Prostheses may be used for foot and hand weakness. Myotonia may be moderately reduced with mexiletine and tocainide, which have been found to be more effective than phenytoin and dysopyramide.

Any strabismus surgery for myotonic dystrophy patients is approached with caution because of the potential for friable and atrophic extraocular muscles.[306] Also any ptosis surgery risks corneal exposure due to lack of Bell's phenomenon in the setting of ophthalmoplegia.

Life expectancy is reduced particularly in the case of early onset disease and proximal muscle involvement. The high mortality rate is due to an increase in deaths from respiratory diseases, cardiovascular diseases, and neoplasms, as well as sudden deaths from cardiac arrhythmias.[320]

Möbius Syndrome

Möbius[328,329] designated congenital, bilateral sixth and seventh nerve palsies as central features of what has come to be known as *Möbius' syndrome*, but subsequent clinical and pathological observations reveal greater complexity. It has become clear that the eponym has been applied to a heterogeneous group of congenital neuromuscular disorders that produce facial weakness in some combination with a variety of other findings (Table 5-10). It has been suggested that the term sequence is more appropriate because a sequence defines a cascade of secondary events after an embryonic insult from heterogeneous causes.[325]

Clinical Features and Systemic Associations

Typically, a short time after birth, an affected infant demonstrates difficulty feeding because of poor sucking and little, if

TABLE 5-10. Manifestations of Möbius Syndrome.

System	*Findings*
Cardinal features	Partial or complete facial paralysis, usually bilateral (may be unilateral)[203,324]
Ocular motor	Straight eyes, esotropia, or exotropia with no horizontal movements and preserved vertical movements[324,407,461]; total ophthalmoplegia[206,324,464]; cocontraction of horizontal recti[61]
Neurological	Unilateral or bilateral palsy of cranial nerves V, VIII, IX, X, or XII[42,475]; autism[325]
Orofacial	Abnormal tongue; bifid uvula; cleft lip/palate; micrognathia, microstomia; external ear defects[324,325]
Musculoskeletal	Syndactyly; brachydactyly; absent or supranumerary digits; arthrogryposis multiplex congenital; talipes; absence of hands or feet[324,325,409,461]
Miscellaneous	Mental retardation[325]; congenital heart defects; absent sternal head of the pectoralis major (second major component of the Poland anomaly)[324,325]; rib defects; Klippel–Feil anomaly; neuroradiologic cerebellar hypoplasia[51,190]; hypogonadotropic hypogonadism with or without anosmia[362,422]

any, facial expression, as a result of the involvement of cranial nerves IX and XII in addition to VII. Generally, horizontal eye movements are clearly abnormal, and vertical eye movements are preserved. If convergence is intact and used for cross-fixation, the ocular motility pattern may resemble that produced by bilateral sixth nerve palsies. On occasion, vertical eye movements may also be affected or total ophthalmoplegia may occur. Crocodile tears, micrognathia, dental anomalies, cleft palate, facial asymmetry, limb malformations, Poland's syndrome, epilepsy, mental retardation, and autism may be present.[325]

Etiology

Fifteen autopsied cases have been classified into four groups based on neuropathological findings in the brainstem.[489] Group I demonstrated absence or hypoplasia of relevant cranial nerve nuclei; group II, in addition to neuronal loss, showed evidence of neuronal degeneration suggesting peripheral nerve injury; group III, in addition to neuronal loss and neuronal generation, had frank necrosis of the tegmentum of the lower pons; group IV revealed no abnormalities in the brainstem and may represent a purely myopathic disorder. Cases of *facio-scapulo-humeral muscular dystrophy* and *congenital centronuclear (myotubular) myopathy* that clinically mimic Möbius syndrome would also presumably belong to group IV.[189,199]

A number of investigators have speculated that disruption of the vascular system causes hypoxia of vulnerable tissues between 4 and 7 weeks gestation.[190,294,396] It has been proposed that Möbius syndrome, the Poland anomaly, and the Klippel–Feil defect all result from a transient interruption during the sixth week of gestation in the development of the subclavian artery and its branches, including the basilar, vertebral, and internal thoracic arteries, which supply the brain, neck, pectoral muscles, and upper limbs; in addition, in Möbius syndrome, the primitive trigeminal artery that supplies the hindbrain during fetal life may regress before the establishment of adequate perfusion from the vertebral or basilar artery and thereby disturb development of the cranial nerve nuclei.[48] Such a mechanism would be consistent with the brainstem necrosis seen in group III Möbius' syndrome patients but would not account for the findings in groups I and II.

Inheritance

As might be expected, most reported cases have been sporadic, and the sexes are affected with equal frequency. At least five families with Möbius' syndrome have been reported without any one consistent chromosomal defect.[206,283,325,531] Chromosomal translocations (1;13 and 1;11), chromosome 13q12.2 deletion, and linkage to chromosome 3q21–22 have been reported by previous authors. The recurrence risk to siblings of isolated cases with these three manifestations appears to be less than 2%.[42]

Treatment and Prognosis

Depending on the severity and types of malformations, the treatment will vary.[325] Initially, sucking problems often require modification in type of bottle used. If lid lag is present from seventh nerve palsy, lubricants are necessary. Refractive errors, amblyopia, and strabismus often need attention.

Maximal medial rectus recessions with or without vertical displacement have been shown to suffice in some cases,[466,516] whereas others have advocated horizontal recess-resections[321,346,490] or vertical muscle transposition.[206,470]

Because of the lack of facial expression, parents and children may have psychological difficulty with bonding and social communication. Plastic surgeries do exist that can improve facial movement.[81,543] Finally, helping families cope by contacting others through a national organization, such as the Möbius Syndrome Foundation, is also important and appreciated, as is the case for other diseases or syndromes mentioned in this chapter.

References

1. Abdul-Rahim AS, et al. Cryptogenic oculomotor nerve palsy. The need for repeated neuroimaging studies. Arch Ophthalmol 1989; 107(3):387–390.
2. Afifi AK, et al. Recurrent lateral rectus palsy in childhood. Pediatr Neurol 1990;6(5):315–318.
3. Afifi AK, Bell WE, Menezes AH. Etiology of lateral rectus palsy in infancy and childhood. J Child Neurol 1992;7(3):295–299.
4. Afifi AK, Bell WE. Tests for juvenile myasthenia gravis: comparative diagnostic yield and prediction of outcome. J Child Neurol 1993; 8(4):403–411.

5. Aguirre-Aquino BI, Rogers DG, Traboulsi EI. A patient with de Morsier and Duane syndromes. J Am Assoc Pediatr Ophthalmol Strabismus 2000;4(4):243–245.
6. Ahn JC, Hoyt WF, Hoyt CS. Tonic upgaze in infancy. A report of three cases. Arch Ophthalmol 1989;107(1):57–58.
7. Aicardi J, et al. Ataxia-ocular motor apraxia: a syndrome mimicking ataxia-telangiectasia. Ann Neurol 1988;24(4):497–502.
8. Al-Din AN, et al. Brainstem encephalitis and the syndrome of Miller Fisher: a clinical study. Brain 1982;105(pt 3):481–495.
9. Aldrich MS, Beck RW, Albers JW. Familial recurrent Bell's palsy with ocular motor palsies. Neurology 1987;37(8):1369–1371.
10. Aleksic S, et al. Congenital ophthalmoplegia in oculoauriculovertebral dysplasia-hemifacial microsomia (Goldenhar–Gorlin syndrome). A clinicopathologic study and review of the literature. Neurology 1976;26(7):638–644.
11. Alfano J. Spasm of fixation. Am J Ophthalmol 1955;40:724–725.
12. Alvarez F, et al. Nervous and ocular disorders in children with cholestasis and vitamin A and E deficiencies. Hepatology 1983;3(3): 410–414.
13. Amit R, Benezra D. Oculomotor ophthalmoplegic migraine in an infant. Headache 1987;27(7):390–391.
14. Anastasopoulos D, et al. Abnormalities of ocular motility in myotonic dystrophy. Brain 1996;119(pt 6):1923–1932.
15. Andrews PI, Massey JM, Sanders DB. Acetylcholine receptor antibodies in juvenile myasthenia gravis. Neurology 1993;43(5):977–982.
16. Andrews PI, et al. Race, sex, and puberty influence onset, severity, and outcome in juvenile myasthenia gravis. Neurology 1994;44(7): 1208–1214.
17. Angelini L, et al. Hallervorden–Spatz disease: clinical and MRI study of 11 cases diagnosed in life. J Neurol 1992;239(8):417–425.
18. Anlar B, et al. Myasthenia gravis in childhood. Acta Paediatr 1996;85(7):838–842.
19. Anlar B. Juvenile myasthenia: diagnosis and treatment. Paediatr Drugs 2000;2(3):161–169.
20. Appukuttan B, et al. Localization of a gene for Duane retraction syndrome to chromosome 2q31. Am J Hum Genet 1999;65(6):1639–1646.
21. Araie M, Ozawa T, Awaya Y. A case of congenital ocular motor apraxia with cerebellospinal degeneration. Jpn J Ophthalmol 1977;21: 355–365.
22. Armstrong MW, Mountain RE, Murray JA. Treatment of facial synkinesis and facial asymmetry with botulinum toxin type A following facial nerve palsy. Clin Otolaryngol 1996;21(1):15–20.
23. Arnold AC, et al. Internuclear ophthalmoplegia in the Chiari type II malformation. Neurology 1990;40(12):1850–1864.
24. Aroichane M, Repka MX. Outcome of sixth nerve palsy or paresis in young children. J Pediatr Ophthalmol Strabismus 1995;32(3):152–156.

25. Asbury AK, Arnason BG, Adams RD. The inflammatory lesion in idiopathic polyneuritis. Its role in pathogenesis. Medicine (Baltim) 1969;48(3):173–215.
26. Aseff AJ, Munoz M. Outcome of surgery for superior oblique palsy with contracture of ipsilateral superior rectus treated by superior rectus recession. Binoc Vs Strabismus Q 1998;13(3):177–180.
27. Ashizawa T, et al. Diagnostic value of ophthalmologic findings in myotonic dystrophy: comparison with risks calculated by haplotype analysis of closely linked restriction fragment length polymorphisms. Am J Med Genet 1992;42(1):55–60.
28. Astle WF, Rosenbaum AL. Familial congenital fourth cranial nerve palsy. Arch Ophthalmol 1985;103(4):532–535.
29. Astle WF, Miller SJ. Acute comitant esotropia: a sign of intracranial disease. Can J Ophthalmol 1994;29(3):151–154.
30. Atwal AJ, Smith BH, Dickenson ES. Letter: Pseudo-internuclear ophthalmoplegia in polyneuritis. Arch Neurol 1976;33(6):457.
31. Avanzini G, et al. Oculomotor disorders in Huntington's chorea. J Neurol Neurosurg Psychiatry 1979;42(7):581–589.
32. Averbuch-Heller L, Leigh RJ. Eye movements. Curr Opin Neurol 1996;9(1):26–31.
33. Awan K. Duane's retraction syndrome and hypertelorism. J Pediatr Ophthalmol Strabismus 1975;12:100–102.
34. Awan K. Flocculi iridis and retraction syndrome: their coexistence and associated ocular anomalies. J Pediatr Ophthalmol Strabismus 1975;12:246–254.
35. Awan KJ. Association of ocular, cervical, and cardiac malformations. Ann Ophthalmol 1977;9(8):1001–1011.
36. Awaya Y, Sugie H, Fukuyama Y. A hereditary variant of spinocerebellar degeneration associated with choreoathetosis and ocular motor apraxia of early onset. Acta Paediatr Jpn 1986;28:271–272.
37. Babel J. Ophthalmological aspects of myotonic dystrophy. In: Huber A, Klein D (eds) Neurogenetics and neuro-ophthalmology. Amsterdam: Elsevier/North Holland, 1981.
38. Bachynski BN, et al. Hyperglycemic acidotic coma and death in Kearns–Sayre syndrome. Ophthalmology 1986;93(3):391–396.
39. Bailey PBD, Ducy PC. Intracranial tumors in infancy and childhood. Chicago: University of Chicago Press, 1939.
40. Bailey TD, et al. Ophthalmoplegic migraine. J Clin Neuroophthalmol 1984;4(4):225–228.
41. Balkan R, Hoyt CS. Associated neurologic abnormalities in congenital third nerve palsies. Am J Ophthalmol 1984;97(3):315–319.
42. Baraitser M. Genetics of Mobius syndrome. J Med Genet 1977;14(6):415–417.
43. Barlow C. Headaches and migraine in childhood. Philadelphia: Lippincott, 1984.
44. Barsoum–Homsy M. Congenital double elevator palsy. J Pediatr Ophthalmol Strabismus 1983;20(5):185–191.

45. Bartkowski SB, et al. Marcus Gunn jaw-winking phenomenon: management and results of treatment in 19 patients. J Craniomaxillofac Surg 1999;27(1):25–29.
46. Barton JJ. Quantitative ocular tests for myasthenia gravis: a comparative review with detection theory analysis. J Neurol Sci 1998;155(1): 104–114.
47. Barton JJ, Fouladvand M. Ocular aspects of myasthenia gravis. Semin Neurol 2000;20(1):7–20.
48. Bavinck JN, Weaver DD. Subclavian artery supply disruption sequence: hypothesis of a vascular etiology for Poland, Klippel–Feil, and Mobius anomalies. Am J Med Genet 1986;23(4):903–918.
49. Beck RW, Meckler RJ. Internuclear ophthalmoplegia after head trauma. Ann Ophthalmol 1981;13(6):671–675.
50. Becker WJ, Watters GV, Humphreys P. Fisher syndrome in childhood. Neurology 1981;31(5):555–560.
51. Beerbower J, et al. Radiographic findings in Moebius and Moebius-like syndromes. AJNR Am J Neuroradiol 1986;7(2):364–365.
52. Bell JA, Fielder AR, Viney S. Congenital double elevator palsy in identical twins. J Clin Neuroophthalmol 1990;10(1):32–34.
53. Benson P. Transient unilateral external rectus muscle in newborn infants. Br Med J 1962;1:1054–1055.
54. Berenberg RA, et al. Lumping or splitting? "Ophthalmoplegia-plus" or Kearns–Sayre syndrome? Ann Neurol 1977;1(1):37–54.
55. Betz R, et al. Children with ocular motor apraxia type Cogan carry deletions in the gene (NPHP1) for juvenile nephronophthisis. J Pediatr 2000;136(6):828–831.
56. Beutler E, Grabowski G. Gaucher disease. In: Scriver C, et al (eds) The metabolic and molecular bases of inherited disease. New York: McGraw-Hill, 1995:2641–2670.
57. Beyer–Machule C, et al. The Marcus–Gunn phenomenon: a review of 80 cases (an update). Orbit 1985;4:15–19.
58. Biedner B, Geltman C, Rothkoff L. Bilateral Duane's syndrome associated with crocodile tears. J Pediatr Ophthalmol Strabismus 1979; 16(2):113–114.
59. Bielschowsky A. Lectures on motor anomalies of the eyes. II. Paralysis of individual muscles. Arch Ophthalmol 1935;13:33–59.
60. Bixenman WW, von Noorden GK. Benigh recurrent VI nerve palsy in childhood. J Pediatr Ophthalmol Strabismus 1981;18(3): 29–34.
61. Blodi FC. Electromyographic evidence for supranuclear gaze palsies. Trans Ophthalmol Soc UK 1970;90:451–469.
62. Bloom JN, Graviss ER, Mardelli PG. A magnetic resonance imaging study of the upshoot-downshoot phenomenon of Duane's retraction syndrome. Am J Ophthalmol 1991;111(5):548–554.
63. Bodensteiner JB, et al. Macrocerebellum: neuroimaging and clinical features of a newly recognized condition. J Child Neurol 1997;12(6): 365–368.

64. Bodziner RA, Singer W, Hedges TR. Bilateral internuclear ophthalmoplegia in meningoencephalitis. Dev Med Child Neurol 1983;25(6): 819–820.
65. Boger WP, et al. Recurrent isolated sixth nerve palsy in children. Ann Ophthalmol 1984;16(3):237–238, 240–244.
66. Boghen D, et al. Primary aberrant third nerve regeneration. Ann Neurol 1979;6(5):415–418.
67. Borchert MS, et al. Congenital ocular motor apraxia in twins. Findings with magnetic resonance imaging. J Clin Neuroophthalmol 1987;7(2):104–107.
68. Bowen J, Daltner C, Troost B. The treatment of ocular myasthenia with plasmapheresis: three case reports. Neuro-Ophthalmology 1986;6:109–112.
69. Breningstall GN, Smith SA, Purple RL. Electroretinography in the evaluation of childhood myotonic dystrophy. Pediatr Neurol 1985; 1(4):238–241.
70. Bresolin N, et al. Clinical and biochemical correlations in mitochondrial myopathies treated with coenzyme Q10. Neurology 1988; 38(6):892–899.
71. Brodsky MC, Frenkel RE, Spoor TC. Familial intracranial aneurysm presenting as a subtle stable third nerve palsy. Case report. Arch Ophthalmol 1988;106(2):173.
72. Brodsky MC, Pollock SC, Buckley EG. Neural misdirection in congenital ocular fibrosis syndrome: implications and pathogenesis. J Pediatr Ophthalmol Strabismus 1989;26(4):159–161.
73. Brodsky MC. Hereditary external ophthalmoplegia synergistic divergence, jaw winking, and oculocutaneous hypopigmentation: a congenital fibrosis syndrome caused by deficient innervation to extraocular muscles. Ophthalmology 1998;105(4):717–725.
74. Buckley SA, Elston JS. Surgical treatment of supranuclear and internuclear ocular motility disorders. Eye 1997;11(pt 3):377–380.
75. Burian H, Miller J. Comitant convergent strabismus with acute onset. Am J Ophthalmol 1968;45:55–64.
76. Butler T. Third nerve paralysis after mumps and chicken-pox. Br Med J 1930;1:1095.
77. Butler T. Ocular paralysis after mumps. Br Med J 1937;1:752–753.
78. Caccavale A, Mignemi L. Acute onset of a bilateral areflexical mydriasis in Miller–Fisher syndrome: a rare neuro-ophthalmologic disease. J Neuroophthalmol 2000;20(1):61–62.
79. Calabrese G, et al. Detection of an insertion deletion of region 8q13–q21.2 in a patient with Duane syndrome: implications for mapping and cloning a Duane gene. Eur J Hum Genet 1998;6(3): 187–193.
80. Calvert P. Personal communication, 2001.
81. Carr MM, Ross DA, Zuker RM. Cranial nerve defects in congenital facial palsy. J Otolaryngol 1996;26(2):80–87.

82. Carroll JE, et al. Depressed ventilatory response in oculocraniosomatic neuromuscular disease. Neurology 1976;26(2):140–146.
83. Cassidy L, Taylor D, Harris C. Abnormal supranuclear eye movements in the child: a practical guide to examination and interpretation. Surv Ophthalmol 2000;44(6):479–506.
84. Catalano RA, Sax RD, Krohel GB. Unilateral internuclear ophthalmoplegia after head trauma. Am J Ophthalmol 1986;101(4):491–493.
85. Catalano RA, et al. Asymmetry in congenital ocular motor apraxia. Can J Ophthalmol 1988;23(7):318–321.
86. Chan CC, Sogg RL, Steinman L. Isolated oculomotor palsy after measles immunization. Am J Ophthalmol 1980;89(3):446–448.
87. Chan TK, Demer JL. Clinical features of congenital absence of the superior oblique muscle as demonstrated by orbital imaging. J Am Assoc Pediatr Ophthalmol Strabismus 1999;3(3):143–150.
88. Charles R, et al. Myocardial ultrastructure and the development of atrioventricular block in Kearns–Sayre syndrome. Circulation 1981;63(1):214–219.
89. Chattha AS, Delong GF. Sylvian aqueduct syndrome as a sign of acute obstructive hydrocephalus in children. J Neurol Neurosurg Psychiatry 1975;38(3):288–296.
90. Christodoulou K, et al. Mapping of the familial infantile myasthenia (congenital myasthenic syndrome type Ia) gene to chromosome 17p with evidence of genetic homogeneity. Hum Mol Genet 1997;6(4):635–640.
91. Christoff N. A clinicopathologic study of vertical eye movements. Arch Neurol 1974;31(1):1–8.
92. Chu BC, et al. MRI of the brain in the Kearns–Sayre syndrome: report of four cases and a review. Neuroradiology 1999;41(10):759–764.
93. Ciafaloni E, et al. Mycophenolate mofetil for myasthenia gravis: an open-label pilot study. Neurology 2001;56(1):97–99.
94. Clausen N, Andersson P, Tommerup N. Familial occurrence of neuroblastoma, von Recklinghausen's neurofibromatosis, Hirschsprung's agangliosis and jaw-winking syndrome. Acta Paediatr Scand 1989;78(5):736–741.
95. Cogan D. Neurology of the ocular muscles. Springfield: Thomas, 1948.
96. Cogan D. A type of congenital ocular motor apraxia presenting jerky head movement. Trans Am Acad Ophthalmol Otolaryngol 1952;56:853–862.
97. Cogan D, et al. A long-term follow-up of congenital ocular motor apraxia: case report. Neuroophthalmology 1980;1:145–147.
98. Cogan DG. Congenital ocular motor apraxia. Can J Ophthalmol 1966;1(4):253–260.
99. Cogan DG. Internuclear ophthalmoplegia, typical and atypical. Arch Ophthalmol 1970;84(5):583–589.
100. Cogan DG, et al. Ocular motor signs in some metabolic diseases. Arch Ophthalmol 1981;99(10):1802–1808.
101. Cooper J, et al. Accommodative and vergence findings in ocular myasthenia: a case analysis. J Neuroophthalmol 2000;20(1):5–11.

102. Coppeto JR, Lessell S. Dorsal midbrain syndrome from giant aneurysm of the posterior fossa: report of two cases. Neurology 1983;33(6):732–736.
103. Couchot J, et al. Guillain–Barre syndrome following varicella. Nouv Presse Med 1978;7(1):47.
104. Coulter DL, Allen RJ. Abrupt neurological deterioration in children with Kearns–Sayre syndrome. Arch Neurol 1981;38(4):247–250.
105. Cox TA, Wurster JB, Godfrey WA. Primary aberrant oculomotor regeneration due to intracranial aneurysm. Arch Neurol 1979;36(9): 570–571.
106. Cross HE, Pfaffenbach DD. Duane's retraction syndrome and associated congenital malformations. Am J Ophthalmol 1972;73(3):442–450.
107. Cruysberg J, et al. Bilateral Duane's syndrome associated with congenital panhypopituitarism. Neuro-Ophthalmology 1986;3:165–168.
108. Cruysberg J, Huygen P. Congenital monocular adduction palsy with synergistic divergence diagnosed in a young infant. Neuro-Ophthalmology 1990;10:253–256.
109. Cruysberg JR, et al. Congenital adduction palsy and synergistic divergence: a clinical and electro-oculographic study. Br J Ophthalmol 1989;73(1):68–75.
110. Cuneo HMRC. Brain tumors of childhood. Springfield: Thomas, 1952.
111. Currie J, Lubin JH, Lessell S. Chronic isolated abducens paresis from tumors at the base of the brain. Arch Neurol 1983;40(4):226–229.
112. Dagi LR, Chrousos GA, Cogan DC. Spasm of the near reflex associated with organic disease. Am J Ophthalmol 1987;103(4):582–585.
113. Daroff R, Hoyt W. Supranuclear disorders of ocular control systems in man: clinical, anatomical, and physiological correlations. In: Bach-y-Rita P, Collins C, Hyde J (eds) The control of eye movements. New York: Academic Press, 1971.
114. Daroff RB, et al. Spongiform encephalopathy with chronic progressive external ophthalmoplegia. Central ophthalmoplegia mimicking ocular myopathy. Neurology 1966;16(2):161–169.
115. Davidson JL, Rosenbaum AL, McCall LC. Strabismus surgery in patients with myasthenia. J Pediatr Ophthalmol Strabismus 1993; 30(5):292–295.
116. Davis TL, Lavin PJ. Pseudo one-and-a-half syndrome with ocular myasthenia. Neurology 1989;39(11):1553.
117. De Graaf J, Cats H, deJager A. Gradenigo's syndrome: a rare complication of otitis media. Clin Neurol Neurosurg 1988;90:237–239.
118. de la Monte SM, et al. Keyhole aqueduct syndrome. Arch Neurol 1986;43(9):926–929.
119. Dehaene I, et al. Guillain–Barre syndrome with ophthalmoplegia: clinicopathologic study of the central and peripheral nervous systems, including the oculomotor nerves. Neurology 1986;36(6): 851–854.
120. Denslow GT, Sims M. Duane's retraction syndrome associated with optic nerve hypoplasia. J Pediatr Ophthalmol Strabismus 1980;17(1): 26–28.

121. Derakhshan I, Lotfi J, Kaufman B. Ophthalmoplegia, ataxia and hyporeflexia (Fisher's syndrome). With a midbrain lesion demonstrated by CT scanning. Eur Neurol 1979;18(6):361–366.
122. DeRespinis PA, et al. Duane's retraction syndrome. Surv Ophthalmol 1993;38(3):257–288.
123. Di Costanzo A, et al. Relative sparing of extraocular muscles in myotonic dystrophy: an electrooculographic study. Acta Neurol Scand 1997;95(3):158–163.
124. Diamond GR, et al. Variations in extraocular muscle number and structure in craniofacial dysostosis. Am J Ophthalmol 1980;90(3): 416–418.
125. Diamond S, Schear HE, Leeds MF. Pseudo-internuclear oculomotor ophthalmoplegia secondary to Guillain–Barre polyneuronitis simulating myasthenia gravis in a air transport pilot. Aviat Space Environ Med 1975;46(2):204–207.
126. Discepola MJ, et al. Autosomal recessive Duane's retraction syndrome. Can J Ophthalmol 1987;22(7):384–386.
127. Dodge P, et al. Myotonic dystrophy in infancy and childhood. Pediatrics 1965;35:3–19.
128. Donahue SP, Lavin PJ, Hamed LM. Tonic ocular tilt reaction simulating a superior oblique palsy: diagnostic confusion with the 3-step test. Arch Ophthalmol 1999;117(3):347–352.
129. Donaldson MD, et al. Familial juvenile nephronophthisis, Jeune's syndrome, and associated disorders. Arch Dis Child 1985;60(5):426–434.
130. Drachman D. Myasthenia gravis: immunobiology of a receptor disorder. Trends Neurosci 1983;6:446–450.
131. Drachman DA. Ophthalmoplegia plus. The neurodegenerative disorders associated with progressive external ophthalmoplegia. Arch Neurol 1968;18(6):654–674.
132. Duffner PK, et al. Survival of children with brain tumors: SEER Program, 1973–1980. Neurology 1986;36(5):597–601.
133. Durkan GP, et al. Recurrent painless oculomotor palsy in children. A variant of ophthalmoplegic migraine? Headache 1981;21(2):58–62.
134. Dyken P. Extraocular myotonia in families with dystrophia myotonica. Neurology 1966;16:738–740.
135. Ebner R. Angiography for IIIrd nerve palsy in children. J Clin Neuroophthalmol 1990;10(2):154–155.
136. Echaniz-Laguna A, et al. The Miller Fisher syndrome: neurophysiological and MRI evidence of both peripheral and central origin in one case. J Neurol 2000;247(12):980–982.
137. Eda I, et al. Computed tomography in congenital ocular motor apraxia. Neuroradiology 1984;26(5):359–362.
138. Edis RH, Mastaglia FL. Vertical gaze palsy in barbiturate intoxication. Br Med J 1977;1(6054):144.
139. Egger J, Lake BD, Wilson J. Mitochondrial cytopathy. A multisystem disorder with ragged red fibres on muscle biopsy. Arch Dis Child 1981;56(10):741–752.

140. Egger J, Wilson J. Mitochondrial inheritance in a mitochondrially mediated disease. N Engl J Med 1983;309(3):142–146.
141. Elizan TS, et al. Syndrome of acute idiopathic ophthalmoplegia with ataxia and areflexia. Neurology 1971;21(3):281–292.
142. Ellis FD, et al. Extraocular muscle responses to orbital cooling (ice test) for ocular myasthenia gravis diagnosis. J Am Assoc Pediatr Ophthalmol Strabismus 2000;4(5):271–281.
143. Emre M, Henn V. Central eye movement disorder in a case of myotonic dystrophy. Neuro-Ophthalmology 1985;5:21–25.
144. Engel A, et al. Molecular basis of congenital myasthenic syndromes: mutations in the acetylcholine receptor. Neuroscientist 1998;4:185–194.
145. Engel AG, et al. A newly recognized congenital myasthenic syndrome attributed to a prolonged open time of the acetylcholine-induced ion channel. Ann Neurol 1982;11(6):553–569.
146. Engel AG. Congenital myasthenic syndromes. J Child Neurol 1988; 3(4):233–246.
147. Eustace P, et al. Congenital ocular motor apraxia: an inability to unlock the vestibulo-ocular reflex. Neuro-Ophthalmology 1994;4: 167–174.
148. Evans JC, et al. Confirmation of linkage of Duane's syndrome and refinement of the disease locus to an 8.8-cM interval on chromosome 2q31. Hum Genet 2000;106(6):636–638.
149. Evoli A, et al. Ocular myasthenia: diagnostic and therapeutic problems. Acta Neurol Scand 1988;77(1):31–35.
150. Evoli A, et al. Therapeutic options in ocular myasthenia gravis. Neuromusc Disord 2001;11(2):208–216.
151. Fenichel GM. Clinical syndromes of myasthenia in infancy and childhood. A review. Arch Neurol 1978;35(2):97–103.
152. Fernandez E, et al. Oculomotor nerve regeneration in rats. Functional, histological, and neuroanatomical studies. J Neurosurg 1987; 67(3):428–437.
153. Fielder AR, et al. Congenital ocular motor apraxia. Trans Ophthalmol Soc UK 1986;105(pt 5):589–598.
154. Fink JK, et al. Clinical spectrum of Niemann–Pick disease type C. Neurology 1989;39(8):1040–1049.
155. Fisher C. An unusual variant of acute idiopathic polyneuritis (syndrome of ophthalmoplegia, ataxia, and areflexia). N Engl J Med 1956;255:57–65.
156. Flynn JT, et al. Hyperglycemic acidotic coma and death in Kearns–Sayre syndrome. Trans Am Ophthalmol Soc 1985;83:131–161.
157. Fox A. Angiography for third nerve palsy in children. J Clin Neuroophthalmol 1989;9:37–38.
158. Gabianelli EB, Klingele TB, Burde RM. Acute oculomotor nerve palsy in childhood. Is arteriography necessary? J Clin Neuroophthalmol 1989;9(1):33–36.
159. Galetta SL, Smith JL. Chronic isolated sixth nerve palsies. Arch Neurol 1989;46(1):79–82.

160. Gallastegui J, et al. Cardiac involvement in the Kearns–Sayre syndrome. Am J Cardiol 1987;60(4):385–388.
161. Gay A, Brodkey J, Miller J. Convergence retraction nystagmus. Arch Ophthalmol 1963;70:456–461.
162. Gentile M, et al. COACH syndrome: report of two brothers with congenital hepatic fibrosis, cerebellar vermis hypoplasia, oligophrenia, ataxia, and mental retardation. Am J Med Genet 1996;64(3):514–520.
163. Giroud M, et al. Miller–Fisher syndrome and pontine abnormalities on MRI: a case report. J Neurol 1990;237(8):489–490.
164. Gittinger JW Jr, Sokol S. The visual-evoked potential in the diagnosis of congenital ocular motor apraxia. Am J Ophthalmol 1982; 93(6):700–703.
165. Gittinger JW Jr, Hughes JP, Suran EL. Medial orbital wall blow-out fracture producing an acquired retraction syndrome. J Clin Neuroophthalmol 1986;6(3):153–156.
166. Glaser J, Bachynski B. Infranuclear disorders of eye movement. In: Glaser J (ed) Neuroophthalmology. Philadelphia: Lippincott, 1990.
167. Glaser JS. Myasthenic pseudo-internuclear ophthalmoplegia. Arch Ophthalmol 1966;75(3):363–366.
168. Glover AT, Powe LK. Ocular motor apraxia and neurofibromatosis. Arch Ophthalmol 1985;103(6):763.
169. Gobin MH. Surgical management of Duane's syndrome. Br J Ophthalmol 1974;58(3):301–306.
170. Goldman HD, Nelson LB. Acute acquired comitant esotropia. Ann Ophthalmol 1985;17(12):777–778.
171. Goldstein JH, Sacks DB. Bilateral Duane's syndrome. J Pediatr Ophthalmol 1977;14(1):12–17.
172. Goldstein JH, Schneekloth BB. Spasm of the near reflex: a spectrum of anomalies. Surv Ophthalmol 1996;40(4):269–278.
173. Golnik KC, et al. An ice test for the diagnosis of myasthenia gravis. Ophthalmology 1999;106(7):1282–1286.
174. Gonatas NK. A generalized disorder of nervous system, skeletal muscle and heart resembling Refsum's disease and Hurler's syndrome. II. Ultrastructure. Am J Med 1967;42(2):169–178.
175. Good WV, et al. Bilateral congenital oculomotor nerve palsy in a child with brain anomalies. Am J Ophthalmol 1991;111(5):555–558.
176. Goodman CR, Chabner E, Guyton DL. Should early strabismus surgery be performed for ocular torticollis to prevent facial asymmetry? J Pediatr Ophthalmol Strabismus 1995;32(3):162–166.
177. Gourdeau A, et al. Central ocular motor abnormalities in Duane's retraction syndrome. Arch Ophthalmol 1981;99(10):1809–1810.
178. Graeber MB, Muller U. Recent developments in the molecular genetics of mitochondrial disorders. J Neurol Sci 1998;153(2):251–263.
179. Green SH. Polyradiculitis (Landry–Guillain–Barre syndrome) with total external ophthalmoplegia: encephalo-myelo-radiculoneuropathy. Dev Med Child Neurol 1976;18(3):369–373.
180. Greer M, Schotland M. Myasthenia gravis in the newborn. Pediatrics 1960;26:101–108.

181. Gresty M, Ell J. Normal modes of head and eye co-ordination and the symptomatology of their disorders. In: Lennestrand G, Zee D, Keller E (eds) Functional basis of ocular motility disorders. New York: Pergamon, 1982;391–405.
182. Griffin JF, Wray SH, Anderson DP. Misdiagnosis of spasm of the near reflex. Neurology 1976;26(11):1018–1020.
183. Grob D, et al. The course of myasthenia gravis and therapies affecting outcome. Ann NY Acad Sci 1987;505:472–499.
184. Grose C, et al. Primary Epstein–Barr virus infections in acute neurologic diseases. N Engl J Med 1975;292(8):392–395.
185. Gross-Tsur V, et al. Oculomotor apraxia: the presenting sign of Gaucher disease. Pediatr Neurol 1090;5(2):128–129.
186. Grunnet ML, Lubow M. Ascending polyneuritis and ophthalmoplegia. Am J Ophthalmol 1972;74(6):1155–1160.
187. Hamed LM, Dennehy PJ, Lingua RW. Synergistic divergence and jaw-winking phenomenon. J Pediatr Ophthalmol Strabismus 1990;27(2):88–90.
188. Hamed LM, et al. Synergistic divergence: saccadic velocity analysis and surgical results. J Pediatr Ophthalmol Strabismus 1992;29(1):30–37.
189. Hanson PA, Rowland LP. Mobius syndrome and facioscapulohumeral muscular dystrophy. Arch Neurol 1971;24(1):31–39.
190. Harbord MG, et al. Moebius' syndrome with unilateral cerebellar hypoplasia. J Med Genet 1989;26(9):579–582.
191. Harley RD. Paralytic strabismus in children. Etiologic incidence and management of the third, fourth, and sixth nerve palsies. Ophthalmology 1980;87(1):24–43.
192. Harper P. Myotonic dystrophy in infancy and childhood. In: Myotonic dystrophy. London: Saunders, 1989.
193. Harrad RA, Graham CM, Collin JR. Amblyopia and strabismus in congenital ptosis. Eye 1988;2(pt 6):625–627.
194. Harris C, Taylor D, Velodi A. Eye movement recording in type 3 Gaucher disease: a preliminary report. Mol Med Ther 1997;5:7–10.
195. Harris CM, et al. Intermittent horizontal saccade failure ('ocular motor apraxia') in children. Br J Ophthalmol 1996;80(2):151–158.
196. Harris CM, et al. Familial congenital saccade initiation failure and isolated cerebellar vermis hypoplasia. Dev Med Child Neurol 1998;40(11):775–779.
197. Harris CM, Taylor DS, Vellodi A. Ocular motor abnormalities in Gaucher disease. Neuropediatrics 1999;30(6):289–293.
198. Harris DJ Jr, et al. Familial congenital superior oblique palsy. Ophthalmology 1986;93(1):88–90.
199. Heckmatt JZ, et al. Congenital centronuclear (myotubular) myopathy. A clinical, pathological and genetic study in eight children. Brain 1985;108(pt 4):941–964.
200. Hedges TR III, et al. Botulin ophthalmoplegia. Clinical and oculographic observations. Arch Ophthalmol 1983;101(2):211–213.

201. Helveston EM, Giangiacomo JG, Ellis FD. Congenital absence of the superior oblique tendon. Trans Am Ophthalmol Soc 1981;79:123–135.
202. Helveston EM, et al. Surgical treatment of superior oblique palsy. Trans Am Ophthalmol Soc 1996;94:315–328.
203. Henderson J. The congenital facial diplegia syndrome. Clinical features, pathology, and aetiology. Brain 1939;62:381–403.
204. Hepler RS, Hoyt WF, Loeffler JD. Paradoxical synkinetic levator inhibition and excitation. An electromyographic study of unilateral oculopalpebral and bilateral mandibulopalpebral (Marcus Gunn) synkineses in a 74-year-old man. Arch Neurol 1968;18(4):416–424.
205. Hertle R. Diagnosis of isolated cyclovertical muscle overaction using a modification of the Parks' Three-Step Test. Strabismus 1993;1:107–120.
206. Hicks A. Congenital paralysis of lateral rotators of the eyes with paralysis of muscles of face. Arch Ophthalmol 1943;30:38–42.
207. Hofmann RJ. Monozygotic twins concordant for bilateral Duane's retraction syndrome. Am J Ophthalmol 1985;99(5):563–566.
208. Holmes JM, Cronin CM. Duane syndrome associated with oculocutaneous albinism. J Pediatr Ophthalmol Strabismus 1992;28(1):32–34.
209. Holmes JM, et al. Pediatric third, fourth, and sixth nerve palsies: a population-based study. Am J Ophthalmol 1999;127(4):388–392.
210. Holtz SJ. Congenital ocular anomalies associated with Duane's retraction syndrome, the nervus of Ota, and axial anisometropia. Am J Ophthalmol 1974;77(5):729–731.
211. Holzman AE, et al. Duane's retraction syndrome in the fetal alcohol syndrome. Am J Ophthalmol 1990;110(5):565.
212. Honda Y, Yoshioka M. Duane's retraction syndrome associated with muscular dystrophy. J Pediatr Ophthalmol Strabismus 1978;15(3):157–159.
213. Hotchkiss MG, et al. Bilateral Duane's retraction syndrome. A clinical-pathologic case report. Arch Ophthalmol 1980;98(5):870–874.
214. Hoyt CS, Billson FA, Alpins N. The supranuclear disturbances of gaze in kernicterus. Ann Ophthalmol 1978;10(11):1487–1492.
215. Hoyt CS, Mousel DK, Weber AA. Transient supranuclear disturbances of gaze in healthy neonates. Am J Ophthalmol 1980;89(5):708–713.
216. Hoyt WF, Nachtigaller H. Anomalies of ocular motor nerves. Neuroanatomic correlates of paradoxical innervation in Duane's syndrome and related congenital ocular motor disorders. Am J Ophthalmol 1965;60(3):443–448.
217. Huber A. Electrophysiology of the retraction syndromes. Br J Ophthalmol 1974;58(3):293–300.
218. Huber A. Botulinum A toxin injections as a new treatment of blepharospasm and strabismus. In: Satoshi I (ed) Highlights in neurophthalmology. Proceedings of the sixth meeting of the

International Neurophthalmology Society. Amsterdam: Aeolus Press, 1897.

219. Hughes J, et al. Congenital vertical ocular motor apraxia. J Clin Neuroophthalmol 1985;5:153–157.
220. Hung TP. A polio-like syndrome in adults following acute hemorrhagic conjunctivitis. Int J Neurol 1981;15(3–4):266–278.
221. Hunt JM, et al. A post-docking role for synaptobrevin in synaptic vesicle fusion. Neuron 1994;12(6):1269–1279.
222. Hurko O, et al. Heteroplasmy in chronic external ophthalmoplegia: clinical and molecular observations. Pediatr Res 1990;28(5):542–548.
223. Iannaccone ST, et al. Familial progressive external ophthalmoplegia and ragged-red fibers. Neurology 1974;24(11):1033–1038.
224. Imes R, Monteiro M, Hoyt W. Ophthalmoplegic migraine with proximal posterior cerebral artery vascular anomaly. J Clin Neuroophthalmol 1984;4:221–223.
225. Ing EB, et al. Oculomotor nerve palsies in children. J Pediatr Ophthalmol Strabismus 1992;29(6):331–336.
226. Inocencio F, Ballecer R. Tuberculosis granuloma in the midbrain causing wall-eyed bilateral internuclear ophthalmoplegia (Webino). J Clin Neuroophthalmol 1985;5:31–35.
227. Inoue A, Koh C, Iwahashi T. Detection of serum anticerebellar antibodies in patients with Miller Fisher syndrome. Eur Neurol 1999; 42(4):230–234.
228. Inoue N, Izumi K, Mawatar S. Congenital ocular motor apraxia and cerebellar degeneration: report of two cases. Jpn J Clin Neurol 1971; 11:855–861.
229. Isenberg S, Urist MJ. Clinical observations in 101 consecutive patients with Duane's retraction syndrome. Am J Ophthalmol 1977; 84(3):419–425.
230. Isenberg S, Blechman B. Marcus Gunn jaw winking and Duane's retraction syndrome. J Pediatr Ophthalmol Strabismus 1983;20(6): 235–237.
231. Jamal GA, et al. Myotonic dystrophy. A reassessment by conventional and more recently introduced neurophysiological techniques. Brain 1986;109(pt 6):1279–1296.
232. Jamal GA, Ballantyne JP. The localization of the lesion in patients with acute ophthalmoplegia, ataxia and areflexia (Miller Fisher syndrome). A serial multimodal neurophysiological study. Brain 1988; 111(pt 1):95–114.
233. James RH. Induction agent sensitivity and ophthalmoplegia plus. Anaesthesia 1986;41(2):216.
234. Jampolsky A. Surgical leashes and reverse leashes in strabismus surgical management. In: Symposium on strabismus. Transactions of the New Orleans Academy of Ophthalmology. St. Louis: Mosby, 1978.
235. Jan JE, et al. Speech, cognition, and imaging studies in congenital ocular motor apraxia. Dev Med Child Neurol 1998;40(2):95–99.

236. Jankowicz E, et al. Familial progressive external ophthalmoplegia with abnormal muscle mitochondria. Eur Neurol 1977;15(6):318–324.
237. Jay WM, Hoyt CS. Abnormal brain stem auditory-evoked potentials in Stilling–Turk–Duane retraction syndrome. Am J Ophthalmol 1980;89(6):814–818.
238. Jimura T, et al. A case of synergistic divergence associated with Horner's syndrome. Folia Ophthalmol Jpn 1983;34:477–480.
239. Johnson LN, Pack WL. Transient oculomotor nerve misdirection in a case of pituitary tumor with hemorrhage. Case report. Arch Ophthalmol 1988;106(5):584–585.
240. Johnson RO, Clay SA, Arnon SS. Diagnosis and management of infant botulism. Am J Dis Child 1979;133(6):586–593.
241. Jones HR Jr. Guillain–Barre syndrome: perspectives with infants and children. Semin Pediatr Neurol 2000;7(2):91–102.
242. Jordan D, Miller D, Anderson R. Acquired oculomotor-abducens synkinesis. Can J Ophthalmol 1990;25:148–151.
243. Kaminski HJ, et al. Why are eye muscles frequently involved in myasthenia gravis? Neurology 1990;40(11):1663–1669.
244. Kaminski HJ, Kusner LL, Block CH. Expression of acetylcholine receptor isoforms at extraocular muscle endplates. Investig Ophthalmol Vis Sci 37(2):345–351.
245. Karpati H, et al. The Kearns–Shy syndrome: a multisystem disease with mitochondrial abnormality demonstrated in skeletal muscle and skin. J Neurol Sci 1973;19:133–151.
246. Katiyar BC, et al. Adult polio-like syndrome following enterovirus 70 conjunctivitis (natural history of the disease). Acta Neurol Scand 1983;67(5):263–274.
247. Kaufman LW, Folk ER, Miller MT. Monozygotic twins discordant for Duane's retraction syndrome. Case report. Arch Ophthalmol 1989;107(3):324–325.
248. Kawano K, Fujita S. Duane's retraction syndrome associated with morning glory syndrome. J Pediatr Ophthalmol Strabismus 1981;18(1):51–54.
249. Keane J. Upward gaze paralysis as the initial sign of Fisher's syndrome. Arch Neurol 1982;32:781–782.
250. Keane JR, Hoyt WF. Myasthenic (vertical) nystagmus. Verification by edrophonium tonography. JAMA 212(7):1209–1210.
251. Keane JR, Davis RL. Pretectal syndrome with metastatic malignant melanoma to the posterior commissure. Am J Ophthalmol 1976;82(6):910–914.
252. Keane JR. Neuro-ophthalmic signs and symptoms of hysteria. Neurology 1982;32(7):757–762.
253. Keane JR. Acute bilateral ophthalmoplegia: 60 cases. Neurology 1986;36(2):279–281.
254. Keane JR. Traumatic internuclear ophthalmoplegia. J Clin Neuroophthalmol 1987;7(3):165–166.

255. Keane JR. The pretectal syndrome: 206 patients. Neurology 1990; 40(4):684–690.
256. Kearns T, Sayre G. Retinitis pigmentosa, external ophthalmoplegia, and complete heart block. Arch Ophthalmol 1958;60:280–289.
257. Keith CG. Oculomotor nerve palsy in childhood. Aust N Z J Ophthalmol 1987;15(3):181–184.
258. Khodadoust AA, von Noorden GK. Bilateral vertical retraction syndrome. A family study. Arch Ophthalmol 1967;78(5):606–612.
259. Khwarg SI, et al. Management of moderate-to-severe Marcus-Gunn jaw-winking ptosis. Ophthalmology 1999;106(6):1191–1196.
260. Kiloh L, Nevin S. Progressive dystrophy of the ocular muscles (ocular myopathy). Brain 1951;74:115–143.
261. Kirkham TH. Cervico-oculo-acusticus syndrome with pseudo-papilloedema. Arch Dis Child 1969;44(236):504–508.
262. Kirkham TH. Duane's syndrome and familial perceptive deafness. Br J Ophthalmol 1969;53(5):335–339.
263. Kirkham TH. Duane's retraction syndrome and cleft palate. Am J Ophthalmol 1970;70(2):209–212.
264. Kirkham TH. Inheritance of Duane's syndrome. Br J Ophthalmol 1970;54(5):323–329.
265. Kirkham TH, Kamin DF. Slow saccadic eye movements in Wilson's disease. J Neurol Neurosurg Psychiatry 1974;37(2):191–194.
266. Kivlin JD, Lundergan MK. Acquired retraction syndrome associated with orbital metastasis. J Pediatr Ophthalmol Strabismus 1985; 22(3):109–112.
267. Knox DL, Clark DB, Schuster FF. Benigh VI nerve palsies in children. Pediatrics 1967;40(4):560–564.
268. Kodsi S. Marcus Gunn jaw winking with trigemino-abducens synkinesis. J Am Assoc Pediatr Ophthalmol Strabismus 2000;4(5): 316–317.
269. Kodsi SR, Younge BR. Acquired oculomotor, trochlear, and abducent cranial nerve palsies in pediatric patients. Am J Ophthalmol 1992; 114(5):568–574.
270. Koeppen AH, Hans MB. Supranuclear ophthalmoplegia in olivopontocerebellar degeneration. Neurology 1976;26(8):764–768.
271. Kommerell GBM. A new type of Duane's syndrome: twitch abduction on attempted upgaze and V-incomitance due to misinnervation of the lateral rectus by superior rectus neurons. Neuro-Ophthalmology 1986;6:159–164.
272. Kommerell G, et al. Oculomotor palsy with cyclic spasms: electromyographic and electron microscopic evidence of chronic peripheral neuronal involvement. Neuro-Ophthalmology 1988;8:9–21.
273. Kompf D, Christen H. Isolated abducens nerve palsy preceding infectious mononucleosis. Neuro-Ophthalmology 1984;4:101–105.
274. Kraft S, Scott W. Masked bilateral superior oblique palsy. Clinical features and diagnosis. J Pediatr Ophthalmol 1986;23:264–272.
275. Kraft S. A surgical approach for Duane syndrome. J Pediatr Ophthalmol Strabismus 1988;25:119–130.

276. Kraft SP, O'Donoghue EP, Roarty JD. Improvement of compensatory head postures after strabismus surgery. Ophthalmology 1992;99(8): 1301–1308.
277. Krohel GB. Blepharoptosis after traumatic third-nerve palsies. Am J Ophthalmol 1979;88(3 pt 2):598–601.
278. Kubis KC, et al. The ice test versus the rest test in myasthenia gravis. Ophthalmology 2000;107(11):1995–1998.
279. Kuncl R, Hoffman P. Myopathies and disorders of neuromuscular transmission. In: Miller N, Newman N (eds) Walsh & Hoyt's clinical neuro-ophthalmology. Baltimore: Williams & Wilkins, 1998.
280. Kushner BJ. The diagnosis and treatment of bilateral masked superior oblique palsy. Am J Ophthalmol 1988;105(2):186–194.
281. Kushner BJ. Errors in the three-step test in the diagnosis of vertical strabismus. Ophthalmology 1989;96(1):127–132.
282. Lambert SR, et al. Joubert syndrome. Arch Ophthalmol 1989;107(5): 709–713.
283. Lammens M, et al. Neuropathological findings in Moebius syndrome. Clin Genet 1998;54(2):136–141.
284. Lavy T, et al. Electrophysiological and eye-movement abnormalities in children with the Bardet–Biedl syndrome. J Pediatr Ophthalmol Strabismus 1995;32(6):364–367.
285. Lebensohn J. Parinaud's syndrome. From obstetric trauma with recovery. Am J Ophthalmol 1955;40:738–740.
286. Lee J, Flynn JT. Bilateral superior oblique palsies. Br J Ophthalmol 1985;69(7):508–513.
287. Lee MS, et al. Sixth nerve palsies in children. Pediatr Neurol 1999;20(1):49–52.
288. Leigh RJ, Zee DS. The neurology of eye movements, 3rd edn. Philadelphia: Davis, 1999.
289. Lepore FE, Glaser JS. Misdirection revisited. A critical appraisal of acquired oculomotor nerve synkinesis. Arch Ophthalmol 1980; 98(12):2206–2209.
290. Lessell S, Coppeto J, Samet S. Ophthalmoplegia in myotonic dystrophy. Am J Ophthalmol 1971;71(6):1231–1235.
291. Leung AK. Transient sixth cranial nerve palsy in newborn infants. Br J Clin Pract 1987;41(4):717–718.
292. Lindstrom JM, et al. Antibody to acetylcholine receptor in myasthenia gravis. Prevalence, clinical correlates, and diagnostic value. Neurology 1976;26(11):1054–1059.
293. Lingua R, Walkoner F. Use of the posterior fixation suture in type I Duane syndrome. J Ocul Ther Surg 1985;4:107–111.
294. Lipson AH, et al. Moebius syndrome: animal model–human correlations and evidence for a brainstem vascular etiology. Teratology 1989;40(4):339–350.
295. Loewenfeld IE, Thompson HS. Oculomotor paresis with cyclic spasms. A critical review of the literature and a new case. Surv Ophthalmol 1975;20(2):81–124.

296. Lubkin V. The inverse Marcus Gunn phenomenon. An electromyographic contribution. Arch Neurol 1978;35(4):249.
297. Lueder GT, et al. Vertical strabismus resulting from an anomalous extraocular muscle. J Am Assoc Pediatr Ophthalmol Strabismus 1998;2(2):126–128.
298. Lyle D. A discussion of ocular motor apraxia with a case presentation. Trans Am Ophthalmol Soc 1961;59:274–285.
299. Lyness RW, et al. Histological appearances of the levator palpebrae superioris muscle in the Marcus Gunn phenomenon. Br J Ophthalmol 1988;72(2):104–109.
300. MacDonald AL, Crawford JS, Smith DR. Duane's retraction syndrome: an evaluation of the sensory status. Can J Ophthalmol 1974;9(4):458–462.
301. MacLennan C, et al. Acetylcholine receptor expression in human extraocular muscles and their susceptibility to myasthenia gravis. Ann Neurol 1997;41(4):423–431.
302. Magoon E. The use of botulinum injection as an alternative to surgery. Contemp Ophthalmic Forum 1987;5:222.
303. Mahadevan M, et al. Myotonic dystrophy mutation: an unstable CTG repeat in the 3′ untranslated region of the gene. Science 1992;255(5049):1253–1255.
304. Mankodi A, et al. Myotonic dystrophy in transgenic mice expressing an expanded CUG repeat. Science 2000;289(5485):1769–1773.
305. Manson JI. Ocular motor apraxia in childhood. Proc Aust Assoc Neurol 1973;10(0):27–29.
306. Marshman WE, Adams GG, Cree I. Extraocular muscle surgery in myotonic dystrophy. J Pediatr Ophthalmol Strabismus 1998;35(3):169–171.
307. Marshman WE, et al. Congenital anomalies in patients with Duane retraction syndrome and their relatives. J Am Assoc Pediatr Ophthalmol Strabismus 2000;4(2):106–109.
308. Maruo T, et al. Duane's syndrome. Jpn J Ophthalmol 1979;23:453–468.
309. Marzetti G, Midulla M, Balducci L. Monolateral paralysis of the 3rd pair of cranial nerves due to A9 Coxsackie virus. Minerva Pediatr 1968;20(18):943–947.
310. Matteuci P. I difetti congenit di abduzione con particolare rifuardo all patogenesi. Rass Ital Ottal 1946;15:345–380.
311. McGettrick P, Eustace P. The w.e.b.i.n.o. syndrome. Neuro-Ophthalmology 1985;5:109–115.
312. McGovern ST, Crompton JL, Ingham PN. Trigemino-abducens synkinesis: an unusual case of aberrant regeneration. Aust N Z J Ophthalmol 1986;14(3):275–279.
313. Mehkri IA, et al. Double vision in a child. Surv Ophthalmol 1999;44(1):45–51; discussion 51–52.
314. Meienberg O, Ryffel E. Supranuclear eye movement disorders in Fisher's syndrome of ophthalmoplegia, ataxia, and areflexia. Report of a case and literature review. Arch Neurol 1983;40(7):402–405.

315. Meienberg O. Lesion site in Fisher's syndrome. Arch Neurol 1984; 41(3):250–251.
316. Meire F, et al. Waardenburg syndrome, Hirschsprung megacolon, and Marcus Gunn ptosis. Am J Med Genet 1987;27(3):683–686.
317. Mellinger J, Gomez M. Agenesis of the cranial nerves. In: Vinken P, Bruyn G (eds) Handbook of clinical neurology. New York: Elsevier, 1977.
318. Melmed C, Karpati G, Carpenter S. Experimental mitochondrial myopathy produced by in vivo uncoupling of oxidative phosphorylation. J Neurol Sci 1975;26(3):305–318.
319. Meola G. Myotonic dystrophies. Curr Opin Neurol 2000;13(5):519–525.
320. Meola G. Clinical and genetic heterogeneity in myotonic dystrophies. Muscle Nerve 2000;23(12):1789–1799.
321. Merz M, Wojtowicz S. The Mobius syndrome. Report of electromyographic examinations in two cases. Am J Ophthalmol 1967; 63(4):837–840.
322. Metz HS, Scott AB, Scott WE. Horizontal saccadic velocities in Duane's syndrome. Am J Ophthalmol 1975;80(5):901–906.
323. Miller MT, et al. Superior oblique palsy presenting in late childhood. Am J Ophthalmol 1970;70(2):212–214.
324. Miller MT, et al. Mobius and Mobius-like syndromes (TTV-OFM, OMLH). J Pediatr Ophthalmol Strabismus 1989;26(4):176–188.
325. Miller MT, Stromland K. The Mobius sequence: a relook. J Am Assoc Pediatr Ophthalmol Strabismus 1999;3(4):199–208.
326. Miller NR. Solitary oculomotor nerve palsy in childhood. Am J Ophthalmol 1977;83(1):106–111.
327. Millichap J, Dodge P. Diagnosis and treatment of myasthenia gravis in infancy, childhood, and adolescence: a study of 51 patients. Neurology 1960;10:1007–1014.
328. Möbius P. Uber angeborene doppelseitige Abducens-Facialis-Lahmung. Munch Med Wochenschr 1888;35:91–108.
329. Möbius P. Uber infantilen Kernschwund. Munch Med Wochenschr 1892;39:17–21.
330. Mohan K, et al. Treatment of congenital adduction palsy with synergistic divergence. J Pediatr Ophthalmol Strabismus 1998;35(3): 149–152.
331. Molarte AB, Rosenbaum AL. Vertical rectus muscle transposition surgery for Duane's syndrome. J Pediatr Ophthalmol Strabismus 1990;27(4):171–177.
332. Moore AT, Taylor DS. A syndrome of congenital retinal dystrophy and saccade palsy—a subset of Leber's amaurosis. Br J Ophthalmol 1984;68(6):421–431.
333. Moore LD, Feldon SE, Liu SK. Infrared oculography of Duane's retraction syndrome (type 1). Arch Ophthalmol 1988;106(7):943–946.
334. Moraes CT, et al. Mitochondrial DNA deletions in progressive external ophthalmoplegia and Kearns–Sayre syndrome. N Engl J Med 1989;320(20):1293–1299.

335. Morimoto T, et al. A case of a rapidly progressive central nervous system disorder manifesting as a pallidal posture and ocular motor apraxia. Brain Dev 1985;7(4):449–453.
336. Mounsey JP, et al. Skeletal muscle sodium channel gating in mice deficient in myotonic dystrophy protein kinase. Hum Mol Genet 2000;9(15):2313–2320.
337. Movaghar M, Slavin ML. Effect of local heat versus ice on blepharoptosis resulting from ocular myasthenia. Ophthalmology 2000; 107(12):2209–2214.
338. Muchnick RS, Aston SJ, Rees TD. Ocular manifestations and treatment of hemifacial atrophy. Am J Ophthalmol 1979;88(5):889–897.
339. Mudgil AV, Repka MX. Ophthalmologic outcome after third cranial nerve palsy or paresis in childhood. J Am Assoc Pediatr Ophthalmol Strabismus 1999;3(1):2–8.
340. Mullaney P, et al. The natural history and ophthalmic involvement in childhood myasthenia gravis at the hospital for sick children. Ophthalmology 2000;107(3):504–510.
341. Mullie MA, et al. The retinal manifestations of mitochondrial myopathy. A study of 22 cases. Arch Ophthalmol 1985;103(12):1825–1830.
342. Muri RM, Meienberg O. The clinical spectrum of internuclear ophthalmoplegia in multiple sclerosis. Arch Neurol 1985;42(9):851–855.
343. Murray R, Steven P. Congenital levator and lateral rectus muscle associated reflex. Neuro-Ophthalmology 1986;6:29–31.
344. Namba T, Brown SB, Grob D. Neonatal myasthenia gravis: report of two cases and review of the literature. Pediatrics 1970;45(3):488–504.
345. Narbona J, Crisci CD, Villa I. Familial congenital ocular motor apraxia and immune deficiency. Arch Neurol 1980;37(5):325.
346. Neimann N, et al. Mobius' syndrome associated with atrophic myopathy. Ann Med Nancy 1965;4:1084–1092.
347. Nellhaus G. Isolated oculomotor nerve palsy in infectious mononucleosis. A report of an unusual case and review of the literature. Neurology 1966;16(2):221–224.
348. Nelson LB. Severe adduction deficiency following a large medial rectus recession in Duane's retraction syndrome. Arch Ophthalmol 1986;104(6):859–862.
349. Nelson S, Kline L. Acquired trigemino-abducens synkinesis. J Clin Neuroophthalmol 1990;10:111–114.
350. Nemet P, Ehrlich D, Lazar M. Benign abducens palsy in varicella. Am J Ophthalmol 1974;78(5):859.
351. Nemet P, Ron S. Ocular saccades in Duane's syndrome. Br J Ophthalmol 1978;62(8):528–532.
352. Nishizaki T, et al. Bilateral internuclear ophthalmoplegia due to hydrocephalus: a case report. Neurosurgery 1985;17(5):822–825.
353. Noel LP, Clarke WN. Adduction deficiency following medial recti recession in Duane's retraction syndrome. Case report. Arch Ophthalmol 1987;105(4):465.

354. Oda K, Shibasaki H. Antigenic difference of acetylcholine receptor between single and multiple form endplates of human extraocular muscle. Brain Res 1988;449(1–2):337–340.
355. O'Day J, Billson F, King J. Ophthalmoplegic migraine and aberrant regeneration of the oculomotor nerve. Br J Ophthalmol 1980;64(7):534–536.
356. Oesterle CS, et al. Eye bobbing associated with jaw movement. Ophthalmology 1982;89(1):63–67.
357. Ogasahara S, et al. Improvement of abnormal pyruvate metabolism and cardiac conduction defect with coenzyme Q10 in Kearns–Sayre syndrome. Neurology 1985;35(3):372–377.
358. Ogasahara S, et al. Treatment of Kearns–Sayre syndrome with coenzyme Q10. Neurology 1986;36(1):45–53.
359. Ogasahara S, et al. Muscle coenzyme Q deficiency in familial mitochondrial encephalomyopathy. Proc Natl Acad Sci USA 1989;86(7):2379–2382.
360. Ohtsuki H, et al. Strabismus surgery in ocular myasthenia gravis. Ophthalmologica 1996;210(2):95–100.
361. Okihiro MM, et al. Duane syndrome and congenital upper-limb anomalies. A familial occurrence. Arch Neurol 1977;34(3):174–179.
362. Olson WH, et al. Moebius syndrome. Lower motor neuron involvement and hypogonadotrophic hypogonadism. Neurology 1970;20(10):1002–1008.
363. O'Malley ER, Helveston EM, Ellis FD. Duane's retraction syndrome—plus. J Pediatr Ophthalmol Strabismus 1982;19(3):161–165.
364. Oohira A, Goto K, Ozawa T. Slow saccades in myogenic and peripheral neurogenic ophthalmoplegia. Late ocular myopathy in myotonic dystrophy. Neuro-Ophthalmology 1985;5:117–123.
365. Oosterhuis HJ. The ocular signs and symptoms of myasthenia gravis. Doc Ophthalmol 1982;52(3–4):363–378.
366. Osher RH, et al. Neuro-ophthalmological complications of enlargement of the third ventricle. Br J Ophthalmol 1978;62(8):536–542.
367. Osher RH, Schatz NJ, Duane TD. Acquired orbital retraction syndrome. Arch Ophthalmol 1980;98(10):1798–1802.
368. Ouhabi H, et al. Bilateral optic neuritis and ponto-mesencephalic involvement shown by MRI in Miller–Fisher syndrome. Rev Neurol (Paris) 1998;154(11):780–782.
369. Ozawa T, Naito M, Takasu T. Disorder of saccadic eye movement in cerebellar degeneration. Jpn J Ophthalmol 1974;18:363–380.
370. Parks M. Isolated cyclovertical muscle palsy. Arch Ophthalmol 1958;60:1027–1035.
371. Pasik P, Pasik T, Bender MB. The pretectal syndrome in monkeys. I. Disturbances of gaze and body posture. Brain 1969;92(3):521–534.
372. Pasik T, Pasik P, Bender MB. The pretectal syndrome in monkeys. II. Spontaneous and induced nystagmus, and "lightning" eye movements. Brain 1969;92(4):871–884.

373. Paysee EA, Coats DK, Plager DA. Facial asymmetry and tendon laxity in superior oblique palsy. J Pediatr Ophthalmol Strabismus 1995;32(3):158–161.
374. Pearse RG, Howeler CJ. Neonatal form of dystrophia myotonica. Five cases in preterm babies and a review of earlier reports. Arch Dis Child 1979;54(5):331–338.
375. Pebbenito R, Cracco J. Congenital ocular motor apraxia. Clin Paediatr 1988;27:27–31.
376. Pesando P, Nuzzi G, Maraini G. Vertical retraction syndrome. Ophthalmologica 1978;177(5):254–259.
377. Pfaffenbach DD, Cross HE, Kearns TP. Congenital anomalies in Duane's retraction syndrome. Arch Ophthalmol 1972;88(6):635–639.
378. Phillips MS, Stewart S, Anderson JR. Neuropathological findings in Miller Fisher syndrome. J Neurol Neurosurg Psychiatry 1984;47(5): 492–495.
379. Pieroni D. Goldenhar's syndrome associated with Duane's retraction syndrome. J Pediatr Ophthalmol Strabismus 1969;6:16–18.
380. Pierrot-Deseilligny C, Gautier JC, Loron P. Acquired ocular motor apraxia due to bilateral frontoparietal infarcts. Ann Neurol 1988;23(2):199–202.
381. Plager DA. Tendon laxity in superior oblique palsy. Ophthalmology 1992;99(7):1032–1038.
382. Polak PE, Zijlstra F, Roelandt JR. Indications for pacemaker implantation in the Kearns–Sayre syndrome. Eur Heart J 1989;10(3): 281–282.
383. Pollard ZF. Aneurysm causing third nerve palsy in a 15-year-old boy. Arch Ophthalmol 1988;106(12):1647–1648.
384. Pollard ZF. Bilateral superior oblique muscle palsy associated with Apert's syndrome. Am J Ophthalmol 1988;106(3):337–340.
385. Pollard ZF. Accommodative esotropia after ocular and head injury. Am J Ophthalmol 1990;109(2):195–198.
386. Poppen JL, Marino R Jr. Pinealomas and tumors of the posterior portion of the third ventricle. J Neurosurg 1968;28(4):357–364.
387. Prasad P, Nair S. Congenital ocular motor apraxia: sporadic and familial. Support for natural resolution. J Neuroophthalmol 1994; 14(2):102–104.
388. Pressman SH, Scott WE. Surgical treatment of Duane's syndrome. Ophthalmology 1986;93(1):29–38.
389. Pruksacholawit K, Ishikawa S. Atypical retraction syndrome: a case study. J Pediatr Ophthalmol Strabismus 1976;13:215–220.
390. Putterman AM. Botulinum toxin injections in the treatment of seventh nerve misdirection. Am J Ophthalmol 1990;110(2):205–206.
391. Raab EL. Clinical features of Duane's syndrome. J Pediatr Ophthalmol Strabismus 1986;23(2):64–68.
392. Ramon Y, Cajal S. Degeneration and regeneration of the nervous system. London: Oxford University Press, 1928.
393. Ramsay J, Taylor D. Congenital crocodile tears: a key to the aetiology of Duane's syndrome. Br J Ophthalmol 1980;64(7):518–522.

394. Rana PV, Wadia RS. The Marin–Amat syndrome: an unusual facial synkinesia. J Neurol Neurosurg Psychiatry 1985;48(9):939–941.
395. Rappaport L, et al. Concurrence of congenital ocular motor apraxia and other motor problems: an expanded syndrome. Dev Med Child Neurol 1987;29(1):85–90.
396. Raroque HG Jr, Hershewe GL, Snyder RD. Mobius syndrome and transposition of the great vessels. Neurology 1988;38(12):1894–1895.
397. Rating D, et al. 4-Hydroxybutyric aciduria: a new inborn error of metabolism. I. Clinical review. J Inherit Metab Dis 1984;7(suppl 1):90–92.
398. Redding FK. Familial congenital ocular motor apraxia. Neurology 1970;20(4):405.
399. Reinecke RD, Thompson WE. Childhood recurrent idiopathic paralysis of the lateral rectus. Ann Ophthalmol 1981;13(9):1037–1039.
400. Reisner SH, et al. Transient lateral rectus muscle paresis in the newborn infant. J Pediatr 1971;78(3):461–465.
401. Ricker K. Myotonic dystrophy and proximal myotonic myopathy. J Neurol 1999;246(5):334–338.
402. Ro A, et al. Duane's retraction syndrome: southwestern Ontario experience. Can J Ophthalmol 1989;24(5):200–203.
403. Ro A, et al. Auditory function in Duane's retraction syndrome. Am J Ophthalmol 1990;109(1):75–78.
404. Roberts NK, Perloff JK, Kark RA. Cardiac conduction in the Kearns–Sayre syndrome (a neuromuscular disorder associated with progressive external ophthalmoplegia and pigmentary retinopathy). Report of 2 cases and review of 17 published cases. Am J Cardiol 1979;44(7):1396–1400.
405. Robertson DM, Hines JD, Rucker CW. Acquired sixth-nerve paresis in children. Arch Ophthalmol 1970;83(5):574–579.
406. Robertson WC, Chun RW, Kornguth SE. Familial infantile myasthenia. Arch Neurol 1980;37(2):117–119.
407. Rodrigues–Alves C, Caldeira J. Moebius' syndrome: a case report with multiple congenital anomalies. J Pediatr Ophthalmol Strabismus 1975;12:103–106.
408. Rodriguez M, et al. Myasthenia gravis in children: long-term follow-up. Ann Neurol 1983;13(5):504–510.
409. Rogers GL, Hatch GF Jr, Gray I. Mobius syndrome and limb abnormalities. J Pediatr Ophthalmol 1977;4(3):134–138.
410. Rogers GL, Bremer DL. Surgical treatment of the upshoot and downshoot in Duanes' retraction syndrome. Ophthalmology 1984;91(11): 1380–1383.
411. Roggenkamper P, et al. Orbicular synkinesis after facial paralysis: treatment with botulinum toxin. Doc Ophthalmol 1994;86(4):395–402.
412. Rollinson RD, Fenichel GM. Relapsing ocular myasthenia. Neurology 1981;31(3):325–326.
413. Ropper A, Wijdicks E, Truax B. Guillain–Barre syndrome. Philadelphia: Davis, 1991.

414. Ropper AH. The CNS in Guillain–Barre syndrome. Arch Neurol 1983;40(7):397–398.
415. Ropper AH. Unusual clinical variants and signs in Guillain–Barre syndrome. Arch Neurol 1986;43(11):1150–1152.
416. Ropper AH. Three patients with Fisher's syndrome and normal MRI. Neurology 1988;38(10):1630–1631.
417. Rosenberg ML, Wilson E. Congenital ocular motor apraxia without head thrusts. J Clin Neuroophthalmol 1987;7(1):26–28.
418. Roses AD, Appel SH. Protein kinase activity in erythrocyte ghosts of patients with myotonic muscular dystrophy. Proc Natl Acad Sci USA 1973;70(6):1855–1859.
419. Rothner AD. The migraine syndrome in children and adolescents. Pediatr Neurol 1986;2(3):121–126.
420. Rowland LP. Molecular genetics, pseudogenetics, and clinical neurology. The Robert Wartenberg lecture. Neurology 1983;33(9):1179–1195.
421. Rozen S, et al. Marfanoid hypermobility syndrome associated with Duane's retraction syndrome. Ann Ophthalmol 1983;15(9):862–864.
422. Rubinstein AE, et al. Moebius syndrome in Kallmann syndrome. Arch Neurol 1975;32(7):480–482.
423. Rush J, Shafrin F. Ocular myasthenia presenting as superior oblique weakness. J Clin Neuroophthalmol 1982;2:125–127.
424. Rush JA, Younge BR. Paralysis of cranial nerves III, IV, and VI. Cause and prognosis in 1,000 cases. Arch Ophthalmol 1981;99(1):76–79.
425. Saavedra J, et al. A cold test for myasthenia gravis. Neurology 1979;29(7):1075.
426. Sakalas R, et al. Chronic sixth nerve palsy. An initial sign of basisphenoid tumors. Arch Ophthalmol 1975;93(3):186–190.
427. Sano K. Trigemino-ocular synkineses. Neurologia 1959;1:29–51.
428. Saraux H, Laroche L, Lacombe H. Congenital horizontal gaze paralysis and ear dysplasia in a boy with Duane's retraction syndrome and seventh nerve palsy. Ophthalmologica 1984;188(4):208–211.
429. Sargent MA, Poskitt KJ, Jan JE. Congenital ocular motor apraxia: imaging findings. AJNR Am J Neuroradiol 1997;18(10):1915–1922.
430. Sarkies NJ, Sanders MD. Convergence spasm. Trans Ophthalmol Soc UK 1985;104(pt 7):782–786.
431. Sarnat HB, McGarry JD, Lewis JE Jr. Effective treatment of infantile myasthenia gravis by combined prednisone and thymectomy. Neurology 1977;27(6):550–553.
432. Sato M. Magnetic resonance imaging and tendon anomaly associated with congenital superior oblique palsy. Am J Ophthalmol 1999;127(4):379–387.
433. Scassellat-Sforzolini G. Una sindroma molto rare: diffeto congenito monolaterale della elevazione con retrazione del globe. Riv Otoneurooftalmol 1958;33:431–439.
434. Schapira AH, Thomas PK. A case of recurrent idiopathic ophthalmoplegic neuropathy (Miller Fisher syndrome). J Neurol Neurosurg Psychiatry 1986;49(4):463–464.

435. Scharf J, Zonis S. Benign abducens palsy in children. J Pediatr Ophthalmol 1975;12:165.
436. Schatz NJ, Savino PJ, Corbett JJ. Primary aberrant aculomotor regeneration. A sign of intracavernous meningioma. Arch Neurol 1977;34(1):29–32.
437. Schmidt D. Prognosis of ocular myasthenia in childhood. Neuro-Ophthalmology 1983;3:117–124.
438. Schneck L, et al. Ophthalmoplegia plus with morphological and chemical studies of cerebellar and muscle tissue. J Neurol Sci 1973;19(1):37–44.
439. Schraeder PL, Cohen MM, Goldman W. Bilateral internuclear ophthalmoplegia associated with fourth ventricular epidermoid tumor. Case report. J Neurosurg 1981;54(3):403–405.
440. Schumacher-Feero LA, et al. Third cranial nerve palsy in children. Am J Ophthalmol 1999;128(2):216–221.
441. Schumm F, et al. Thymectomy in patients with pure ocular symptoms. J Neurol Neurosurg Psychiatry 1985;48:332–337.
442. Scott A. Botulinum toxin treatment for strabismus. Am Orthop J 1985;35:28.
443. Scott AB, Wong GY. Duane's syndrome. An electromyographic study. Arch Ophthalmol 1971;87(2):140–147.
444. Scott AB, Kraft SP. Botulinum toxin injection in the management of lateral rectus paresis. Ophthalmology 1985;92(5):676–683.
445. Seaber J, Nashold B. Comparison of ocular motor effects of unilateral stereotactic midbrain lesions in man. Neuro-Ophthalmology 1980;1:95–99.
446. Sharf B, Hyams S. Oculomotor palsy following varicella. J Pediatr Ophthalmol 1972;9:245–247.
447. Sharpe JA, Johnston JL. Ocular motor paresis versus apraxia. Ann Neurol 1989;25(2):209–210.
448. Shauly Y, Weissman A, Meyer E. Ocular and systemic characteristics of Duane syndrome. J Pediatr Ophthalmol Strabismus 1993; 30(3):178–183.
449. Shaunak S, et al. Saccades and smooth pursuit in myotonic dystrophy. J Neurol 1999;246(7):600–606.
450. Shawkat FS, et al. Neuroradiological and eye movement correlates in children with intermittent saccade failure: "ocular motor apraxia." Neuropediatrics 1995;26(6):298–305.
451. Shawkat FS, et al. The role of ERG/VEP and eye movement recordings in children with ocular motor apraxia. Eye 1996;10(pt 1):53–60.
452. Shoffner JM, et al. Spontaneous Kearns–Sayre/chronic external ophthalmoplegia plus syndrome associated with a mitochondrial DNA deletion: a slip-replication model and metabolic therapy. Proc Natl Acad Sci USA 1989;86(20):7952–7956.
453. Shulman LM, Gallo BV, Weiner WJ. Acquired abducens-trigeminal synkinesis. Neurology 1998;50(5):1507–1508.
454. Sibony PA, Lessell S. Transient oculomotor synkinesis in temporal arteritis. Arch Neurol 1984;41(1):87–88.

455. Sibony PA, Lessell S, Gittinger JW Jr. Acquired oculomotor synkinesis. Surv Ophthalmol 1984;28(5):382–390.
456. Sibony PA, Evinger C, Lessell S. Retrograde horseradish peroxidase transport after oculomotor nerve injury. Investig Ophthalmol Vis Sci 1986;27(6):975–980.
457. Simcock PR, Kelleher S, Dunne JA. Neuro-ophthalmic findings in botulism type B. Eye 1994;8(pt 6):646–648.
458. Simpson LL. The origin, structure, and pharmacological activity of botulinum toxin. Pharmacol Rev 1981;33(3):155–188.
459. Slavin ML. Gaze palsy associated with viral syndrome. Am J Ophthalmol 1985;100(3):468–473.
460. Slavin ML. Transient comitant esotropia in a child with migraine. Am J Ophthalmol 1989;107(2):190–191.
461. Smith C. Nuclear and infranuclear ocular motility disorders. In: Miller N, Newman N (eds) Clinical neuro-ophthalmology. Baltimore: Williams & Wilkins, 1999:1238–1240.
462. Snead OC III, et al. Juvenile myasthenia gravis. Neurology 1980;30(7 pt 1):732–739.
463. Soliven BC, et al. Seronegative myasthenia gravis. Neurology 1988;38(4):514–517.
464. Spatz H, Ullrich O. Klinischer und anatomischer Beitrag zu den angeborenen Beweglichkeitsdefekten im Hirnnervenbereich. Z Kinderheilkd 1931;51:579–597.
465. Spielmann A, Richter J. Oculomotor surgery in Parinaud's syndrome. Ophtalmologie 1989;3(2):157–159.
466. Spierer A, Barak A. Strabismus surgery in children with Mobius syndrome. J Am Assoc Pediatr Ophthalmol Strabismus 2000;4(1):58–59.
467. Spiro AJ, et al. A cytochrome-related inherited disorder of the nervous system and muscle. Arch Neurol 1970;23(2):103–112.
468. Spooner JW, Baloh RW. Eye movement fatigue in myasthenia gravis. Neurology 1979;29(1):29–33.
469. Stamler J, Nerad J, Keech R. Acquired pseudo-Duane's retraction syndrome secondary to acute orbital myositis. Binoc Vision 1989;4: 103–108.
470. Stansbury J. Moebius's syndrome. Am J Ophthalmol 1952;35:256–261.
471. Starr A. A disorder of rapid eye movements in Huntington's chorea. Brain 1967;90(3):545–564.
472. Steinlin M, et al. Congenital oculomotor apraxia: a neurodevelopmental and neuroradiological study. Neuro-Ophthalmology 1990;10: 27–32.
473. Stell R, et al. Ataxia telangiectasia: a reappraisal of the ocular motor features and their value in the diagnosis of atypical cases. Mov Disord 1989;4(4):320–329.
474. Sternberg I, Ronen S, Arnon N. Recurrent, isolated, post-febrile abducens nerve palsy. J Pediatr Ophthalmol Strabismus 1980;17(5): 323–324.

475. Sudarshan A, Goldie WD. The spectrum of congenital facial diplegia (Moebius syndrome). Pediatr Neurol 1985;1(3):180–184.
476. Sullivan S. Benign recurrent isolated VI nerve palsy of childhood. Clin Pediatr 1985;24:160–161.
477. Summers CG, MacDonald JT, Wirtschafter JD. Ocular motor apraxia associated with intracranial lipoma. J Pediatr Ophthalmol Strabismus 1987;24(5):267–269.
478. Swick HM. Pseudointernuclear ophthalmoplegia in acute idiopathic polyneuritis (Fisher's syndrome). Am J Ophthalmol 1974;77(5):725–728.
479. Sydnor CF, Seaber JH, Buckley EG. Traumatic superior oblique palsies. Ophthalmology 1982;89(2):134–138.
480. Tamura EE, Hoyt CS. Oculomotor consequences of intraventricular hemorrhages in premature infants. Arch Ophthalmol 1987;105(4):533–535.
481. Taylor MJ, Polomeno RC. Further observations on the auditory brainstem response in Duane's syndrome. Can J Ophthalmol 1983;18(5):238–240.
482. Tekkok IH, et al. Bilateral intranuclear ophthalmoplegia associated with fourth ventricular dermoid tumor. J Clin Neuroophthalmol 1989;9(4):254–257.
483. Teller J, Karmon G, Savir H. Long-term follow-up of traumatic unilateral superior oblique palsy. Ann Ophthalmol 1988;20(11):424–425.
484. Ter Bruggen JP, et al. Disorders of eye movement in myotonic dystrophy. Brain 1990;113(pt 2):463–473.
485. Terranova W, Palumbo JN, Breman JG. Ocular findings in botulism type B. JAMA 1979;241(5):475–477.
486. Thomas R, et al. Bilateral synergistic divergence. J Pediatr Ophthalmol Strabismus 1993;30(2):122–123.
487. Tjissen C, Goor C, van Woerkom T. Spasm of the near reflex: functional or organic disorder? Neuro-Ophthalmology 1983;3:59–64.
488. Toshniwal P. Demyelinating optic neuropathy with Miller–Fisher syndrome. The case for overlap syndromes with central and peripheral demyelination. J Neurol 1987;234(5):353–358.
489. Towfighi J, et al. Mobius syndrome. Neuropathologic observations. Acta Neuropathol (Berl) 1979;48(1):11–17.
490. Traboulsi EI, Maumenee IH. Extraocular muscle aplasia in Moebius syndrome. J Pediatr Ophthalmol Strabismus 1986;23(3):120–122.
491. Tredici TD, von Noorden GK. Are anisometropia and amblyopia common in Duane's syndrome? J Pediatr Ophthalmol Strabismus 1985;22(1):23–25.
492. Tripp JH, et al. Juvenile Gaucher's disease with horizontal gaze palsy in three siblings. J Neurol Neurosurg Psychiatry 1977;40(5):470–478.
493. Trobe JD, Glaser JS, Post JD. Meningiomas and aneurysms of the cavernous sinus. Neuro-ophthalmologic features. Arch Ophthalmol 1978;96(3):457–467.
494. Trobe JD. Cyclodeviation in acquired vertical strabismus. Arch Ophthalmol 1984;102(5):717–720.

495. Trobe JD. Third nerve palsy and the pupil. Footnotes to the rule. Arch Ophthalmol 1988;106(5):601–602.
496. Troost BT, et al. Upbeat nystagmus and internuclear ophthalmoplegia with brainstem glioma. Arch Neurol 1980;37(7):453–456.
497. Tsai L, et al. Oculomotor apraxia in a case of Gaucher's disease with homozygous T1448C mutation. Chung Hua Min Kuo Hsiao Erh Ko I Hsueh Hui Tsa Chih 1996;37:52–55.
498. Vajsar J, et al. Arthrogryposis multiplex congenita due to congenital myasthenic syndrome. Pediatr Neurol 1995;12(3):237–241.
499. Valbuena O, et al. Ataxia telangiectasia: review of 13 new cases. Rev Neurol 1996;24(125):77–80.
500. Valmaggia C, Zaunbauer W, Gottlob I. Elevation deficit caused by accessory extraocular muscle. Am J Ophthalmol 1996;121(4):444–445.
501. Vassella F, Lutschg J, Mumenthaler M. Cogan's congenital ocular motor apraxia in two successive generations. Dev Med Child Neurol 1972;14(6):788–796.
502. Velez FG, Clark RA, Demer JL. Facial asymmetry in superior oblique muscle palsy and pulley heterotopy. J Am Assoc Pediatr Ophthalmol Strabismus 2000;4(4):233–239.
503. Versino M, et al. Lateral gaze synkinesis on downward saccade attempts with paramedian thalamic and midbrain infarct. J Neurol Neurosurg Psychiatry 1999;67(5):696–697.
504. Victor DI. The diagnosis of congenital unilateral third-nerve palsy. Brain 1976;99(4):711–718.
505. Vincent C, et al. A proposed new contiguous gene syndrome on 8q consists of branchio-oto-renal (BOR) syndrome, Duane syndrome, a dominant form of hydrocephalus and trapeze aplasia; implications for the mapping of the BOR gene. Hum Mol Genet 1994;3(10):1859–1866.
506. Vincent FM, Vincent T. Relapsing Fisher's syndrome. J Neurol Neurosurg Psychiatry 1986;49(5):604–606.
507. Vivian A, Harris C, Kriss A. Oculomotor signs in infantile Gaucher disease. Neuro-Ophthalmology 1993;13:151–155.
508. von Ludinghausen M. Bilateral supernumerary rectus muscles of the orbit. Clin Anat 1998;11(4):271–277.
509. von Ludinghausen M, Miura M, Wurzler N. Variations and anomalies of the human orbital muscles. Surg Radiol Anat 1999;21(1):69–76.
510. von Noorden GK, Murray E. Up- and downshoot in Duane's retraction syndrome. J Pediatr Ophthalmol Strabismus 1986;23(5):212–215.
511. von Noorden GK. A magnetic resonance imaging study of the upshoot-downshoot phenomenon of Duane's retraction syndrome. Am J Ophthalmol 1991;112(3):358–359.
512. Wadia NH, Swami RK. A new form of heredo-familial spinocerebellar degeneration with slow eye movements (nine families). Brain 1971;94(2):359–374.

513. Wadia NH, et al. A study of the neurological disorder associated with acute haemorrhagic conjunctivitis due to enterovirus 70. J Neurol Neurosurg Psychiatry 1983;46(7):599–610.
514. Wagner RS, Caputo AR, Frohman LP. Congenital unilateral adduction deficit with simultaneous abduction. A variant of Duane's retraction syndrome. Ophthalmology 1987;94(8):1049–1053.
515. Walsh F, Hoyt W. Clinical neuro-ophthalmology. Baltimore: Williams & Wilkins, 1969.
516. Waterhouse WJ, Enzenauer RW, Martyak AP. Successful strabismus surgery in a child with Moebius syndrome. Ann Ophthalmol 1993; 25(8):292–294.
517. Weeks CL, Hamed LM. Treatment of acute comitant esotropia in Chiari I malformation. Ophthalmology 1999;106(12):2368–2371.
518. Weinacht S, Huber A, Gottlob I. Vertical Duane's retraction syndrome. Am J Ophthalmol 1996;122(3):447–449.
519. Weinberg DA, Lesser RL, Vollmer TL. Ocular myasthenia: a protean disorder. Surv Ophthalmol 1994;39(3):169–210.
520. Weintraub MI. External ophthalmoplegia, ataxia, and areflexia complicating acute infectious polyneuritis. Am J Ophthalmol 1977;83(3): 355–357.
521. Welch R. Chicken-pox and the Guillain–Barre syndrome. Arch Dis Child 1962;37:557–559.
522. Werner DB, Savino PJ, Schatz NJ. Benign recurrent sixth nerve palsies in childhood. Secondary to immunization or viral illness. Arch Ophthalmol 1983;101(4):607–608.
523. Whitsel EA, Castillo M, D'Cruz O. Cerebellar vermis and midbrain dysgenesis in oculomotor apraxia: MR findings. AJNR Am J Neuroradiol 1995;16(suppl 4):831–834.
524. Wieacker P, et al. A new X-linked syndrome with muscle atrophy, congenital contractures, and oculomotor apraxia. Am J Med Genet 1985;20(4):597–606.
525. Wilcox LM Jr, Gittinger JW Jr, Breinin GM. Congenital adduction palsy and synergistic divergence. Am J Ophthalmol 1981;91(1):1–7.
526. Williams AS, Hoyt CS. Acute comitant esotropia in children with brain tumors. Arch Ophthalmol 1989;107(3):376–378.
527. Willison HJ, O'Hanlon GM. The immunopathogenesis of Miller Fisher syndrome. J Neuroimmunol 1999;100(1–2):3–12.
528. Wilson ME, Hoxie J. Facial asymmetry in superior oblique muscle palsy. J Pediatr Ophthalmol Strabismus 1993;30(5):315–318.
529. Wilson RS, Landers JH. Anomalous duplication of inferior oblique muscle. Am J Ophthalmol 1982;93(4):521–522.
530. Wise GA, McQuillen MP. Transient neonatal myasthenia. Clinical and electromyographic studies. Arch Neurol 1970;22(6):556–565.
531. Wishnick M, et al. Mobius syndrome and limb abnormalities with dominant inheritance. Ophthalmic Pediatr Genet 1983;2:77–81.
532. Woods CG, Taylor AM. Ataxia telangiectasia in the British Isles: the clinical and laboratory features of 70 affected individuals. Q J Med 1992;82(298):169–179.

533. Woody R, Reynolds J. Association of bilateral internuclear ophthalmoplegia and myelomeningocele with Arnold–Chiari malformation type II. J Clin Neuroophthalmol 1985;5:124–126.
534. Woody RC, Blaw ME. Ophthalmoplegic migraine in infancy. Clin Pediatr (Phila) 1986;25(2):82–84.
535. Wright PW, Strauss GH, Langford MP. Acute hemorrhagic conjunctivitis. Am Fam Physician 1992;45(1):173–178.
536. Wybar K. Disorders of ocular motility in brain stem lesions in children. Ann Ophthalmol 1971;3(6):645–647.
537. Yang MC, et al. Electrooculography and discriminant analysis in Duane's syndrome and sixth-cranial-nerve palsy. Graefe's Arch Clin Exp Ophthalmol 1991;229(1):52–56.
538. Yeh JH, et al. Miller Fisher syndrome with central involvement: successful treatment with plasmapheresis. Ther Apher 1999;3(1):69–71.
539. Yuki N. Pathogenesis of Guillain–Barre and Miller Fisher syndromes subsequent to *Campylobacter jejuni* enteritis. Jpn J Infect Dis 1999;52(3):99–105.
540. Zaret CR, Behrens MM, Eggers HM. Congenital ocular motor apraxia and brainstem tumor. Arch Ophthalmol 1980;98(2):328–330.
541. Zasorin NL, Yee RD, Baloh RW. Eye-movement abnormalities in ophthalmoplegia, ataxia, and areflexia (Fisher's syndrome). Arch Ophthalmol 1985;103(1):55–58.
542. Zee DS, Yee RD, Singer HS. Congenital ocular motor apraxia. Brain 1977;100(3):581–599.
543. Zuker RM. Facial paralysis in children. Clin Plast Surg 1990;17(1): 95–99.

6

Congenital Optic Nerve Abnormalities

Paul H. Phillips and Michael C. Brodsky

The ophthalmologist is frequently called upon to evaluate infants and children with decreased vision related to congenital abnormalities of the optic nerve. Such evaluation necessitates a detailed understanding of the ophthalmoscopic features, associated neuro-ophthalmic findings, current theories of pathogenesis, and appropriate ancillary studies in each condition. This chapter examines congenital optic nerve abnormalities, discusses current controversies surrounding their pathogeneses, and reviews associated neuroradiologic findings that may predicate the general medical management of affected patients.

Certain general principles apply to the evaluation and management of the child with congenital optic nerve abnormalities.

1. Children who have bilateral optic disc anomalies generally present with poor vision and nystagmus in infancy; those with unilateral disc anomalies typically present with sensory strabismus.

2. Small optic discs are associated with a wide variety of central nervous system (CNS) malformations involving the cerebral hemispheres, pituitary infundibulum, and midline intracranial structures (septum pellucidum, corpus callosum). A trans-sphenoidal basal encephalocele is common in patients with large discs of the morning glory variety. The presence of a basal encephalocele can often be predicted clinically by the finding of midfacial anomalies (hypertelorism, flat nasal bridge, cleft lip or palate).[62] Large optic discs with a colobomatous configuration may be associated with systemic anomalies in a variety of coloboma syndromes. Magnetic resonance imaging

(MRI) is advisable in all children with small optic discs, and in children with large optic discs who either have facial characteristics suggestive of basal encephalocele or neurodevelopmental deficits.

3. Color vision is typically normal in an eye with a congenitally anomalous optic disc (i.e., limited only by the visual acuity), in contradistinction to the severe dyschromatopsia that characterizes most acquired optic abnormalities.

4. A structural ocular abnormality that reduces visual acuity often leads to superimposed amblyopia. A trial of occlusion therapy is therefore warranted in most patients with unilateral optic disc anomalies and decreased vision. The findings of an afferent pupillary defect should not discourage this effort.

5. The finding of a discrete V- or tongue-shaped zone of infrapapillary retinochoroidal depigmentation in an eye with an anomalous optic disc should prompt a search for a transsphenoidal encephalocele.[14]

OPTIC NERVE HYPOPLASIA

Incidence

Optic nerve hypoplasia, once considered a rare anomaly, is now the most common congenital optic anomaly encountered in pediatric ophthalmic practice. Part of the increased prevalence may reflect a greater recognition of optic nerve hypoplasia on the part of clinicians. To the uninitiated observer, the small size of the hypoplastic disc is not readily apparent, and the disc may be interpreted as atrophic or even normal.[9] Many cases of optic nerve hypoplasia were undoubtedly misdiagnosed in the past. On the other hand, some authors have suggested that drug and alcohol abuse, both of which have become more widespread in recent years, may account in part for the increased number of cases.[46]

Clinical Features

Ophthalmoscopically, the hypoplastic disc appears as an abnormally small optic nerve head (Fig. 6-1). It may appear gray or pale in color and is often surrounded by a yellowish, mottled peripapillary halo, bordered by a dark pigment ring (*double-ring sign*).[35] Retinal vascular tortuosity is commonly seen. Histolog-

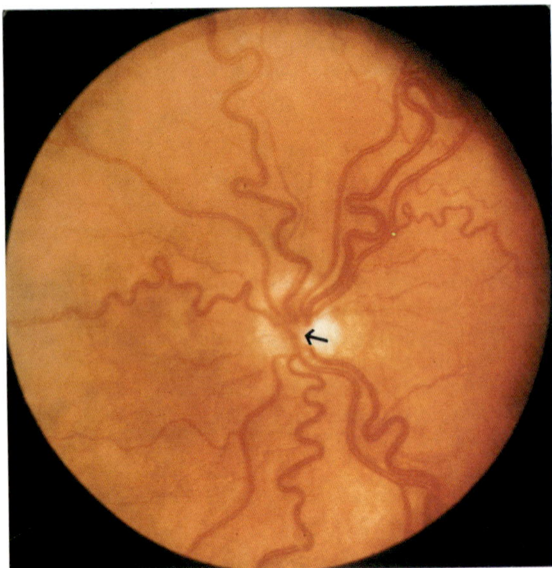

FIGURE 6-1. Optic nerve hypoplasia with double-ring sign. *Arrow* denotes true margin of the hypoplastic disc. (From Lambert SR, Hoyt CS, Narahara MH. Optic nerve hypoplasia. Surv Ophthalmol 1987;32:1–9, with permission.[46])

ically, optic nerve hypoplasia is characterized by a subnormal number of optic nerve axons with normal mesodermal elements and glial supporting tissue.[35] Visual acuity ranges from 20/20 to no light perception, and affected eyes invariably show localized visual field defects, often combined with a general constriction of the visual fields.[27] Because visual acuity is determined primarily by the integrity of the papillomacular nerve fiber bundle, it does not necessarily correlate with the overall size of the disc.

It is now appreciated that some forms of optic nerve hypoplasia are segmental (Fig. 6-2). A pathognomonic superior segmental hypoplasia with an inferior visual field defect occurs in some children of insulin-dependent diabetic mothers.[15,43] Conversely, colobomatous malformations of the optic disc produce an inferior segmental hypoplasia.[7] Intrauterine insults to the retina, optic nerve, optic tract, or occipital lobe are associated with hypoplasia of the affected portions of each optic nerve.[57]

Patients with *periventricular leukomalacia* (PVL) often have a unique form of optic nerve hypoplasia characterized by an abnormally large cup and a thin neuroretinal rim contained within a normal-sized optic disc.[8,39] This morphological appearance has been attributed to bilateral injury to the optic radiations with retrograde transsynaptic degeneration of retinogeniculate axons after the scleral canals have established normal diameter. Optic disc cupping in patients with PVL may cause diagnostic confusion with glaucoma.[8] Therefore, a history of prematurity and neurodevelopmental delay should be sought in children who have abnormally large optic cups and normal intraocular pressures. Neuroimaging is necessary to confirm the diagnosis.

Associated Features

Optic nerve hypoplasia is often associated with other CNS malformations. *Septo-optic dysplasia (de Morsier's syndrome)* refers

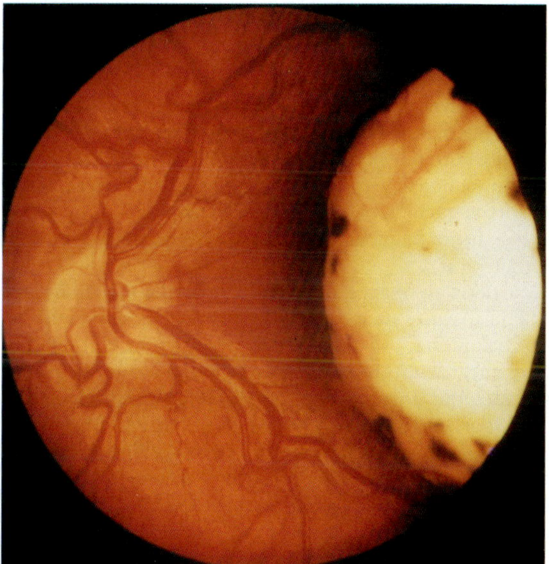

FIGURE 6-2. Segmental optic nerve hypoplasia associated with macular coloboma. Note focal absence of temporal optic disc with corresponding temporal nerve fiber layer defect. (From Novakovic P, Taylor DSI, Hoyt WF. Localizing patterns of optic nerve hypoplasia: retina to occipital lobe. Br J Ophthalmol 1988;72:176–182, with permission.[57])

to the constellation of small anterior visual pathways, absence of the septum pellucidum, and agenesis or thinning of the corpus callosum.[22] The clinical association of septo-optic dysplasia and pituitary dwarfism was documented by Hoyt et al. in 1970.[36] MRI is the optimal noninvasive neuroimaging modality for delineating congenital CNS malformations in patients with septo-optic dysplasia.[13] Because MRI provides high-contrast resolution and multiplanar imaging capability, the anterior visual pathways can be visualized as distinct, well-defined structures. Coronal and sagittal MRI consistently demonstrate a reduction in the intracranial optic nerve diameter in optic nerve hypoplasia (Fig. 6-3). In bilateral optic nerve hypoplasia, coronal MRI shows diffuse thinning of the optic chiasm (chiasmal hypoplasia). When MRI demonstrates a reduction in intracranial optic nerve size accompanied by other midline CNS features of septooptic dysplasia, the presumptive diagnosis of optic nerve hypoplasia can be made neuroradiologically.[13]

In addition to septo-optic dysplasia, MRI may demonstrate cerebral hemispheric migration anomalies (*schizencephaly*, cortical heterotopias) or intrauterine or perinatal hemispheric injury (periventricular leukomalacia, encephalomalacia). These abnormalities occur in approximately 45% of patients with optic nerve hypoplasia and are highly predictive of neurodevelopmental deficits.[12] Absence of the septum pellucidum alone does not portend neurodevelopmental deficits or pituitary hormone deficiency.[72] Thinning or agenesis of the corpus callosum is predictive of neurodevelopmental problems only by virtue of its frequent association with cerebral hemispheric abnormalities.

Magnetic resonance imaging demonstrates neurohypophyseal abnormalities in approximately 15% of patients with optic nerve hypoplasia.[12] In normal subjects, high-resolution cranial MRI delineates the pituitary infundibulum, anterior pituitary gland, and the posterior pituitary gland, which appears as a "bright spot" in the sella. The "posterior pituitary bright spot" has been attributed to the posterior pituitary hormones as well as the phospholipid content of the vesicles containing these hormones. In patients with optic nerve hypoplasia, absence of the infundibulum and posterior pituitary ectopia is associated with endocrine dysfunction.[12,61,66] When the pituitary infundibulum and its surrounding portal venous system are absent, the hypothalamus is unable to stimulate the anterior pituitary gland, resulting in anterior pituitary hormone deficiency. *Posterior*

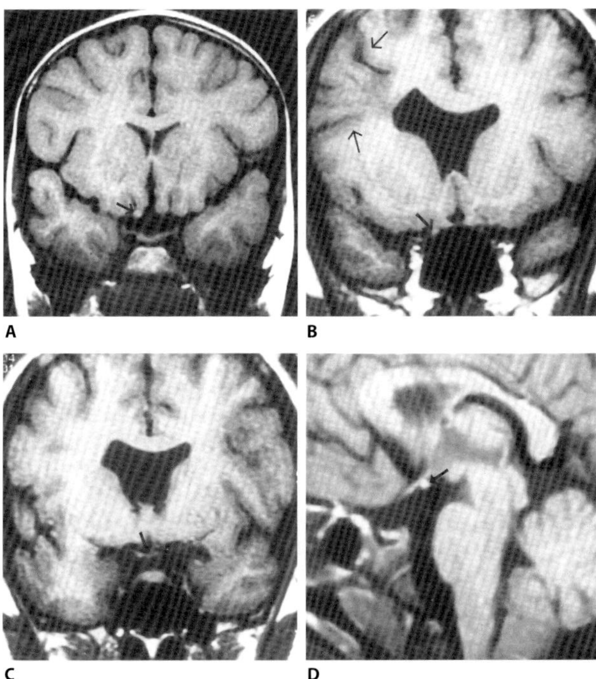

FIGURE 6-3A–D. Magnetic resonance imaging in optic nerve hypoplasia. (**A**) Left optic nerve hypoplasia. T_1-weighted coronal MR image shows normal right optic nerve (*arrow*) and no visible signal corresponding to the left optic nerve. (**B**) Septo-optic dysplasia. Clinically, this patient had mild right optic nerve hypoplasia and severe left optic nerve hypoplasia. T_1-weighted coronal MR image shows thinning and signal attenuation of the left optic nerve compared to the right (*lower arrow*, right optic nerve). Also note absence of the septum pellucidum and squaring of the right frontal horn contiguous to an area of schizencephaly (*long thin arrows*). (**C**) Chiasmal hypoplasia in a patient with septo-optic dysplasia. T_1-weighted coronal MR image demonstrates absence of the septum pellucidum and diffuse thinning of the optic chiasm. *Arrow* denotes thin hypoplastic chiasm. (**D**) Posterior pituitary ectopia. T_1-weighted sagittal MRI shows abnormal hyperintense nodule (*upper arrow*) at median eminence with absence of normal signal corresponding to the infundibulum (*lower arrow*). (**A–C:** From Brodsky MC, Glasier CM, Pollock SC, et al. Optic nerve hypoplasia: identification by magnetic resonance imaging. Arch Ophthalmol 1990;108:1562–1567, with permission. **D:** From Brodsky MC. Septo-optic dysplasia: a reappraisal. Semin Ophthalmol 1991;6:227–232, with permission.[9])

pituitary ectopia (see Fig 6-3) denotes the formation of an ectopic bright spot where the proximal infundibulum is normally located. Injury to the infundibulum disrupts transport of posterior pituitary hormones, which are synthesized in the hypothalamus. The posterior pituitary hormones accumulate proximal to the site or injury and form an ectopic nodule, visible as a bright spot on T_1-weighted MRI. Hormones secretion from the ectopic gland is often sufficient to maintain adequate posterior pituitary function. However, this ectopic bright spot is a marker of infundibular dysgenesis, and is virtually pathognomonic of anterior pituitary hormone deficiency.[12,61] MRI therefore provides crucial prognostic information in infants with optic nerve hypoplasia.

Growth hormone deficiency is the most common endocrinological abnormality associated with septo-optic dysplasia.[9,46] Hypothyroidism, hypocortisolism, panhypopituitarism, hyperprolactinemia, and diabetes insipidus may also occur.[2,35,38,52] Clinical signs of growth hormone deficiency include decreased growth rate and neonatal hypoglycemia. Reduced growth rate from growth hormone deficiency may not be clinically apparent during the first 4 years of life because high prolactin levels can stimulate normal growth during this period.[21] Clinical signs of hypothyroidism include prolonged neonatal jaundice, decreased growth rate, and developmental delay. Clinical signs of hypocortisolism include neonatal hypoglycemia, hypotension, recurrent infections, seizures, and developmental delay. Low corticotropin levels are particularly dangerous because they place children at risk for sudden death during physical stress such as febrile illnesses.[11] This clinical deterioration is caused by an impaired ability to increase corticotropin secretion to maintain blood pressure and blood sugar in response to the physical stress of infection. Corticotropin-deficient children may also have poikilothermia (impaired temperature regulation) and develop high fevers or have unusually low body temperatures during healthy periods.

Children with optic nerve hypoplasia and anterior pituitary hormone deficiency may have coexistent *diabetes insipidus*, which further increases the risk of life-threatening clinical deterioration in response to physical stress.[11] The absence of the pituitary infundibulum and the posterior pituitary bright signal (normal or ectopic) on MRI portends posterior pituitary deficiency with consequent diabetes insipidus.[11,61,66] Clinical signs of diabetes insipidus include polydipsia, polyuria, and hypernatremia.

TABLE 6-1. Systemic and Teratogenic Associations with Optic Nerve Hypoplasia.

Systemic associations
Albinism
Aniridia
Duane's syndrome
Median facial cleft syndrome
Klippel–Trenauney–Weber syndrome
Goldenhar's syndrome
Linear sebaceous nevus syndrome
Meckel's syndrome
Hemifacial atrophy
Blepharophimosis
Osteogenesis imperfecta
Chondrodysplasia punctata
Aicardi's syndrome
Apert syndrome
Trisomy 18
Potter's syndrome
Chromosome 13q−
Neonatal isoimmune thrombocytopenia
Fetal alcohol syndrome
Dandy–Walker syndrome
Delleman syndrome
Teratogenic agents
Dilantin
Quinine
PCP
LSD
Alcohol
Maternal diabetes

Source: Modified from Zeki SM, Dutton GV. Optic nerve hypoplasia in children. Br J Ophthalmol 1990;74:300–304, with permission.

Children with diabetes insipidus often become dehydrated during illness, which hastens the development of shock. These children may have coexistent hypothalamic thermoregulatory disturbances, characterized by episodes of hypothermia during well periods and high fevers during illnesses, that may cause life-threatening hyperthermia. Optic nerve hypoplasia is associated with numerous systemic conditions and teratogenic agents (Table 6-1).

Etiology

Early investigators attributed optic nerve hypoplasia to a primary failure of retinal ganglion differentiation at the 13- to 15-mm stage of embryonic life (4–6 weeks gestation).[65] This hypothesis fails to account for the frequent coexistence of optic nerve hypoplasia with other CNS malformations. More recently, it has been suggested that an encephaloclastic process involving the afferent visual pathways in utero could cause direct axonal injury, leading to subsequent degeneration. The frequent association of cerebral hemispheric anomalies with optic nerve hypoplasia suggests that some cases of optic nerve hypoplasia may result from a diffuse disruption of neuronal guidance mechanisms that regulate the migration of both cerebral hemispheric neurons and optic nerve axons in utero. Toxic substances or structural abnormalities may augment the usual process by which superfluous optic nerve axons are eliminated between the 16th and 31st gestational weeks and thereby result in optic nerve hypoplasia. In some cases, optic nerve hypoplasia may occur secondary to retrograde transsynaptic degeneration of retinogeniculate axons secondary to a prenatal injury to the optic radiations.[8,39,57] This mechanism may be responsible for the optic nerve cupping that occurs in children with periventricular leukomalacia.[39]

Clinical Assessment

The detection of hypopituitarism is an essential component of the evaluation of children with optic nerve hypoplasia because children with endocrinological deficiency are at risk for impaired growth, hypoglycemia, developmental delay, seizures, and death.[11] Early pituitary hormone replacement may prevent or ameliorate these complications. Parents should be asked about protracted neonatal jaundice (which suggests hypothyroidism) and previous episodes of hypoglycemia in the neonatal period or during periods of illness (which suggest hypocortisolism).

Magnetic resonance imaging is an integral part of the diagnostic evaluation of children with optic nerve hypoplasia. Cerebral hemispheric anomalies are predictive of neurodevelopmental deficits, and neurohypophyseal abnormalities are predictive of endocrinological deficiency.[12,61] Children with neurohypophyseal abnormalities or clinical signs of hypopituitarism require diagnostic endocrinological evaluation.[61] Conversely, children with a normal neurohypophysis are at low risk for hypopituitarism. Parents, pediatricians, and neurologists can be informed of this potential risk, and these children can be followed for clinical signs of hypopituitarism including monitoring of their growth rate. If these children do not manifest clinical signs or symptoms of hypopituitarism, further endocrinological investigation is not warranted.[61]

Inheritance

Usually sporadic.

Natural History

Infants with optic nerve hypoplasia may have superimposed delayed visual maturation. Therefore, infants who initially appear to be blind may have improvement of their vision during the first several months of life. In children with unilateral or asymmetric optic nerve hypoplasia, superimposed amblyopia may further reduce vision. Children with hypopituitarism are at risk for growth retardation, developmental delay, hypoglycemia, seizures, and death.[11]

Treatment

Superimposed amblyopia should be treated with a trial of occlusion therapy. Children with hypopituitarism are treated with pituitary hormone replacement.

Prognosis

Occlusion therapy may improve vision in children with superimposed amblyopia. Treatment of children with endocrinological deficiency with pituitary hormone replacement should prevent or ameliorate complications of hypopituitarism noted previously.

EXCAVATED OPTIC DISC ANOMALIES

Optic disc coloboma, morning glory disc anomaly, and peripapillary staphyloma fall within the category of excavated anomalies involving the optic disc. In the latter two conditions, an excavation of the posterior globe surrounds and incorporates the optic disc. Pollock has elegantly detailed the clinical features that distinguish the excavated optic disc anomalies.[63] He points out that the terms morning glory disc, optic disc coloboma, and peripapillary staphyloma are often transposed in clinical reports and review articles, which has propagated confusion about their diagnostic clinical features, associated findings, and pathogenesis. From his analysis, it is clear that optic disc colobomas, morning glory optic discs, and peripapillary staphylomas constitute distinct clinical entities, each with a specific embryologic origin, and not simple clinical variants along a broad phenotypic spectrum.

MORNING GLORY DISC ANOMALY

Incidence

Unknown.

Clinical Features

The morning glory anomaly is a congenital, funnel-shaped excavation of the posterior fundus that incorporates the optic disc.[63] It was so named by Kindler in 1970[44] because of its resemblance to the morning glory flower (Fig. 6-4). The disc is markedly

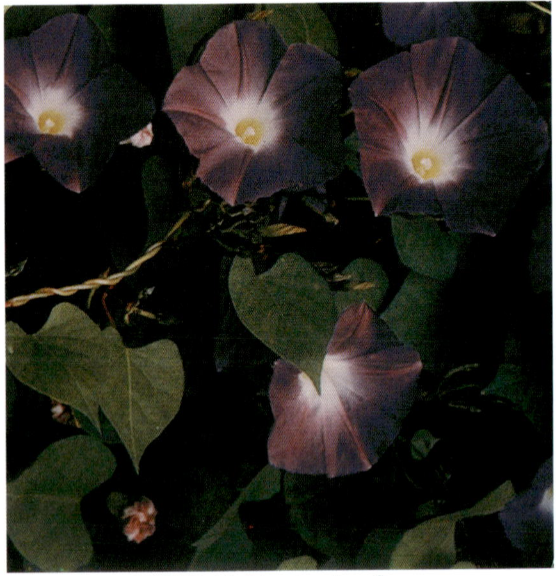

FIGURE 6-4. Morning glory flower.

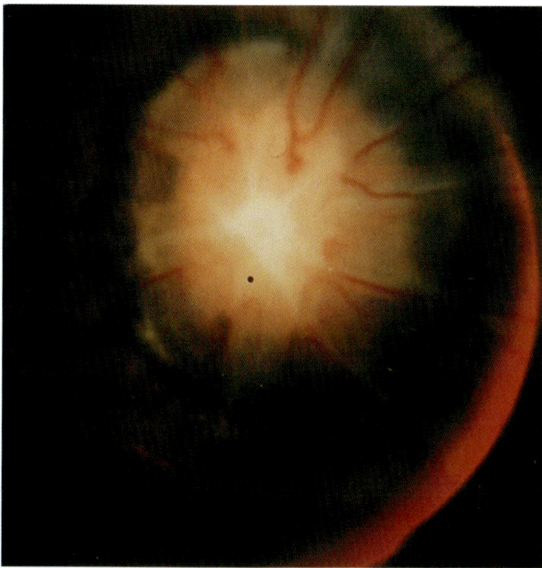

FIGURE 6-5. Morning glory optic disc. The disc is large with a surrounding zone of pigmentary disturbance. The retinal vessels appear increased in number as they emerge from the disc and have an abnormally straight, radial configuration. A central glial bouquet overlies the disc. (From Pollock S. The morning glory disc anomaly: contractile movement, classification, and embryogenesis. Doc Ophthalmol 1987;65:439–460, with permission.[63])

enlarged, orange or pink in color, and typically situated within a funnel-shaped excavation (Fig. 6-5). Surrounding the excavation is a variably elevated annular zone of altered retinal pigmentation. A white tuft of glial tissue overlies the recessed central portion of the lesion. The blood vessels appear increased in number and arise from the periphery of the disc. They run an abnormally straight course over the peripapillary retina and tend to branch at acute angles. It is often difficult to distinguish arterioles from venules. The macula may be incorporated into the excavation (macular capture) (Fig. 6-6). Computed tomography (CT) scanning shows a funnel-shaped enlargement of the distal optic nerve at its junction with the globe[6,50] (Fig. 6-7).

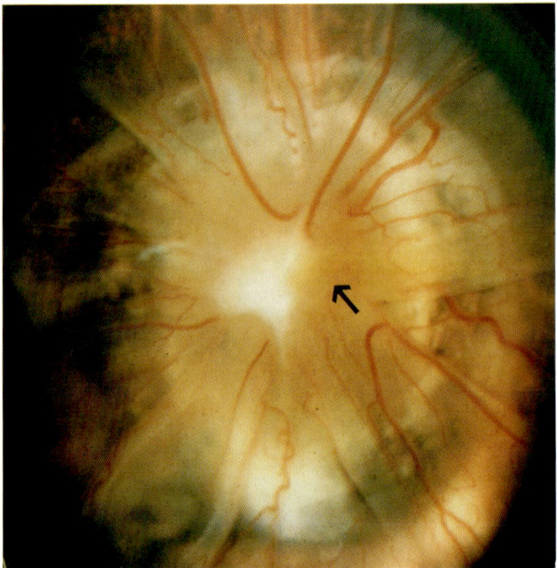

FIGURE 6-6. Morning glory optic disc. *Arrow* denotes focal yellowish discoloration that corresponds to macula lutea pigment (macular capture). (From Goldhammer Y, Smith JL. Optic nerve anomalies in basal encephalocele. Arch Ophthalmol 1975;93:115–118, with permission[28])

Visual acuity generally ranges between 20/200 and finger counting, but cases with 20/20 vision and others with no light perception have been reported. Although most cases are unilateral, several bilateral cases with 20/20 to 20/70 vision have been reported, suggesting that functional amblyopia may be an important mechanism of visual loss in unilateral cases.[6] Morning glory discs are more common in females and rare in blacks.[30]

Natural History

Serous retinal detachments are reported to occur in 26% to 38% of eyes with morning glory discs and usually involve the peripapillary retina.[63] In addition, careful fundus examination reveals nonattachment and radial folding of the retina within the excavated zone in a substantial percentage of the remaining cases. The source of subretinal fluid is unknown. Pathological findings in one case showed that the vitreous, subarachnoid space, and subretinal space were interconnected.[37] Rarely, contractile movements of the optic disc have been observed and have been attributed to fluctuations in subretinal fluid volume and the degree of retinal separation within the confines of the excavation.[63]

Associated Features

The association of the morning glory disc anomaly with *basal encephalocele* in patients with midfacial anomalies (hypertelorism, cleft lip, cleft palate, depressed nasal bridge, midline upper lid notch) is well established.[6]

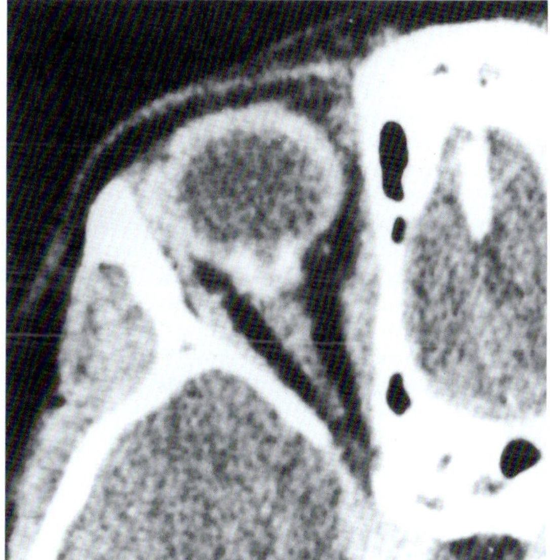

FIGURE 6-7. CT scan of morning glory disc anomaly. Note calcified, funnel-shaped enlargement of the distal optic nerve at its junction with the globe.

Clinical Assessment

Magnetic resonance imaging is indicated for patients with mid-facial anomalies and neurological deficits because these patients are at high risk for an associated basal encephalocele.

Inheritance

Generally sporadic, rarely familial.

Etiology

The embryologic defect leading to the morning glory disc anomaly is unknown.[71] Histopathological reports have unfortunately lacked clinical confirmation. Some authors have proposed that the morning glory disc anomaly is but one phenotypic form of a colobomatous (i.e., embryonic fissure-related) defect.[23] Others have interpreted the central glial tuft, vascular anomalies, and scleral defect to signify a primary mesodermal abnormality. Dempster et al. have attempted to reconcile these views by proposing that the basic defect is mesodermal but that some clinical features of the defect may result from a dynamic imbalance between the relative growth of mesoderm and ectoderm.[23]

Pollock has proposed that the initial embryologic defect leading to the development of the morning glory disc anomaly is an abnormal funnel-shaped enlargement of the distal optic stalk at its junction with the primitive optic vesicle.[63] When this occurs, invagination of the optic vesicle leads to formation of the embryonic fissure that extends from the newly formed optic cup into the expanded distal optic stalk. Closure of the embryonic fissure occurs normally, but because of the increased dimensions of the distal optic stalk, this process of closure fails to obliterate the space within the distal stalk, resulting in a persistent excavated defect at the site of entry of the optic nerve into the eye. According to this hypothesis, glial and vascular abnormalities develop later in embryogenesis and reflect abnormal development of mesodermal elements in a setting of primary neuroectodermal dysgenesis.[63]

Treatment

Superimposed amblyopia should be treated with a trial of occlusion therapy. Patients with a basal encephalocele should be evaluated for surgical repair.

Prognosis

Most patients have vision less than 20/200, although cases with 20/20 vision and others with no light perception have been reported.

OPTIC DISC COLOBOMA

Incidence

Unknown.

Clinical Features

In optic disc coloboma, a sharply delimited, glistening white, bowl-shaped excavation occupies an enlarged optic disc (Fig. 6-8).

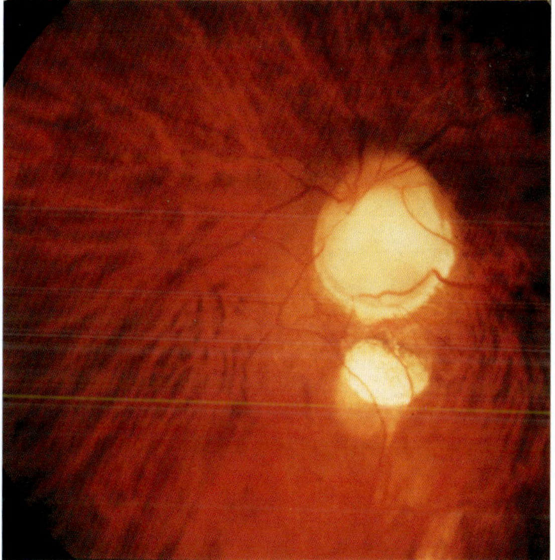

FIGURE 6-8. Optic disc coloboma. The disc is enlarged, and a white excavation is contained within the inferior aspect of the disc. The retinal vessels line the margins of the excavation as they emerge, but are otherwise normal in configuration. A small, discrete retinochoroidal coloboma is seen below the disc. Note absence of peripapillary pigment disturbance. (Courtesy of Dr. S.C. Pollock)

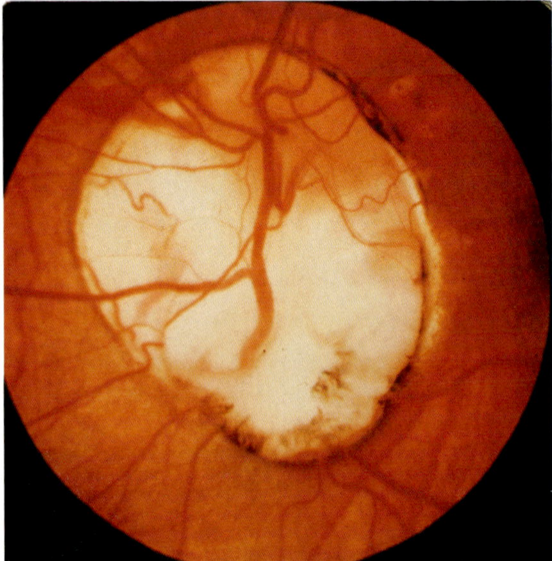

FIGURE 6-9. Optic disc coloboma. The superior disc substance is spared. The inferior aspect of the disc appears as a white excavation that merges into a retinochoroidal coloboma. (Courtesy of Dr. K. Packo)

The excavation is decentered inferiorly, so that the superior neuroretinal rim is often spared, reflecting the position of the embryonic fissure relative to the primitive epithelial papilla.[63] In some instances, the entire disc is excavated, but the colobomatous nature of the defect can still be appreciated ophthalmoscopically because the excavation is deeper inferiorly. The defect may extend further inferiorly to involve the adjacent choroid and retina (Fig. 6-9), in which case microphthalmia is frequently present.[26] Iris and ciliary colobomas often coexist. Histopathological examination in optic disc coloboma has demonstrated the presence of smooth muscle strands oriented concentrically around the distal optic nerve.[73] This pathological finding accounts for the contractility observed clinically in rare cases of optic disc coloboma. Visual acuity may be mildly or severely decreased and is difficult to predict from the optic disc appearance. Unilateral and bilateral optic disc colobomas occur with approximately equal frequency. Magnetic resonance imaging shows hypoplasia of the ipsilateral intracranial optic nerve, corresponding to the inferior segmental hypoplasia observed ophthalmoscopically.[7]

Natural History

Isolated optic disc colobomas are prone to develop serous macular detachments (in contrast to the rhegmatogenous retinal detachments that complicate retinochoroidal colobomas).[47]

Associated Features

Ocular colobomas may also be accompanied by multiple systemic abnormalities in a number of conditions such as the CHARGE association, Walker–Warburg syndrome, Goltz focal dermal hypoplasia, Goldenhar's sequence, basal encephalocele, and linear sebaceous nevus syndrome.[59]

Clinical Assessment

Patients with ocular colobomas should be evaluated for associated genetic syndromes. Family members should be examined to identify subclinical cases of ocular colobomas and establish autosomal dominant inheritance.

Inheritance

As with all ocular colobomas, optic disc colobomas may arise sporadically or be inherited in an autosomal dominant fashion.[64]

Etiology

Optic disc coloboma results from incomplete or abnormal coaptation of the proximal end of the embryonic fissure (also see Chapter 1).

Treatment

Superimposed amblyopia should be treated with a trial of occlusion therapy.

Prognosis

Visual acuity may be mildly or severely decreased and is difficult to predict from the optic disc appearance.

PERIPAPILLARY STAPHYLOMA

Incidence

Extremely rare.

Clinical Features

Peripapillary staphyloma is an extremely rare, usually unilateral, anomaly in which a deep fundus excavation surrounds the optic disc. The disc is seen at the bottom of the excavated defect and appears normal or nearly so (Fig. 6-10). The walls and margin of the defect may show atrophic pigmentary changes in the retinal pigment epithelium (RPE) and choroid. Unlike the morning glory optic disc, however, there is no central glial tuft

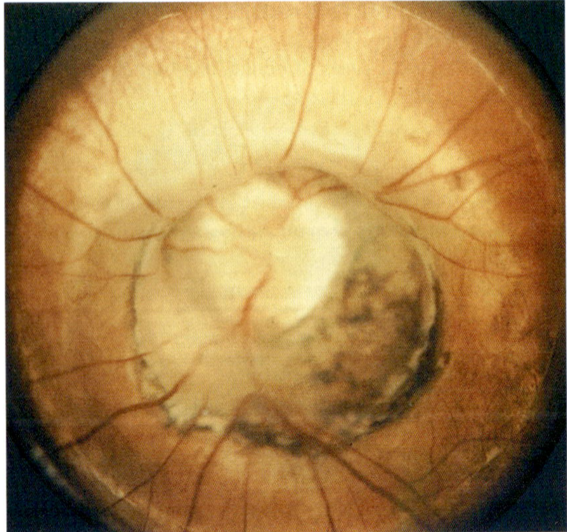

FIGURE 6-10. Peripapillary staphyloma. A relatively normal disc is seen within the recess of a deep peripapillary excavation. The normal optic disc appearance, absence of vascular anomalies, absence of a central glial tuft, and depth of the lesion distinguish this condition from the morning glory optic disc. (From Apple DJ, Rabb MF, Walsh PM. Congenital anomalies of the optic disc. Surv Ophthalmol 1982;27:3–41, with permission.[1])

TABLE 6-2. Ophthalmoscopic Findings That Distinguish Isolated Optic Disc Coloboma from Morning Glory Disc Anomaly.

Isolated optic disc coloboma	*Morning glory disc anomaly*
Excavation inferiorly decentered and contained within the disc	Disc contained centrally within the excavation; radial retinal folds
No central glial tuft	Central glial bouquet
Minimal if any peripapillary pigment disturbance	Marked peripapillary pigment disturbance
Normal retinal vasculature outside of colobomas; other ocular colobomas	Anomalous retinal vasculature

overlying the disc, and the retinal vascular pattern is normal, apart from reflecting the essential contour of the lesion. In peripapillary staphyloma, the excavation surrounding the disc is much deeper than in the morning glory disc anomaly. Several cases of contractile peripapillary staphyloma have been reported.[45]

Visual acuity may be mildly or severely decreased. Affected eyes are usually slightly myopic, although high myopia has been reported in isolated cases.[76] Eyes with decreased vision frequently have centrocecal scotomas. Although peripapillary staphyloma, morning glory disc anomaly, and optic disc coloboma are clinically and embryologically distinct, these conditions have often been confused in the literature. Tables 6-2, 6-3, and 6-4 contrast ophthalmoscopic features and associated findings that distinguish these three entities.

Associated Features

Rarely associated with basal encephalocele in patients with midfacial anomalies.[33]

TABLE 6-3. Associated Findings That Distinguish Isolated Optic Disc Coloboma from Morning Glory Disc Anomaly.

Isolated optic disc coloboma	*Morning glory disc anomaly*
Associated colobomas	No associated colobomas
Bilaterality common	Bilaterality rare
May be familial	Rarely familial
Associated with coloboma syndromes	No association with coloboma syndromes
Associated with basal encephalocele: rare	Associated with basal encephalocele

TABLE 6-4. Ophthalmoscopic Findings That Distinguish Peripapillary Staphyloma from Morning Glory Disc Anomaly.

Peripapillary staphyloma	*Morning glory disc anomaly*
Deep cup-shaped excavation	Relatively shallow funnel-shaped excavation
Relatively normal, well-defined optic disc	Anomalous poorly defined optic disc
Absence of glial and vascular alterations	Central glial bouquet; anomalous vascular pattern; retinal folds

Natural History

Several cases of contractile peripapillary staphyloma have been reported.[45]

Clinical Assessment

Magnetic resonance imaging is indicated for patients with midfacial anomalies because these patients are at risk for an associated basal encephalocele.[33]

Inheritance

Usually sporadic.

Etiology

The relatively normal appearance of the optic disc and retinal vessels in peripapillary staphyloma suggests that the development of these structures is complete before the onset of the staphylomatous process.[63] The clinical features of peripapillary staphyloma are consistent with diminished peripapillary structural support, perhaps resulting from incomplete differentiation of sclera from posterior neural crest cells in the fifth month of gestation. Staphyloma formation presumably occurs when establishment of normal intraocular pressure leads to herniation of unsupported ocular tissues through the defect. Thus, peripapillary staphyloma and the morning glory disc anomaly appear to be pathogenetically distinct both in timing of the insult (5 months gestation versus 6 to 8 weeks gestation), as well as the embryologic site of structural dysgenesis (posterior sclera versus distal optic stalk).

Treatment

Superimposed amblyopia should be treated with a trial of occlusion therapy. Patients with a basal encephalocele should be evaluated for surgical repair.

Prognosis

Visual acuity may be mildly or severely decreased.

MEGALOPAPILLA

Incidence

Unknown. A high prevalence of megalopapilla has been observed in natives of the Marshall Islands.[51]

Clinical Features

Megalopapilla is a condition in which the optic disc diameter is abnormally large (greater than 2.1 mm).[16,25,68] This finding is often associated with an increased cup-to-disc ratio (Fig. 6-11), and affected patients often are evaluated for normal-tension

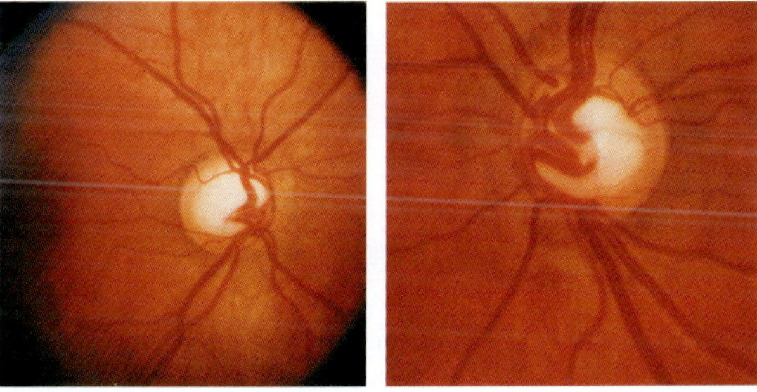

FIGURE 6-11A,B. Megalopapilla. (**A**) The right optic disc is enlarged with a large cup. Unlike glaucoma, the cup is horizontally oval with an intact neuroretinal rim, and there is no nasalization of vessels as they emerge from the disc. (**B**) Left optic disc from the same patient under higher magnification shows similar appearance.

glaucoma. In megalopapilla, however, the optic cup is round or horizontally oval, and there is no vertical notching or encroachment. Thus, despite the increased cup-to-disc ratio, the quotient of horizontal to vertical cup to disc ratio is normal, in contradistinction to the decreased quotient that characterizes glaucomatous optic atrophy.[41] Cilioretinal arteries are seen more commonly in large optic discs.[41] Unilateral cases of megalopapilla appear to be more common than bilateral cases.[54]

Visual acuity is often normal, but it may be slightly decreased in some cases. Visual fields are usually normal except for blind spot enlargement, allowing the examiner to effectively rule out low-tension glaucoma or compressive optic atrophy. Aside from glaucoma, the differential diagnosis of megalopapilla includes orbital optic glioma, which can rarely cause an acquired progressive optic disc enlargement.[29]

Associated Features

Generally none. There is one report of a basal encephalocele in a child with megalopapilla.

Clinical Assessment

Although there is one report of basal encephalocele in a child with megalopapilla,[28] neuroimaging is unwarranted unless midline facial anomalies (hypertelorism, cleft palate, cleft lip, depressed nasal bridge) coexist.

Inheritance

Usually sporadic.

Etiology

Pathogenetically, some cases of megalopapilla may simply represent a statistical variant of normal while other cases may result from altered axonal migration, as evidenced by a report of megalopapilla in a child with basal encephalocele.[28]

Treatment

Superimposed amblyopia should be treated with a trial of occlusion therapy.

Prognosis

Visual acuity is often normal, but it may be mildly decreased in some cases.

OPTIC PIT

Incidence

Unknown.

Clinical Features

An optic pit is a round or oval, gray, white, or yellowish depression in the optic disc (Fig. 6-12). Optic pits commonly involve

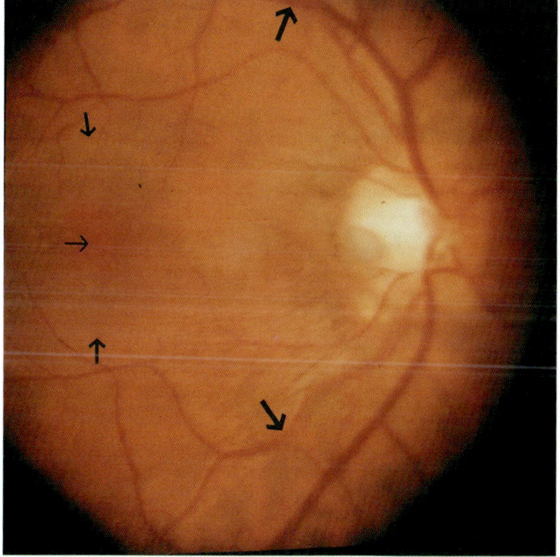

FIGURE 6-12. Optic pit with associated retinoschisis cavity (*large thick arrows*), outer layer detachment (*small thick arrows*), and macular hole (*small thin arrow*). From Lincoff H, Lopez R, Kressig I, et al. Retinoschisis associated with optic nerve pits. Arch Ophthalmol 1988;106:61–67, with permission.[48]

the temporal optic disc but may be situated in any sector.[16] Temporally located optic pits are often accompanied by adjacent peripapillary pigment epithelial changes. A cilioretinal artery is found in 59% of eyes with optic pits. Although optic pits are typically unilateral, bilateral pits are identified in 15% of cases.[16] In unilateral cases, the involved disc is slightly larger than the normal disc. Acquired optic pits have been documented in low-tension glaucoma.[40]

Natural History

Approximately 45% of eyes with congenital optic pits develop serous macular elevations. Until recently, these elevations were thought to represent serous retinal detachments. Lincoff et al. have proposed that careful serial stereoscopic examination of the macula demonstrates the following progression of events[48]:

1. An inner layer retinoschisis cavity initially forms in direct communication with the optic pit.
2. An outer layer macular hole develops beneath the boundaries of the retinoschisis cavity.
3. An outer layer retinal detachment develops around the macular hole (presumably from influx of fluid from the retinoschisis cavity). This outer layer detachment ophthalmoscopically can be mistaken for a pigment epithelial detachment, but it does not hyperfluoresce on fluorescein angiography.
4. The outer layer detachment eventually enlarges and obliterates the retinoschisis cavity. At this stage, it becomes clinically indistinguishable from a primary serous macular detachment.

Figures 6-12 and 6-13 depict the retinal changes that take place in the evolution of optic pit-associated macular detachment.

Optic pit-associated macular retinoschisis/detachments generally occur in the third and fourth decade of life. The risk of an eye developing a retinoschisis/detachment is greater with large pits and with temporally located pits.[17] Laser photocoagulation to block the flow of fluid from the optic pit to the macula has been largely unsuccessful, perhaps owing to the inability of laser photocoagulation to seal a retinoschisis cavity. The combination of internal gas tamponade, vitrectomy, and laser photocoagulation has been shown to improve acuity by displacing subretinal fluid away from the macula.[49,53]

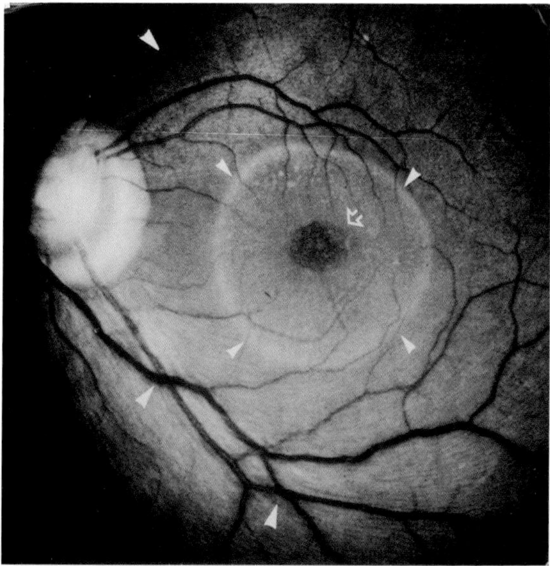

FIGURE 6-13. Optic pit with retinoschisis cavity (*large arrowheads*), macular hole (*open arrowhead*), and outer layer sensory detachment (*small arrowheads*). (Courtesy of Dr. H. Lincoff)

The source of intraretinal fluid is controversial. Possible sources include (1) vitreous cavity via the pit, (2) the subarachnoid space, (3) blood vessels at the base of the pit, and (4) choroidal blood vessels.[16] Optic pits do not generally leak fluorescein, and there is no extension of fluorescein into the subretinal space toward the macula.[1] In collie dogs, active flow of fluid from the vitreous cavity through the pit to the subretinal space has been demonstrated.[18] This mechanism has never been conclusively demonstrated in humans.

Visual acuity is typically normal in the absence of subretinal fluid. Visual field defects are variable and frequently do not correlate predictably with the location of the pit.[1] Histologically, the lamina cribrosa is defective in the area of the pit. Retinal fibers descend into the pit then reemerge before entering the optic nerve. Some optic pits extend into the subarachnoid space.

Clinical Evaluation

Ophthalmologic examination to detect associated retinoschisis/detachment.

Inheritance

Generally sporadic. Rarely familial, with autosomal dominant inheritance.[67]

Etiology

The pathogenesis of optic pits is unclear. Some authors believe that they represent the mildest variant in the spectrum of optic disc colobomas[1]; they substantiate this by pointing out that optic pits and colobomas have occurred together in rare patients (Fig. 6-14). Problems with this putative mechanism include the following:

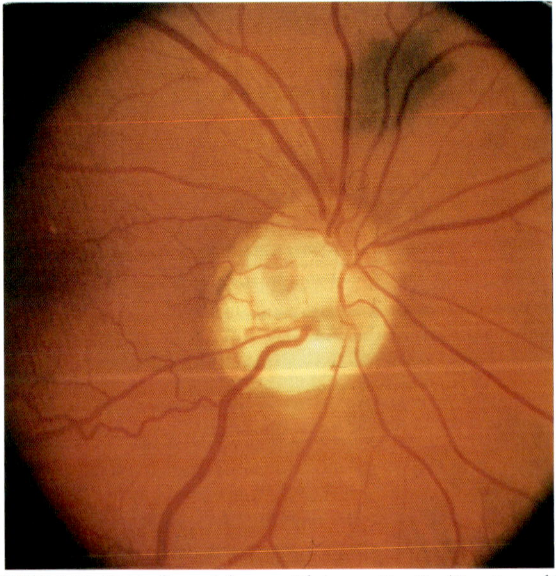

FIGURE 6-14. Optic disc coloboma with two optic pits. (Courtesy of Dr. S.C. Pollock)

1. Optic pits often occur in locations unrelated to the embryonic fissure.
2. Optic pits are usually unilateral, sporadic, and unassociated with systemic anomalies. Colobomas are bilateral as often as unilateral, commonly autosomal dominant, and may be associated with a variety of multisystem disorders.
3. Optic pits do not accompany iris or retinal colobomas.

While it is true that colobomas may contain focal crater-like deformations that resemble optic pits, and that the distinction between an inferiorly located pit and a small optic disc coloboma can at times be difficult, there appears to be sufficient evidence to conclude that most optic pits are fundamentally distinct from colobomas in their pathogenesis. The presence of one or more cilioretinal arteries emerging from the majority of optic pits suggests that these two findings must somehow be pathogenetically related.

Treatment

Associated macular retinoschisis/detachments may be treated as noted previously.

Prognosis

Visual acuity is typically normal in the absence of subretinal fluid. Approximately 45% of eyes with optic pits develop serous macular elevations.

CONGENITAL TILTED DISC SYNDROME

Incidence

Unknown.

Clinical Features

In the tilted disc syndrome, the superotemporal optic disc is elevated and the inferonasal disc is posteriorly displaced, resulting in an oval-appearing optic disc, with its long axis obliquely oriented (Fig. 6-15). This configuration is accompanied by situs

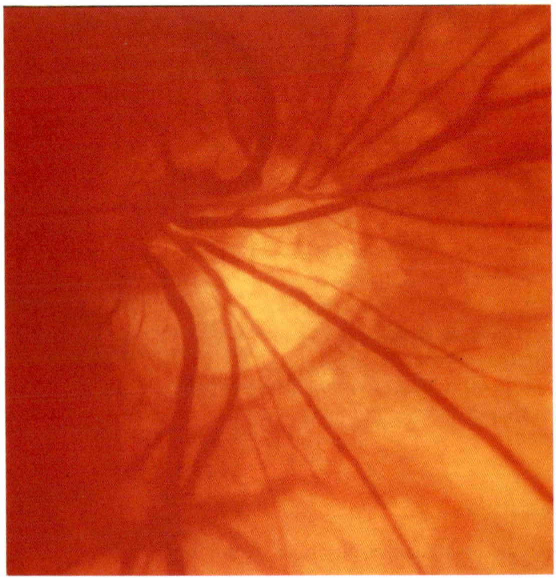

FIGURE 6-15. Congenitally tilted right optic disc. The disc substance appears obliquely oval. There is elevation of the superonasal disc and posterior displacement of the inferonasal disc. Note inferonasal peripapillary crescent, albinotic appearance confined to the inferonasal retina, and situs inversus of the vessels as they emerge from the disc. (Courtesy of Dr. W.F. Hoyt)

inversus of the retinal vessels, congenital inferonasal conus, thinning of the inferonasal RPE and choroid, and bitemporal hemianopia.[74] The anomalous optic disc appearance is secondary to a posterior ectasia of the inferonasal fundus and optic disc. Because of the regional fundus ectasia, affected patients have myopic astigmatism, with the plus axis oriented parallel to the ectasia.

Familiarity with the tilted disc syndrome is crucial because affected patients may present with bitemporal hemianopia and optic disc elevation.[1] The bitemporal hemianopia, which is typically incomplete and involves the superior quadrants, represents a refractive scotoma, secondary to regional myopia localized to the inferonasal retina (Figs. 6-15, 6-16). Unlike the visual field loss accompanying chiasmal lesions, the field defects seen in the tilted disc syndrome do not respect the vertical meridian on careful Goldmann kinetic perimetry. Furthermore, large and small isopters are fairly normal, whereas medium-sized isopters are selectively constricted, owing to the marked ectasia of the midperipheral fundus (Fig. 6-17). Repeating the Goldmann visual field after placement of a −1.50 to −3.00 lens over the patient's glasses will often eliminate the visual field abnormality, confirming the refractive nature of the defect. In some cases retinal sensitivity may be decreased in the area of the ectasia, so that the defect persists to some degree despite appropriate refractive correction.[74] It should be emphasized, however, that if a patient with the tilted disc syndrome has a bitemporal hemianopia that respects the vertical meridian, intracranial MRI is mandatory because congenitally tilted discs have rarely been reported in patients with both congenital and acquired suprasellar tumors.[42,58,69]

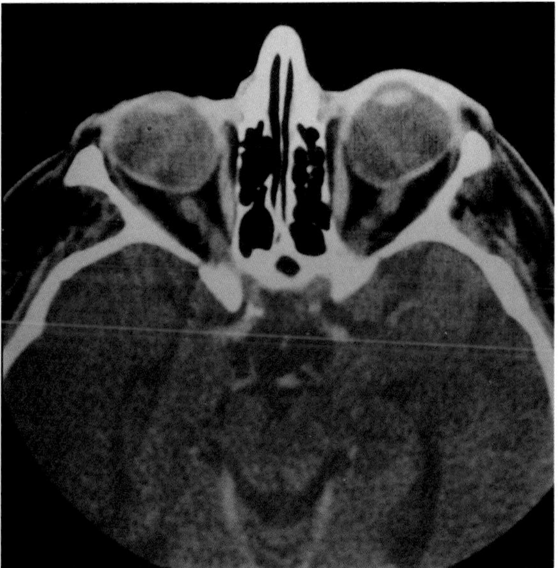

FIGURE 6-16. Axial CT scan through lower aspect of globes. The nasal aspect of both globes protrudes posteriorly.

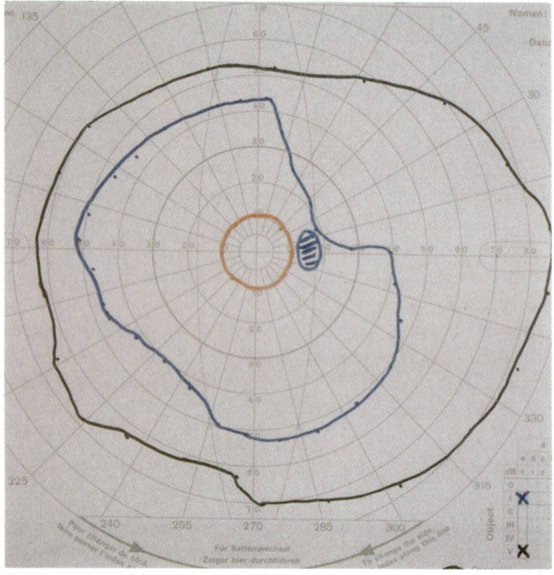

FIGURE 6-17. Goldmann visual field (right eye) in a patient with congenitally tilted discs. A superotemporal visual field defect is confined to the midperipheral isopter and does not respect the vertical meridian.

Associated Conditions

Congenitally tilted discs have rarely been reported in patients with both congenital and acquired suprasellar tumors.[42,58] In patients with nystagmus, the finding of tilted discs should suggest the possibility of X-linked congenital stationary night blindness.[32]

Clinical Assessment

Patients with tilted optic discs and visual field deficits that do not respect the vertical meridian do not require neuroimaging. However, patients with a bitemporal hemianopia that respects the vertical meridian require cranial MRI to detect suprasellar tumors, which are rarely associated with congenitally tilted discs as noted previously.[42,58,69] Patients with nystagmus should be evaluated with an electroretinogram to detect congenital stationary night blindness.[32]

Inheritance

Usually sporadic.

Etiology

The cause of the condition is unknown, but the inferonasal or inferior location of the excavation is at least vaguely suggestive of a pathogenic relationship to retinochoroidal coloboma.[1]

Prognosis

Visual acuity is typically normal.

CONGENITAL OPTIC DISC PIGMENTATION

Incidence

Unknown.

Clinical Features

Congenital optic disc pigmentation is a condition in which melanin deposition anterior to or within the lamina cribrosa imparts a gray appearance to the optic disc (Fig. 6-18). True congenital optic disc pigmentation is extremely rare, but it has been described in a child with an interstitial deletion of chromosome 17[10] and in *Aicardi's syndrome.*[70] Congenital optic disc pigmentation is compatible with good visual acuity but may be associated with coexistent optic disc anomalies that decrease vision.

Most cases of gray optic discs are not caused by congenital optic disc pigmentation. For reasons that are poorly understood, optic discs of infants with delayed visual maturation and albinism may have a diffuse gray tint when viewed ophthalmoscopically (Fig. 6-19). In these conditions, the gray tint disappears within the first year of life without visible pigment migration. Beauvieux observed gray optic discs in premature infants and albinotic infants who were apparently blind but who later developed good vision as the gray color disappeared.[4,5]

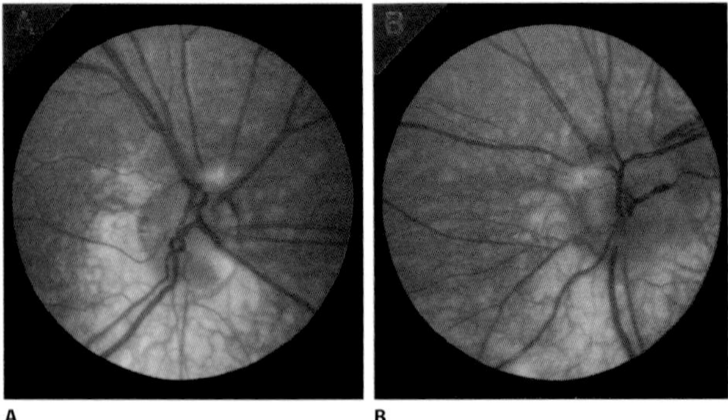

A B

FIGURE 6-18A,B. Congenital optic disc pigmentation. **(A)** Right optic disc. A circular area of patchy pigment surrounds a severely hypoplastic, elevated, central tuft of optic nerve substance, producing a gray optic disc. Arteries and veins overlying the disc are anomalous. **(B)** Left optic disc. There is a uniform, gray discoloration of the optic disc. The peripheral disc appears elevated. An anomalous venous trunk extends along the temporal disc at 2 o'clock. (From Brodsky MC, Buckley EG, McConkie-Rosell A. The case of the gray optic disc. Surv Ophthalmol 1989;33:367–372, with permission.[10])

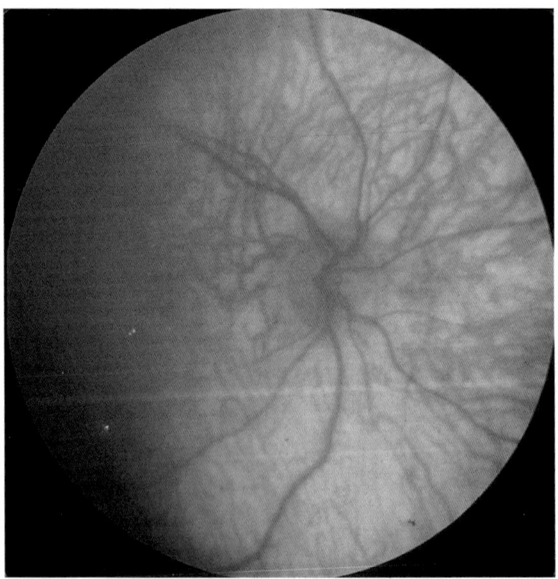

FIGURE 6-19. Diffuse gray cast to the optic disc in an infant with albinism.

Beauvieux attributed the gray appearance of these neonatal discs to delayed optic nerve myelination with preservation of the "embryonic tint." However, gray optic discs may also be seen in normal neonates and are therefore a nonspecific finding of little diagnostic value, except when accompanied by other clinical signs of delayed visual maturation or albinism.

Patients with "optically gray optic discs" have unfortunately been lumped together, in many reference books, with patients who have congenital optic disc pigmentation. These two conditions can usually be distinguished ophthalmoscopically, because melanin deposition in true congenital optic disc pigmentation is often discrete, irregular, and granular in appearance.

Associated Features

Congenital optic disc pigmentation has been described in a child with an interstitial deletion of chromosome 17[10] and in Aicardi's syndrome.[70]

AICARDI'S SYNDROME

Incidence

Unknown.

Clinical Features

Aicardi's syndrome is a cerebroretinal disorder of unknown etiology. The salient clinical features of Aicardi's syndrome are infantile spasms, agenesis of the corpus callosum, and a pathognomonic optic disc appearance consisting of multiple depigmented "chorioretinal lacunae" clustered around the disc[19,34] (Fig. 6-20). Histologically, chorioretinal lacunae consist of well-circumscribed, full-thickness defects limited to the RPE and choroid. The overlying retina remains intact but is often histologically abnormal.[19]

Congenital optic disc anomalies including optic disc coloboma, optic nerve hypoplasia, and congenital optic disc pigmentation may accompany chorioretinal lacunae. Other ocular abnormalities include microphthalmos, retrobulbar cyst,

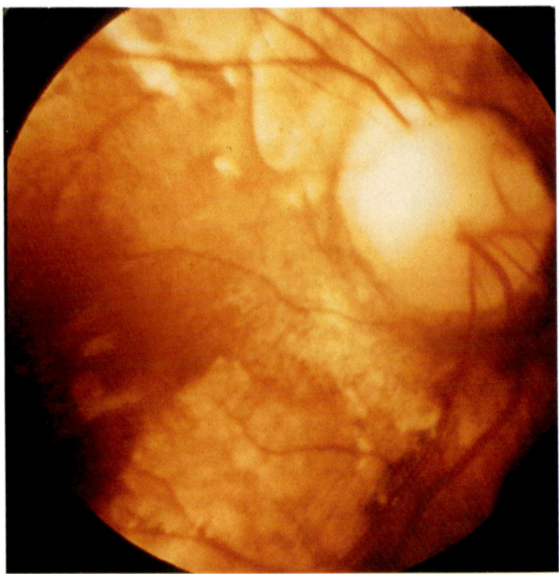

FIGURE 6-20. Aicardi's syndrome. A cluster of peripapillary lacunae surround an enlarged, anomalous right optic disc. (Courtesy of Dr. J.R. Buncic)

pseudoglioma, retinal detachment, macular scars, cataract, pupillary membranes, iris synechiae, and iris colobomas.

Associated Features

The most common systemic findings associated with Aicardi's syndrome are vertebral malformations (fused vertebrae, scoliosis, spina bifida) and costal malformations (absent ribs, fused or bifurcated ribs). Other systemic associations include muscular hypotonia, microencephaly, dysmorphic facies, and auricular anomalies. The intriguing association between choroid plexus papilloma and Aicardi's syndrome has been documented in five patients. Severe mental retardation is almost invariable.[19]

Magnetic resonance abnormalities in Aicardi's syndrome include agenesis of the corpus callosum, cortical migration anomalies (pachygyria, polymicrogyria, cortical heterotopias), and multiple structural CNS malformations (cerebral hemispheric asymmetry, Dandy–Walker variant, colpocephaly, midline arachnoid cysts).[3,31] An overlap between Aicardi's syndrome and septo-optic dysplasia has been recognized in several patients.[19]

Clinical Assessment

Magnetic resonance imaging is indicated to detect associated CNS abnormalities. Neurological assessment and electroencephalogram are indicated to evaluate patients for characteristic seizure activity.

Inheritance

Aicardi's syndrome is thought to result from an X-linked mutational event that is lethal in males.[24,56] Chevrie and Aicardi have suggested that all cases of Aicardi's syndrome represent fresh gene mutations because no cases of affected siblings have been reported.[20] However, a recent report of Aicardi's syndrome in two sisters challenges the notion that Aicardi's syndrome always results from a de novo mutation in the affected infant and indicates that germline mosaicism for the mutation may be an additional mechanism of inheritance.[55]

Etiology

Although early infectious CNS insults can lead to severe CNS anomalies, tests for infective agents have been consistently negative. No teratogenic drug or other toxin has yet been associated with Aicardi's syndrome. Based on the pattern of cerebroretinal malformations on Aicardi's syndrome, it is speculated that an insult to the CNS must take place between the fourth and eighth weeks of gestation.[20]

Treatment

Medications for associated seizures are used.

Prognosis

Vision is variable. Systemic prognosis is dependent on associated malformations and seizure activity.

V- OR TONGUE-SHAPED INFRAPAPILLARY DEPIGMENTATION

Incidence

Five cases reported.

Clinical Features

A discrete infrapapillary zone of V- or tongue-shaped retinochoroidal depigmentation has been described in five patients with dysplastic optic discs and transsphenoidal encephalocele.[14] These juxtapapillary defects differ from typical retinochoroidal colobomas, which widen inferiorly and are not associated with basal encephalocele. Unlike the typical retinochoroidal coloboma, this distinct juxtapapillary defect is associated with minimal scleral excavation and no visible disruption in the integrity of the overlying retina.

Associated Features

Transsphenoidal encephalocele as previously noted.

Inheritance

Usually sporadic.

Clinical Assessment

In patients with anomalous optic discs, the finding of this V- or tongue-shaped infrapapillary retinochoroidal anomaly should prompt neuroimaging to look for transsphenoidal encephalocele.[14]

Etiology

Unknown.

PAPILLORENAL SYNDROME

Incidence

Unknown. Twenty-two families are reported in the literature.[60] This syndrome may be underrecognized as patients are often misdiagnosed as having glaucoma, colobomas, or atypical morning glory anomalies.

Clinical Features

Ophthalmoscopically, the disc appears excavated with multiple peripheral cilioretinal arteries.[60] The central retinal vasculature is often absent or rudimentary. When central retinal vessels are observed ophthalmoscopically, Doppler ultrasonography often reveals entry of these central vessels into the nerve near the globe, indicating their origin as aberrant cilioretinal vessels. Patients often have superonasal visual field defects that correspond with inferotemporal areas of hypoplastic retina with anomalous retinal and choroidal perfusion.[60] Peripapillary serous retinal detachments may occur.

Associated Features

Associated renal anomalies include renal hypoplasia, renal hypertension, renal failure, and recurrent pyelonephritis.[60] Renal disease may be subclinical.

Etiology

Unknown. Parsa et al.[60] hypothesized that a primary deficiency in vascular development compromises growth of the ocular and renal circulations.

Inheritance

Autosomal dominant. Some pedigrees harbor the PAX2 mutation.[60]

Clinical Assessment

Renal function studies followed by Doppler spectral studies of renal blood flow if conventional studies are normal.[60] Renal angiography may also be indicated.[60]

Treatment

Prophylactic reduction of systemic blood pressure should be considered if resistance to renal blood flow is abnormally high.[60]

Prognosis

Unknown.

Acknowledgment. This work was supported in part by a grant from Research to Prevent Blindness, Inc.

References

1. Apple DJ, Rabb MF, Walsh PM. Congenital anomalies of the optic disc. Surv Ophthalmol 1982;27:3–41.
2. Arslanian SA, Rothfus WE, Foley TP, Becker DJ. Hormonal, metabolic, and neuroradiologic abnormalities associated with septo-optic dysplasia. Acta Endocrinol 1984;107:282–288.
3. Baieri P, Markl A, Thelen M, et al. MR imaging in Aicardi syndrome. ANJR 1988;9:805–806.
4. Beauvieux J. La cecite apparente chez le nouveau-ne: la psuedoatrophie grise du nerf optique. Arch Ophthalmol (Paris) 1947;7:241–249.
5. Beauvieux J. La pseudo-atrophie optique des nouveaunes (dysgenesie myelinique des voies optiques). Ann Ocul (Paris) 1926;163:881–921.
6. Beyer WB, Quencer RM, Osher RH. Morning glory syndrome: a functional analysis including fluorescein angiography, ultrasonography, and computerized tomography. Ophthalmology 1982;89:1362–1364.
7. Brodsky MC. Magnetic resonance imaging of colobomatous optic hypoplasia. Br J Ophthalmol 1999;83:755–756.
8. Brodsky MC. Periventricular leukomalacia: an intracranial cause of pseudoglaucomatous cupping. Arch Ophthalmol 2001;119:626.
9. Brodsky MC. Septo-optic dysplasia: a reappraisal. Semin Ophthalmol 1991;6:227–232.
10. Brodsky MC, Buckley EG, McConkie-Rosell A. The case of the gray optic disc! Surv Ophthalmol 1989,33:367–372.
11. Brodsky MC, Conte FA, Taylor D, et al. Sudden death in septo-optic dysplasia. Report of 5 cases. Arch Ophthalmol 1997;115:66–70.
12. Brodsky MC, Glasier CM. Optic nerve hypoplasia: clinical significance of associated central nervous system abnormalities on magnetic resonance imaging. Arch Ophthalmol 1993;111:66–74.
13. Brodsky MC, Glasier CM, Pollock SC, et al. Optic nerve hypoplasia: identification by magnetic resonance imaging. Arch Ophthalmol 1990;108:562–567.
14. Brodsky MC, Hoyt WF, Hoyt CS, et al. Atypical retinochoroidal coloboma in patients with dysplastic optic discs and transsphenoidal encephalocele. Arch Ophthalmol 1995;113:624–628.

15. Brodsky MC, Schroeder GT, Ford R. Superior segmental optic hypoplasia in identical twins. J Clin Neuroophthalmol 1993;13:152–154.
16. Brown G, Tasman W. Congenital anomalies of the optic disc. New York: Grune & Stratton, 1983.
17. Brown GC, Shields JA, Goldberg RE. Congenital pits of the optic nerve head. II. Clinical studies in humans. Ophthalmology 1980;87: 51–65.
18. Brown GC, Shields JA, Patty BE, et al. Congenital pits of the optic nerve head. I. Experimental studies in collie dogs. Arch Ophthalmol 1979;97:1341–1344.
19. Carney SH, Brodsky MC, Good WV, et al. Aicardi syndrome: more than meets the eye. Surv Ophthalmol 1993;37:419–424.
20. Chevrie JJ, Aicardi J. The Aicardi syndrome. In: Pedley TA, Meldrum BS (eds) Recent advances in epilepsy. New York: Churchill Livingston, 1986.
21. Costin G, Murphree AL. Hypothalamic-pituitary dysfunction in children with optic nerve hypoplasia. AJDC (Am J Dis Child) 1985;139:249–254.
22. De Morsier G. Etudes sur les dysraphies cranio-encephaliques. III. Agenesis du septum lucidum avec malformation du tractus optique. La dysplasie septo-optique. Schweitz Arch Neurol Psychiatry 1956; 77:267–292.
23. Dempster AG, Lee WR, Forrester JV, et al. The 'morning glory syndrome': a mesodermal defect? Ophthalmologica 1983;187:222–230.
24. Donnenfield AE, Packer RJ, Zackai EH, et al. Clinical, cytogenetic and pedigree findings in 18 cases of Aicardi syndrome. Am J Med Genet 1989;32:461–467.
25. Franceschetti A, Bock RH. Megalopapilla. A new congenital anomaly. Am J Ophthalmol 1950;33:227–235.
26. Francois J. Colobomatous malformations of the ocular globe. Int Ophthalmol Clin 1968;8:797–816.
27. Frisen L, Holmegaard L. Spectrum of optic nerve hypoplasia. Br J Ophthalmol 1975;62:7–15.
28. Goldhammer Y, Smith JL. Optic nerve anomalies in basal encephalocele. Arch Ophthalmol 1975;93:115–118.
29. Grimson BS, Perry DD. Enlargement of the optic disc in childhood optic nerve tumors. Am J Ophthalmol 1984;97:627–631.
30. Haik BG, Greenstein SH, Smith ME, et al. Retinal detachment in the morning glory disc anomaly. Ophthalmology 1984;91:1638–1647.
31. Hall-Craggs MA, Harbord MG, Finn JP, et al. Aicardi syndrome: MR assessment of brain structure myelination. AJNR (Am J Neuroradiol) 1990;11:532–536.
32. Hittner HM, Borda RP, Justice J. X-linked recessive congenital stationary night blindness, myopia, and tilted discs. J Pediatr Ophthalmol Strabismus 1981;18:15–20.
33. Hodgkins P, Lees M, Lawson J, et al. Optic disc anomalies and frontonasal dysplasia. Br J Ophthalmol 1998;82:290–293.

34. Hoyt CS, Billson F, Ouvrier R, et al. Ocular features of Aicardi's syndrome. Arch Ophthalmol 1978;96:291–295.
35. Hoyt CS, Billson FA. Optic nerve hypoplasia: Changing perspectives. Aust NZ J Ophthalmol 1986;14:325–331.
36. Hoyt WF, Kaplan SL, Grumback MM, et al. Septo-optic dysplasia and pituitary dwarfism. Lancet 1970;2:893–894.
37. Irvine AR, Crawford JB, Sullivan JH. The pathogenesis of retinal detachment with morning glory disc and optic pit. Retina 1986; 6:146–150.
38. Izenberg N, Rosenblum M, Parks JS. The endocrine spectrum of septo-optic dysplasia. Clin Pediatr 1984;23:632–636.
39. Jacobson L, Hellstrom A, Flodmark O. Large cups in normal-sized optic discs: a variant of optic nerve hypoplasia in children with periventricular leukomalacia. Arch Ophthalmol 1997;115:1263–1269.
40. Javitt JC, Spaeth GL, Katz LJ, et al. Acquired pits of the optic nerve. Ophthalmology 1990;97:1038–1044.
41. Jonas JB, Zach F, Gusek GC, et al. Pseudoglaucomatous physiologic optic cups. Am J Ophthalmol 1989;107:137–144.
42. Keane JR. Suprasellar tumors and incidental optic disc anomalies: diagnostic problems in two patients with hemianopic temporal scotomas. Arch Ophthalmol 1977;2180–2183.
43. Kim RY, Hoyt WF, Lessell S, Narahara MH. Superior segmental optic hypoplasia: a sign of maternal diabetes. Arch Ophthalmol 1989;107: 1312–1315.
44. Kindler P. Morning glory syndrome: unusual congenital optic disc anomaly. Am J Ophthalmol 1970;69:376–384.
45. Kral K, Svarc D. Contractile peripapillary staphyloma. Am J Ophthalmol 1971;71:1092–1094.
46. Lambert SR, Hoyt CS, Narahara MH. Optic nerve hypoplasia. Surv Ophthalmol 1987;32:1–9.
47. Lin CCL, Tso MOM, Vygantas CM. Coloboma of optic nerve associated with serous maculopathy: a clinicopathologic correlative study. Arch Ophthalmol 1984;102:1651–1654.
48. Lincoff H, Lopez R, Kreissig I, et al. Retinoschisis associated with optic nerve pits. Arch Ophthalmol 1988;106:61–67.
49. Lincoff H, Yanuzzi L, Singerman L, et al. Improvement in visual function after displacement of the retinal elevations emanating from optic pits. Arch Ophthalmol 1993;111:1071–1079.
50. Mafee MF, Jampol LM, Langer BG, et al. Computed tomography of optic nerve colobomas, morning glory anomaly, and colobomatous cyst. Radiol Clin North Am 1987;25:693–699.
51. Maisel JM, Pearlstein CS, Adams WH, et al. Large optic discs in the Marshallese population. Am J Ophthalmol 1989;107:145–150.
52. Margalith D, Tze WJ, Jan JE. Congenital optic nerve hypoplasia with hypothalamic-pituitary dysplasia. AJDC (Am J Dis Child) 1985;139: 361–366.

53. McDonald HR, Schatz H, Johnson RN. Treatment of retinal detachment associated with optic nerve pits. Int Ophthalmol Clin 1992; 32:35–42.
54. Miller NR. Walsh and Hoyt's clinical neuro-opthalmology, 4th edn, vol I. Baltimore: Williams & Wilkins, 1982.
55. Molina JA, Mateos F, Merino M, et al. Aicardi syndrome in two sisters. J Pediatr 1980;115:282–283.
56. Neidich JA, Nussbaum RL, Packer RJ, et al. Heterogeneity of clinical severity and molecular lesions in Aicardi syndrome. J Pediatr 1990;116:911–917.
57. Novakovic P, Taylor DSI, Hoyt WF. Localizing patterns of optic nerve hypoplasia—retina to occipital lobe. Br J Ophthalmol 1988; 72:176–182.
58. Osher RH, Schatz NJ. A sinister association of the congenital tilted disc syndrome with chiasmal compression. In: Smith JL (ed) Neuro-ophthalmology focus 1980. New York: Masson, 1979.
59. Pagon RA. Ocular coloboma. Surv Ophthalmol 1981;25:223–236.
60. Parsa CF, Silva ED, Sundin OH, et al. Redefining papillorenal syndrome: an underdiagnosed cause of ocular and renal morbidity. Ophthalmology 2001;108:738–749.
61. Phillips PH, Speer C, Brodsky MC. Magnetic resonance diagnosis of congenital hypopituitarism in children with optic nerve hypoplasia. J Am Assoc Pediatr Ophthalmol Strabismus 2001;5(5):275–280.
62. Pollack JA, Newton JH, Hoyt WF. Transsphenoidal and transethmoidal encephaloceles: a review of clinical and roentigen features in 8 cases. Radiology 1968;90:442–453.
63. Pollock S. The morning glory disc anomaly: contractile movement, classification, and embryogenesis. Doc Ophthalmol 1988;65:439–460.
64. Savell J, Cook JR. Optic nerve colobomas if autosomal dominant heredity. Arch Ophthalmol 1976;94:395–400.
65. Scheie HG, Adler FH. Aplasia of the optic nerve. Arch Ophthalmol 1941;26:61–70.
66. Sorkin JA, Davis PC, Meacham LR, et al. Optic nerve hypoplasia: absence of posterior pituitary bright signal on magnetic resonance imaging correlates with diabetes insipidus. Am J Ophthalmol 1996; 122:717–723.
67. Stefko ST, Campochiaro P, Wang P, et al. Dominant inheritance of optic pits. Am J Ophthalmol 1997;124:112–113.
68. Streiff B. Uber Megalopapillae. Klin Monatsbl Augenheilkd 1961;139: 824–827.
69. Taylor D. Congenital tumors of the anterior visual pathways. Br J Ophthalmol 1982;66:455–463.
70. Taylor D. Pediatric ophthalmology, 1st edn. London: Blackwell, 1990.
71. Traboulsi EI, O'Neill JF. The spectrum of the so-called "morning glory disc anomaly." J Pediatr Ophthalmol Strabismus 1988;25: 93–98.

72. Williams J, Brodsky MC, Greibel M. Septo-optic dysplasia: clinical insignificance of an absent septum pellucidum. Dev Med Child Neurol 1993;35:490–501.
73. Willis R, Zimmerman LE, O'Grady R, et al. Heterotopic adipose tissue and smooth muscle in the optic disc, association with isolated colobomas. Arch Ophthalmol 1972;88:139–146.
74. Young Se, Walsh FB, Knox DL. The tilted disc syndrome. Am J Ophthalmol 1976;82:16–23.

7

Cortical Visual Impairment

Susan M. Carden and William V. Good

Cortical visual impairment (CVI) is the most common cause of bilateral visual impairment in children in the developed world.[1] In less-affluent countries, the incidence is increasing because the survival rate of premature babies is improving. As a consequence, the mortality of children with complex medical problems has begun to decline.[18] Retinopathy of prematurity (ROP) is also a major cause of visual handicap: its rate is increasing, and it may become the commonest cause of visual impairment in children. A risk factor for CVI is prematurity, which is also a risk for ROP. Thus, these two disease processes often coexist.

CVI is defined as visual impairment caused by damage to the central nervous system. Visual acuity is reduced as a result of a disease process that does not involve the ocular structures.[9]

HISTORICAL PERSPECTIVE

CVI has come into prominence recently partly because of its increasing incidence and also the greater understanding that is being developed of the pathophysiology. Whiting, Jan, and Wong first coined the term cortical visual impairment in 1985[19]; before then, the problem was referred to as cortical blindness. Cortical blindness is a term more relevant to adults who experience a devastating injury to their occipital cortices. Infants and children who experience such insults tend not to be blind but rather impaired. Their brains are still growing, and as a consequence some aspects of their vision improve over time.

INCIDENCE

Cortical visual impairment is now recognized as the most frequent cause of bilateral visual impairment in the Western world. The Blind Babies Foundation of Northern California has found that, in children under 5 years of age with visual impairment, CVI is the most prominent causative factor.[15] The Oxford Registry of Early Childhood Impairments found that nearly 30% of children with bilaterally poor vision had CVI.[16] In Liverpool (U.K.), it was found that in children with neurological disorders and visual impairment, CVI was the most common cause of poor vision.[17] A study in 1996 in the Nordic countries found that brain damage is causing an increasing number of children to have visual impairment.[18]

ETIOLOGY: PATHOPHYSIOLOGY, HISTOPATHOLOGY

The cause of CVI can be diverse: hypoxia-ischemia; congenital brain malformation (*schizencephaly*, *holoprosencephaly*, *lissencephaly*)[3]; central nervous system infection (meningitis, encephalitis); blockage of a ventriculo-peritoneal shunt; head injury, particularly that resulting from child abuse[10]; or metabolic derangements.[12]

Hypoxia-Ischemia

The most common cause of CVI is an hypoxic-ischemic event. The consequence of an hypoxic-ischemic event can best be assessed by the age at which the insult occurred. At each age level, a different area of the brain is more susceptible to damage in an hypoxic-ischemic event.

In premature babies, the *germinal matrix* is most at risk of being damaged.[6] The germinal matrix is a watershed area of the brain, but only in preterm babies. It is situated in the walls of the lateral ventricles. The optic radiations are supplied with blood from the germinal matrix, as are the long motor tracts. Thus, the preterm baby who suffers CVI is very likely to also have cerebral palsy.[1] Periventricular leukomalacia ensues after an hypoxic-ischemic event in preterm babies (Fig. 7-1).

In the term infant, an hypoxic-ischemic insult is more likely to affect the watershed area of the brain, which is now an area

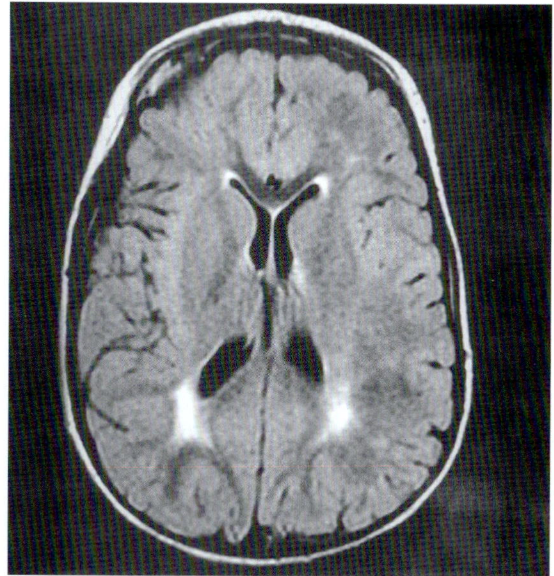

FIGURE 7-1. Preterm infant brain with periventricular leukomalacia.

including the striate cortex (see Fig. 7-2). In term children, an hypoxic-ischemic insult causing permanent CVI is much less common.

Shunt Blockage

Ventriculoperitoneal shunt blockage has been described as a cause of CVI.[4] The occipital lobes become infarcted because the posterior cerebral arteries are compressed against the edge of the tentorium.[13]

Twin Pregnancy

A risk factor for CVI is twin pregnancy.[6] Twin pregnancy increases the risk of premature birth, which is a risk factor for CVI in itself. There is an even higher chance of prematurity if the twins are monozygotic.[2] Twin–twin transfusion syndrome can occur if the twins are monozygous and also share one pla-

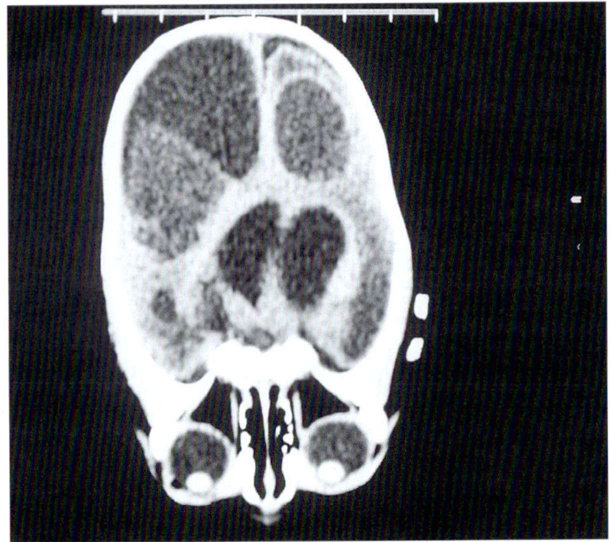

FIGURE 7-2. Term infant with multicystic encephalomalacia.

centa (monochorionic).[5] If one twin dies, then there may be an acute twin–twin transfusion of blood to the dead fetus. The surviving fetus may become hypovolemic and develop neurological abnormalities as a consequence. Emboli and thromboplastin from the dead fetus may enter the survivor's circulation and induce disseminated intravascular coagulation.[14] The developing brain is then exposed to hypoxia-ischemia.

CLINICAL FEATURES

Neurobehavioral characteristics, or mannerisms, exhibited by children with CVI are helpful in deciding the position of a lesion in the visual pathways. These behaviors tend to be adaptations to the anatomic defect.[7]

Differential Diagnosis

The differential diagnoses of CVI are varied, and include conditions in which the child appears to have poor vision but either improves later (delayed visual maturation); has a poor motor response (oculomotor apraxia); or has no apparent interest in their surroundings, as may be exhibited in autism.[9]

CLINICAL ASSESSMENT: WORKUP, EXAMINATION TECHNIQUE, LABORATORY, PATHOLOGY

The child who presents with CVI can usually be diagnosed with a clinical examination. In pure cases the ocular examination is normal. It should be remembered that ocular and cortical abnormalities can coexist. Children with CVI have poor visual function and do not exhibit eye contact. They also do not regard a face. Parents may comment that sometimes the child sees better than other times; variability in visual performance is a characteristic of CVI.

SYSTEMIC ASSOCIATIONS

Any child who is diagnosed with CVI will have an associated neurological abnormality.[11] Most children with CVI have a coexistent ocular problem.[19] An example of this is the child who is extremely premature and has a risk of developing retinopathy of prematurity. In this child, the anterior (ROP) and posterior (CVI) visual pathways are involved, causing the visual impairment.

INHERITANCE

CVI is usually the result of an insult to the developing brain, often an episode of hypoxia-ischemia. Thus inheritance is not considered to be a major factor in the causation. Nevertheless, some clinical features suggest a partial genetic cause. Some children have a remarkable recovery from a neurological insult, and this invulnerability might be genetically determined.

NATURAL HISTORY

CVI improves with time, although full, normal vision is rarely achieved.[8] It is more usual for gradual improvement to occur over months and years. Visual behavior can change from hour to hour depending on fatigue or distractibility of the child, so it is important for parents to realize that the best vision which they observe is more indicative of the child's potential.

Visual improvement after an hypoxic-ischemic event seldom regresses. Parents need not be concerned that the vision will decrease unless there is a progressive neurodegenerative disorder, or unless some other neurological event occurs that interferes with vision (e.g., intractable seizures).

TREATMENT: MEDICAL OR SURGICAL

Surgical: Indication, Technique, and Complications

Surgical treatment is seldom helpful in CVI. Exceptions include a shunt blockage that needs to be relieved or a tumor that requires resection. Cerebral edema or hemorrhage secondary to trauma may require relieving.

Medical: Specific Medication and Dose

Medical treatment for CVI is limited. In the preterm baby, the amount of oxygen delivered needs to be carefully regulated as it could affect other disease processes such as retinopathy of prematurity (ROP). Some children with CVI have epilepsy as a result of their structural brain abnormality. Caregivers sometimes believe that treating the epilepsy or treating the abnormal EEG will help vision, but this is usually not the case. If epileptic seizures are present, then they should be treated, but simply treating the EEG will not improve vision.

PROGNOSIS: OUTCOME OF TREATMENT

The prognosis is dependent on the age at which the insult was sustained and the extent of the insult. Associated neurological abnormalities are also an important factor to be considered. Rehabilitation improves outcome significantly, and it is important that the approach is multidisciplinary as the child rarely has purely an ocular disorder. The preterm infant who receives an hypoxic-ischemic insult tends not to improve as much as the term infant.[11]

In general, there is visual improvement over time with CVI. However, in prognosticating whether there will be significant improvement, it is important to note the cause of the CVI (some causes have a worse prognosis for improvement than others) and also the age of the child when the insult occurred. Involvement of the optic radiations has a worse prognosis than involvement of the striate cortex.[12] If *periventricular leukomalacia* is found on neuroimaging, the prognosis is thus poorer, as it suggests optic radiation damage. Visual recovery from CVI caused by bacterial meningitis is known to be poor.[3]

FUTURE RESEARCH

Research is focused on assessment of children with CVI as well as treatment. It is difficult to assess what a child with CVI sees. Electrophysiological tests (visual evoked potential) are helpful in indicating different qualities of sight. The use of functional magnetic resonance imaging (fMRI) in diagnosis of CVI is being investigated, but there are major limitations in children because the technique requires the subject to be alert, still, and cooperative.[8]

References

1. Ahmann P, Lazzara A, Dykes F, Brann A, Schwartz J. Intraventricular hemorrhage in the high-risk preterm infant: incidence and outcome. Ann Neurol 1980;7:118–124.
2. Benirschke K. Twin placenta in perinatal mortality. NY State J Med 1961;61:1499–1508.
3. Chen T, Weinberg M, Catalano R, Simon J, Wagle W. Development of object vision in infants with permanent cortical visual impairment. Am J Ophthalmol 1992;114:575–578.
4. Connelly M, Jan J, Cochrane D. Rapid recovery from cortical visual impairment following correction of prolonged shunt malfunction in congenital hydrocephalus. Arch Neurol 1991;48:956–957.
5. Galea P, Scott J, Goel K. Feto-fetal transfusion syndrome. Arch Dis Child 1982;57:781–783.
6. Good W, Brodsky M, Angtuaco T, Ferriero M, Stephens D III, Khakoo M. Cortical visual impairment caused by twin pregnancy. Am J Ophthalmol 1996;122:709–716.
7. Good W, Hoyt C. Behavioral correlates of poor vision in children. Int Ophthalmol Clin 1989;29:57–59.
8. Good W, Jan J, Burden S, Skoczenski A, Candy R. Recent advances in cortical visual impairment. Dev Med Child Neurol 2001;43:56–60.

9. Good W, Jan J, DeSa L, Barkovich J, Groenveld M, Hoyt C. Cortical visual impairment in children. Surv Ophthalmol 1994;38:351–364.
10. Groenveld M, Jan J, Leader P. Observations on the habilitation of children with cortical visual impairment. J Visual Impair Blindness 1990;84:11–15.
11. Jan J. Neurological causes and investigations. In: Fielder A, Best A, Bax M (eds) The management of visual impairment in childhood. Cambridge: Cambridge University Press, 1993:48–63.
12. Lambert S, Hoyt C, Jan J, Barkovich J, Flodmark O. Visual recovery from hypoxic cortical blindness during childhood. Arch Ophthalmol 1987;105:1371–1377.
13. Meyer A. Herniation of the brain. Arch Neurol Psychiatry 1920;4: 387–400.
14. Moore C, McAdams M, Sutherland J. Intrauterine disseminated intravascular coagulation: a syndrome of multiple pregnancy with a dead twin fetus. J Pediatr 1969;74:523–528.
15. Murphy D, Good W. The epidemiology of blindness in children, vol 157. San Francisco: American Academy of Ophthalmology, 1997.
16. Oxford register of early childhood impairments. Annual report. Oxford: National Perinatal Epidemiology Unit, Radcliffe Infirmary, 1988:32–36.
17. Rogers M. Visual impairment in Liverpool: prevalence and morbidity. Arch Disabled Child 1996;74:299–300.
18. Rosenberg T, Flage T, Hansen E, et al. Incidence of registered visual impairment in the Nordic child population. Br J Ophthalmol 1996; 80:49–53.
19. Whiting S, Jan J, Wong P, Flodmark O, Farrell K, McCormick A. Permanent cortical visual impairment in children. Dev Med Child Neurol 1985;27:730–739.

Brain Lesions with Ophthalmologic Manifestations

Michael X. Repka

Abnormalities of the brain often manifest with problems of either the afferent or efferent visual systems. Many of the disorders discussed in this chapter portend a guarded prognosis and often require urgent or even emergent therapy. This chapter discusses congenital abnormalities of brain development, hydrocephalus, infections, and tumor. The importance of the ophthalmologic examination in each of these clinical settings cannot be overestimated. For example, one-half of intracranial tumors present with ocular signs or symptoms.[17] Thus, the physician must maintain a high index of suspicion that an abnormality that varies from the typical appearance of amblyopia or strabismus might be produced by intracranial abnormalities.

The important ophthalmologic signs and symptoms include nystagmus, ocular motor dysfunction, reduced visual acuity, visual field deficits, dyschromatopsia, an afferent pupillary defect, anisocoria, optic atrophy, or papilledema. Other more subtle motor or sensory disturbances include agnosias, dysmetric eye movements, or visual hallucinations. These latter signs and symptoms are uncommonly mentioned by a child.

CONGENITAL ABNORMALITIES

The embryologic development of the brain may be divided into three distinct phases. The period from 0 to 60 days of gestation is the *induction phase*. During this period, precursor brain structures are formed. The brain is exquisitely sensitive to insult throughout this time. The timing of the insult during this period rather than the nature of the agent leads to the particular defect or family of defects observed. Thus, insults at 15 days gestation, no matter the cause, are phenotypically the same. Most of the congenital abnormalities of the brain discussed in this section result from an insult during this stage of development.

The second phase of brain development occurs from 60 days gestation through the immediate postnatal period. This is the phase of *cellular proliferation*. There is a tremendous proliferation of cells throughout the brain. In addition, the proliferating cells also migrate as they mature from the deeper layers to the more superficial layers, which occurs in both the cerebrum and the cerebellum.

The third phase of brain development occurs from 25 weeks of gestation to 4 years of age; this is the period of *synapse formation and myelination*.

Brief description follows of some of the common congenital abnormalities affecting vision, ordered by the timing of insult.

Induction Disorders

1. *The Chiari malformation* consists of cerebellar elongation and protrusion through the foramen magnum into the cervical spinal canal (Fig. 8-1). The clinical features of this group of disorders have been divided into four types. Type II is the most common form to present in childhood. In addition to the cerebellar protrusion, there is a malformation of the skull and/or the cervical spine and cerebellar hypoplasia. The ophthalmological features of the Chiari malformation include papilledema because of increased intracranial pressure, Horner's syndrome (oculosympathetic paresis) produced from syringomyelia, and downbeat nystagmus. The treatment of a symptomatic Chiari malformation consists of decompressing the protruding cerebellar tissue by removing cervical laminae and a portion of the occipital bone. A secondary approach is utilized when there appears to be traction on the cauda equina. In this instance, the neurosurgeon severs the filum terminale, thus releasing the tethering of the spinal cord from the sacrum.

2. *Holoprosencephaly* is a malformation caused by an insult occurring just before 23 days gestation. The brain, rather than dividing into two halves, develops a single large ventricular cavity. Subsequently, there is poor cortical and thalamic development, whereas the brainstem is usually normal (Fig. 8-2).

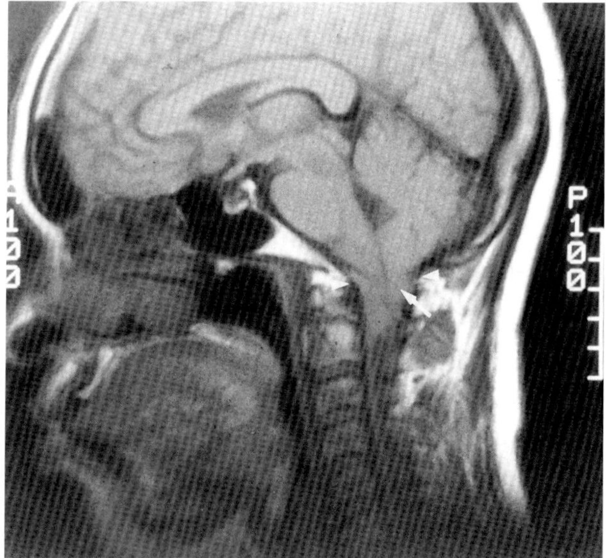

FIGURE 8-1. Sagittal MRI of a type II Chiari malformation. The cerebellar tonsils (*arrow*) are below the foramen magnum (*arrowheads*) within the spinal canal. Syringomyelia is also present.

There may be multiple associated midline facial defects. This abnormality may be associated with trisomy 13, trisomy 18, maternal diabetes mellitus, syphilis, cytomegalovirus (CMV), and toxoplasmosis.[3] The visual prognosis is usually quite poor because of substantial damage to the visual cortex.

3. *Septo-optic dysplasia* likely represents a mild form of holoprosencephaly.[9] The features include agenesis of the septum pellucidum, hypoplasia of the optic nerves and chiasm, hypoplasia of the infundibulum, and diabetes insipidus (Fig. 8-3). Suggested causes include maternal diabetes, anticonvulsants, and CMV.[6,22] In most cases, no specific identifiable cause is present. The features include widely variable reductions of visual acuity and nystagmus. A paradoxical pupillary response may be seen (dilation to light). Hypopituitarism is frequently present, manifest most often by thyroid hormone and growth hormone deficiencies. Patients with bilateral anomalies need endocrine evaluation. If vision is poor, neuroimaging is recommended to be certain there is not a superimposed abnormality of the visual pathway from tumor.

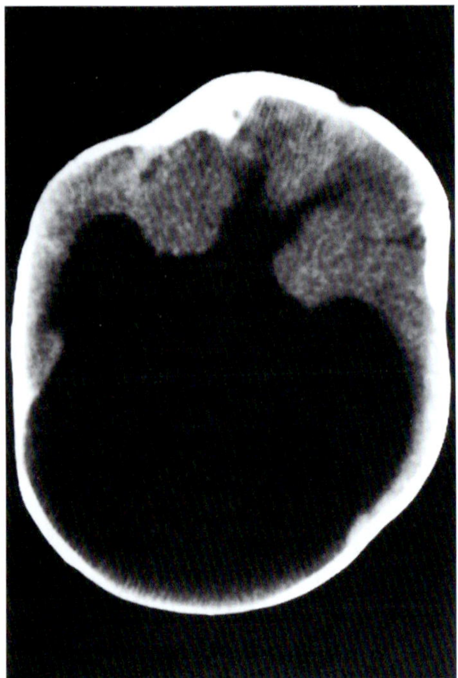

FIGURE 8-2. Coronal MRI of a 1-week-old patient with holoprosencephaly. There is a single ventricular cavity with a very thin cortical rim. This patient had a shunt placed with a dramatic increase in the cortical tissue present.

Disorders of Cellular Migration and Proliferation

This period is dominated by increasing numbers of cortical cells and migration of those cells peripherally in the brain. A number of common developmental abnormalities of the brain are produced by insults during this period: these include the fetal alcohol syndrome, the fetal hydantoin syndrome, and some of the phakomatoses. These disorders are discussed in the disease-specific sections of this text. An insult that leads to impaired cellular proliferation and cellular migration produces several characteristic brain morphologies.

Lissencephaly (agyria) is a malformation in which the surface of the brain is smooth. There are no cortical surface sulci present because there was no elaboration of cortical structure as cells failed to proliferate and subsequently migrate. The diagnosis is readily made with magnetic resonance imaging (MRI).

Macrogyria (pachygyria) is produced by abnormal migration in which only a few broad *gyria* are seen. Patients with lissencephaly and pachygyria have seizure disorders and severe cortical visual loss.

Microcephaly is produced by a variety of insults from radiation exposure, infections in utero, and chemical agents, particularly during the proliferation period. There are also frequent genetic associations. Microcephaly may also occur on a familial basis as an autosomal recessive. Patients with chromosomal abnormalities may manifest microcephaly.[27] Chromosomal defects include trisomies, deletions, and translocations. Microcephaly may also occur in several inherited syndromes with ocular findings (Cornelia de Lange, Hallermann–Streiff). The external skull has a receding forehead, flat occipit, pointed

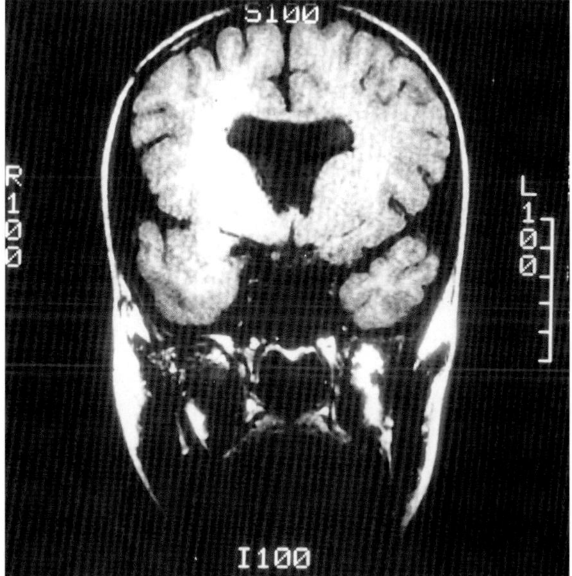

FIGURE 8-3. Coronal MRI of the suprasellar region of a patient with septo-optic dysplasia. The corpus callosum is poorly defined; the septum pellucidum is absent.

vortex, and head circumference more than 3 standard deviations less than the age-adjusted norm.

Other Congenital Abnormalities of the Brainstem and Cerebellum

Möbius syndrome is characterized by congenital paralysis of the facial muscles and impairment of ocular movements, most often abduction. This disorder often presents in the differential diagnosis of infantile esotropia. There is complete or partial absence of facial nuclei as well as other brainstem nuclei. In addition to ocular abduction weakness and poor lid closure, corneal hypoesthesia is frequently present. The ophthalmologist should monitor the integrity of the cornea.

Joubert syndrome is a rare autosomal recessive syndrome. The disorder consists of cerebellar vermis hypoplasia, nystagmus, poor ocular saccades, reduced visual acuity,[23] and breathing irregularity (Fig. 8-4). The breathing abnormalities are

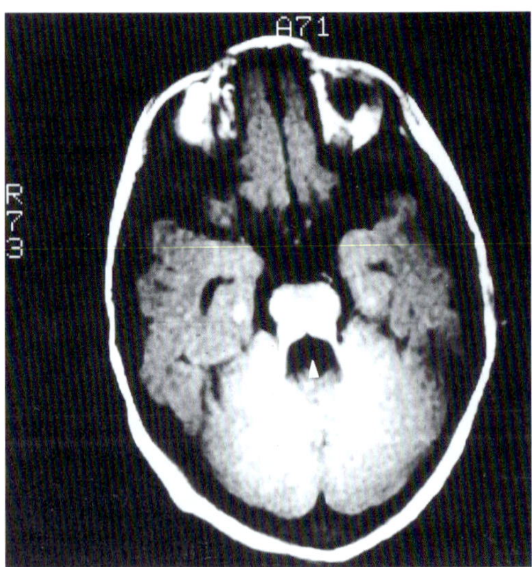

FIGURE 8-4. Axial MRI of Joubert syndrome demonstrates cerebellar vermis hypoplasia. Radiologists often describe the resultant enlargement of the fourth ventricle as a "butterfly" (*arrowhead*). This finding was associated, in this 10-month-old patient, with nystagmus, poor vision, and a reduced ERG.

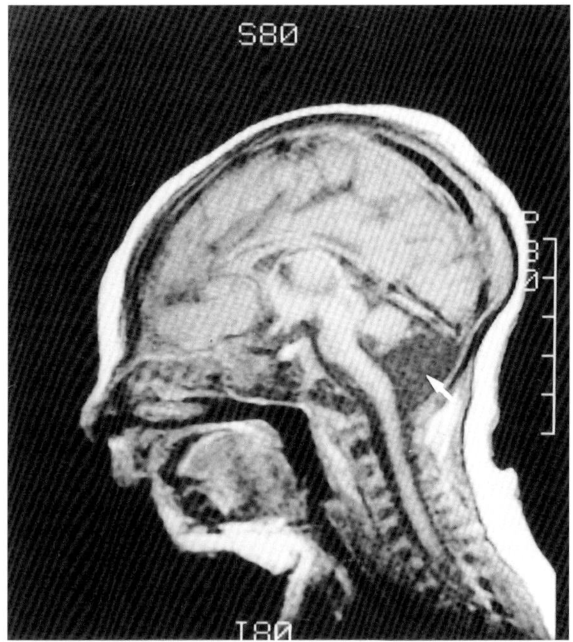

FIGURE 8-5. Sagittal MRI of a Dandy–Walker cyst. A lucent cyst (CSF density) is seen dorsal to the brainstem, producing a mass effect in the posterior fossa pushing the brain forward (*arrow*).

generally seen during infancy. The poor vision appears to be due to an associated retinal dystrophy that shows progressive deterioration.

Dandy–Walker cyst is a malformation in which the fourth ventricle is dilated with the caudal herniation of a glial-covered cyst, which separates the cerebellar hemispheres (Fig. 8-5). The cerebellar vermis and choroid plexus in this area of the brain are poorly developed. The foramina of the fourth ventricle are usually open but atretic. Hydrocephalus may be caused by either a mass effect in the posterior fossa, or less often from obstruction of cerebrospinal fluid (CSF) flow by the atretic foramina. Hydrocephalus may be manifest with papilledema and ocular motor neuropathies, most often abducens nerve pareses, though trochlear palsies have been infrequently reported.[38]

MACROCEPHALY

Macrocephaly is a head circumference 2 standard deviations above the mean for age, race, and sex. Hydrocephalus is the most important cause of macrocephaly. Hydrocephalus is most simply defined as an enlargement of the head produced by increased ventricular volume. The other major cause of macrocephaly is megalencephaly, which is an enlargement of the brain caused by an abnormally large amount of brain constituents. Such a situation may be produced by increased numbers of cells or excessive storage of metabolites. The latter condition may be manifested by seizures and mental retardation. Many patients being evaluated for head size or seizure disorder without evidence of hydrocephalus will be sent to the ophthalmologist for evidence of associated ocular disorders, particularly optic atrophy and nerve fiber layer loss. For example, some patients may have optic atrophy secondary to a leukodystrophy (accumulation of very long chain fatty acids) or neurofibromatosis type I (increased number of brain cells). Strabismus is frequently seen in these patients, most often on a sensory basis. Exotropia is a frequent ophthalmologic sign of adrenoleukodystrophy.[41] Retinal changes might be seen in Tay–Sachs disease and corneal changes in mucopolysaccharidosis. The ocular findings are discussed in the appropriate section of this volume. In my experience, however, only very rarely is a diagnosis made on the basis of the ophthalmologic examination in this clinical setting. In all circumstances, neuroimaging is necessary to eliminate hydrocephalus as a cause of macrocephalus.

Hydrocephalus with increased intraventricular volume may be caused by excessive secretion, impaired flow, or impaired resorption of CSF (Fig. 8-6). CSF is produced by the choroid plexus, located in each of the ventricles. CSF passes from the lateral ventricles through the foramen of Monro into the third ventricle, then via the cerebral aqueduct into the ventricle. CSF passes into the subarachnoid space through the two foramina of Luschka into the pontine cisterns at the apex of the fourth ventricle. CSF also exits the fourth ventricle from a single midline foramen Magendie into the cisterna magna.

Production of CSF involves carbonic anhydrase in one of the secretory steps. Thus, carbonic anhydrase inhibitors are used to treat increased CSF production and hydrocephalus. Eighty percent of CSF resorption occurs in the subarachnoid space by the arach-

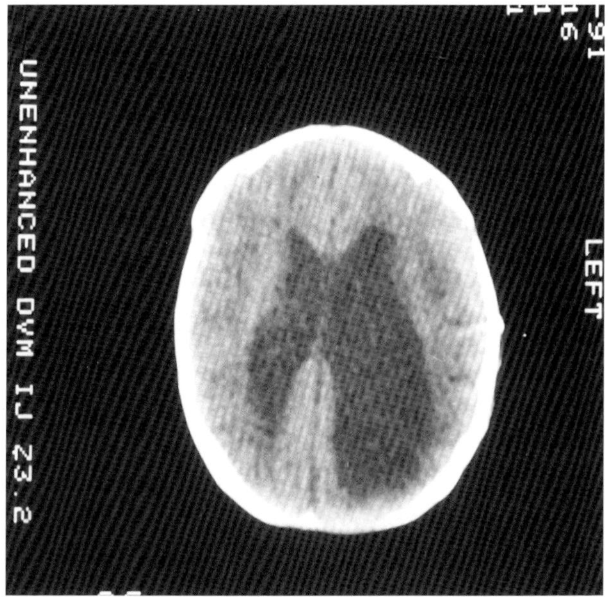

FIGURE 8-6. An axial unenhanced CT of a 5-day-old patient with obstructive hydrocephalus. Note the large lateral ventricles.

noidal villi, which are associated with the large venous sinuses of the skull. Twenty percent of CSF passes into the spinal canal from where it is resorbed. Normal lumbar CSF pressure of a child is up to 180 mm water.[28]

Hydrocephalus is classically divided into communicating and noncommunicating types. In noncommunicating hydrocephalus, the obstruction to CSF flow may be at any point within the ventricular system. In the communicating form, CSF flows freely to the subarachnoid space. At that point, flow is obstructed by meningeal scarring or by a blockage of resorption. Meningeal scarring is most often caused by subarachnoid hemorrhage or bacterial meningitis. There is an additional form of hydrocephalus, hydrocephalus ex vacuo, in which there is increased ventricular volume, but this increase is caused solely by atrophy of cortex.

The only significant cause of excessive CSF secretion is a papilloma of the choroid plexus. These tumors most commonly present with signs of increased intracranial pressure, including papilledema, abduction deficiencies, headache, and vomiting (see later section on Tumors).

The causes of obstruction within the ventricular system include occlusion of the foramina, space-occupying lesions, aqueductal stenosis, Chiari malformation, and the Dandy–Walker syndrome. The malformations of the fourth ventricle, Chiari and Dandy–Walker, account for 40% of all causes of hydrocephalus in childhood.[24] The Dandy–Walker syndrome may present as a posterior fossa mass lesion in addition to a presentation from CSF flow obstruction. Posterior fossa eye signs as described here most likely accompany the signs of increased intracranial pressure; these also include downbeat nystagmus.

Aqueductal stenosis is responsible for 20% of cases of obstructive hydrocephalus. It has an incidence of approximately 1 per 1000 births. Although congenital, it may present insidiously at almost any age from birth to adulthood. The cerebral aqueduct may also become compromised from scarring following meningitis or intraventricular hemorrhage.

The two major causes of decreased absorption of CSF are sequelae of meningitis and infection. Meningitis damages the arachnoidal granulations, thus blocking resorption of CSF into the dural sinuses. Carcinomas may also infiltrate the meninges, blocking subarachnoid CSF flow. Lymphoma and leukemia, if widely metastatic to the meninges, may produce a communicating hydrocephalus by this mechanism.

The age of a patient's presentation with hydrocephalus allows some generalizations to be made. Hydrocephalus presenting in infancy is usually associated with major CNS anomalies (e.g., holoprosencephaly, Chiari, Dandy–Walker). A minority of cases may be a result of intrauterine or postpartum meningoencephalitis. The major eye findings include impaired upgaze from damage to the posterior commissure, abduction weakness, nystagmus, pupillary light–near dissociation, and optic atrophy. Papilledema is uncommon, but increasing head circumference is common. Other clinical findings are specific to the malformation. Gaston has evaluated a large series of children with hydrocephalus and spina bifida.[13] In addition to the ocular motor signs just listed, 73% were believed to have abnormal afferent visual systems.

Childhood-onset hydrocephalus is usually caused by tumor or infection. The typical findings include papilledema, abduction weakness and early morning headache. The treatment of hydrocephalus depends on the particular cause of the hydrocephalus, which is best elucidated with MRI. Infection may produce hydrocephalus by obstructing CSF flow, but it may also produce a thrombosis in a dural sinus, thus secondarily blocking resorption. A classic example is otitic hydrocephalus, produced by a thrombosis of the transverse sinus from an adjacent otitis media.

Patients with mass lesion or obstruction of CSF flow are not treated with medication but are treated surgically with ventriculoperitoneal shunts, ventriculovascular shunts, or lumboperitoneal shunts. Hydrocephalus may also be treated indirectly with resection of a mass lesion.

PERINATAL INJURIES

The developing brain may be injured in the perinatal period by trauma during delivery, by asphyxia before, during, and after delivery, or by hemorrhage.

Mechanical

Mechanical trauma to the brain itself usually induces subdural hemorrhage by inducing lacerations of the tentorium or falx cerebri. Such injuries appear to be of decreasing frequency.

Asphyxia

Asphyxia is a significant cause of brain injury, both before and after delivery. About half of asphyxic insults occur before delivery, 40% during delivery, and 10% after delivery.[6]

There are several distinct patterns of postasphyxic injury. The most devastating is that of cystic encephalomalacia, which occurs in an infant who suffers acute total asphyxia. These patients develop bilateral symmetrical lesions of the thalamus and brainstem nuclei. There is extensive cystic degeneration of the cortex with formation of cystic cavities in the white matter of the brain (Fig. 8-7).

Partial asphyxia produces a syndrome known as periventricular leukomalacia. Bilateral symmetrical areas of necrosis

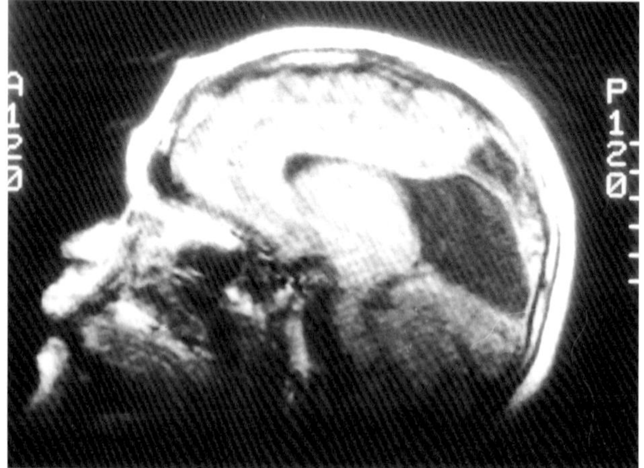

FIGURE 8-7. Sagittal MRI of an antenatal asphyxic insult of the left posterior cerebral artery leading to cortical blindness. Two large cystic areas are seen in the region of the occipital lobe.

develop in the periventricular area, probably the most common brain abnormality seen in premature infants following prolonged asphyxia. It appears that the areas of involvement represent the vascular watershed zones prone to hypoperfusion producing thrombotic infarction. The clinical findings in a patient will depend on the extent of necrosis. In the term infant, the cortex is the site of most of the injury. Such damage occurs most often in the posterior parietal and occipital regions. Thus, one of the most frequent abnormalities associated with asphyxic brain damage is visual dysfunction.

Asphyxia may also damage areas of the basal ganglia, the cerebellum, and brainstem. The particular visual abnormalities, usually of the efferent system associated with such abnormalities, depend on the precise sites involved. There is a high incidence of strabismus, particularly esotropia. Neuroimaging and clinical evaluation are necessary to document the extent of disease.

The syndrome of delayed visual maturation may be more common in infants following mild asphyxic injury. Delayed visual maturation occurs without a distinct cortical injury. There is delayed development of normal visual acuity in some infants.[11] These infants may represent the mildest form of injury.

Intracranial Hemorrhage

Intracranial hemorrhage may result from mechanical trauma, which usually results in subdural or subarachnoid bleeding; this may be accidental or as part of the shaken baby syndrome. Periventricular and intraventricular hemorrhages are more likely associated with prematurity, asphyxia, or other metabolic disturbances leading to significant brain injury. The precise location of the hemorrhage is usually dependent on the age of the patient. A preterm infant will bleed from the germinal matrix, an area of the developing cortex just outside the ependymal lining of the ventricle. Such bleeding leads to periventricular hemorrhage. A term infant, on the other hand, generally bleeds from the choroid plexus, the vascular CSF-secreting tissue within the ventricle. Hemorrhage from this location produces an intraventricular hemorrhage.

Hemorrhage in the preterm and term infant generally occurs 24 to 48 h after an asphyxic insult. Risk factors include prematurity, respiratory distress, and overall health. The brain injury produced by the hemorrhage may result from the asphyxia itself, the hemorrhage itself, or secondary vasospasm of the surrounding vascular supply. The brain injury will ultimately lead to cystic degeneration in that area. Intraventricular and periventricular hemorrhages have been occasionally associated with an increased risk of retinopathy of prematurity. These patients with hemorrhagic brain injury commonly develop ocular abnormalities. Strabismus may develop in up to 50% of patients.

Cranial Neuropathies

Cranial nerves may be damaged by perinatal injury, usually trauma. The most commonly involved cranial nerve is the facial nerve. There is evidence of deficit in up to 6% of newborns. The problem is most often self-limited, and therapy is maintenance of corneal integrity until recovery of facial muscle function. The abducens and ocular motor nerves may also be damaged. As with facial nerve paresis, most do recover.

The cervical sympathetics may be damaged if the lower portion of the brachial plexus is stretched during delivery. Such damage will produce an oculosympathetic paresis with anisocoria and heterochromia iridis. Congenital Horner's syndrome, however, may occur in the absence of obstetrical trauma, probably because of an unidentified insult earlier in pregnancy.

INFECTION

Congenital Infection

There are five organisms most frequently associated with congenital neurologic infection: rubella, cytomegalovirus (CMV), varicella, toxoplasma, and herpes simplex. The congenital rubella syndrome is the one postinfectious syndrome that often presents with ophthalmologic features. The infection rate is highest early in pregnancy, declining as the duration of pregnancy increases. The major ocular findings include chorioretinitis, cataract, and glaucoma. Other signs include deafness, congenital heart disease, congenital malformations of the brain including microcephaly, hydrocephalus, spina bifida, and developmental delay. The chorioretinitis is described as a "salt-and-pepper" depigmentation.[12] Affected patients may have a seizure disorder, mental retardation, and spasticity.

The pediatric ophthalmologist is often asked to evaluate a patient in the newborn nursery or following discharge for evidence of current or previous CMV infection. A patient with congenital CMV has jaundice, hepatomegaly, thrombocytopenia, and severe anemia. Typically, there is microcephaly, hydrocephalus, and microgyria. Multiple ocular abnormalities have been reported in this condition including chorioretinitis, optic disc anomalies, microphthalmia, and cataract. Radiologic support for the diagnosis of CMV (although not pathognomonic) is the demonstration of periventricular calcifications.

Toxoplasma gondii affects approximately 1 in 1000 newborn infants. The infection is acquired during the second and third trimesters of pregnancy, usually from an asymptomatic mother. The clinical picture includes chorioretinitis, which is usually bilateral, as well as anemia, pleocytosis, and seizures. Most patients affected have significant neurological disease. CNS calcification may be present. In one study, 90% of the affected children had mental retardation and 40% had severely impaired visual acuity.[8] Neurological and retinal manifestations of this disease may be absent at birth but may develop progressively as the child grows.

Infection with herpes simplex virus usually occurs at the time of birth. The use of cesarean section has reduced the rate of infection, but many cases continue to occur because many mothers are asymptomatic. A wide range of neurological abnormalities may exist. The ophthalmologic abnormalities include microphthalmia and retinal scarring.

Congenital infection with varicella rarely produces ophthalmologic findings. Acquired infection is responsible for many cases of tonic pupil. Careful monitoring of amblyopia is necessary in affected patients due to deficient accommodation.

Acquired Infection

Bacterial meningitis may be responsible for infection of the fetal or child's brain. Infection of the developing brain is responsible for multiple defects, yet it usually incites far less inflammatory response than the same infection would in a child's brain. The inflammatory response, responsible for much of the damage following infection, is attenuated in the fetus. The infection of the neonate is accompanied by few clinical signs. However, the infection of the child is associated with fever, headache, nausea, vomiting, nuchal rigidity, cranial nerve pareses, loss of vision, and rarely papilledema. The most commonly involved cranial nerves are III, IV, and VI, presumably from inflammation of the perineurium. Optic atrophy and cranial nerve palsy are ophthalmologic sequelae of meningitis.[32] The most common sequela is hearing loss.

Bacteria may also form a brain abscess (Fig. 8-8), which generally occurs 2 to 4 weeks after gaining access to the brain.[5] The initial stage is a cerebritis that often lacks symptoms. Ophthalmologic signs and symptoms are produced only when there is sufficient brain necrosis or mass effect to produce visual loss or papilledema. For example, Wohl and colleagues reported a 13-year-old girl with an occipital lobe abscess and a dense hemianopsia 2 weeks following a dental cleaning.[43] Diagnosis required MRI, followed by neurosurgical drainage.

Many viruses may infect a child's central nervous system. They gain entry through the blood, the peripheral nerves, or the olfactory system. Enteroviruses may cause an acute paralytic syndrome of ocular motor nerve or inflammation of the optic nerve(s). Most cases of childhood optic neuritis are thought to be viral related. Enterovirus type 70 produces a hemorrhagic conjunctivitis followed by motor paralysis.[42]

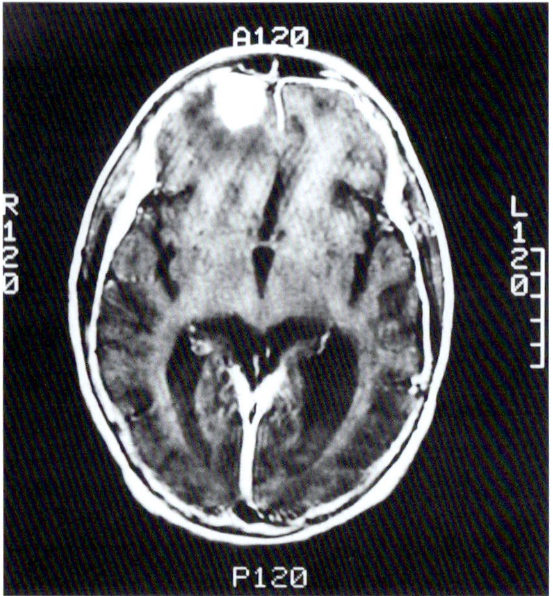

FIGURE 8-8. A 12-year-old patient with a brain abscess in the right frontal lobe.

Polio virus and some strains of vaccine have produced frequent involvement of ocular motor nerves. Adenoviruses, responsible for many cases of conjunctivitis, only rarely have produced a meningoencephalitis.

TUMORS

An ophthalmologist is only rarely confronted by a patient in whom they establish the diagnosis of an intracranial neoplasm. They are much more often asked to consult on the signs, symptoms, and ophthalmologic management of a previously diagnosed tumor patient. The specific signs and symptoms that a patient may present vary depending on the particular tumor and its location. The duration of signs and symptoms bears a direct relationship to the type of tumor and often to the prognosis for that tumor. Rapid onset is typical of aggressive tumors.

Many patients will complain of headache, particularly if there is increased intracranial pressure. This sign is of no localizing value. Ophthalmologic signs specific for a tumor are rare. Acquired nystagmus, diplopia, ocular motor dysfunction, and papilledema are suggestive of progressive intracranial neoplasm and demand emergent evaluation. These symptoms may be of nontumor etiology.

This survey is divided into tumors of glial origin, neural origin, meningeal origin, and congenital origin.

Tumors of Glial Origin

Gliomas are tumors that arise from neuroglial cells. These cells provide support for neural tissue. In childhood, gliomas comprise 75% or more of primary intracranial tumors.[35] Gliomas include astrocytomas, oligodendrogliomas, ependymomas, choroid plexus papillomas, and colloid cysts.

Astrocytomas develop in several areas of the brain: the brainstem, cerebrum, optic pathway, and cerebellum. The tumors in each of these areas have specific biological behaviors. In addition to topographic nomenclature based on the site of origin, astrocytomas have also been divided on the basis of histological differences. The most common type of tumor is a fibrillary astrocytoma. A grading system with the three levels is commonly employed to describe the histological characteristics of fibrillary astrocytomas. Grade 1 is a well-differentiated astrocytoma, grade 2 is an anaplastic, more cellular astrocytoma, and grade 3 is glioblastoma multiforme, which is the most aggressive form with the worst prognosis.[7]

Most fibrillary astrocytomas during childhood occur in the cerebellum, brainstem, or hypothalamus. These tumors as a rule infiltrate normal brain tissue, preserving functions until late in the disease course. This tendency frequently leads to a delay in diagnosis.

Some fibrillary astrocytomas assume an appearance of parallel tumor cell growth and orientation termed pilocytic. The juvenile form of the pilocytic astrocytoma occurs in children and has a very benign prognosis. This tumor type is particularly common in the optic pathway.

Astrocytoma of the cerebellum is one of the most common childhood brain tumors. These tumors arise from either the vermis or the lateral lobes of the cerebellum. They are well circumscribed and often develop a large cyst. Often the tumor is just a small nodule in the midline (Fig. 8-9). The majority of these tumors have a benign histological appearance with a pilocytic growth pattern. Treatment of a cerebellar astrocytoma is complete surgical excision when possible. Adjunct radiotherapy is suggested for patients with incomplete resection. The prognosis for the majority of these patients with benign histology is remarkably good. A 25-year survival rate greater than 90% has been reported.[34] Occasional recurrences have been reported, as many as 40 years after initial diagnosis.

Astrocytomas of brainstem are usually bilateral in involvement, originating in the pons. The tumor produces a diffuse enlargement of the brainstem, occasionally with occlusion of the fourth ventricle and noncommunicating hydrocephalus (Fig. 8-10). About one in four will have papilledema.[19] These tumors appear to initially have a slow growth pattern, infiltrating normal structures without destroying them. Treatment for this tumor is radiation therapy because complete surgical resection in the brainstem is impossible. Treatments that are more recent include enhanced

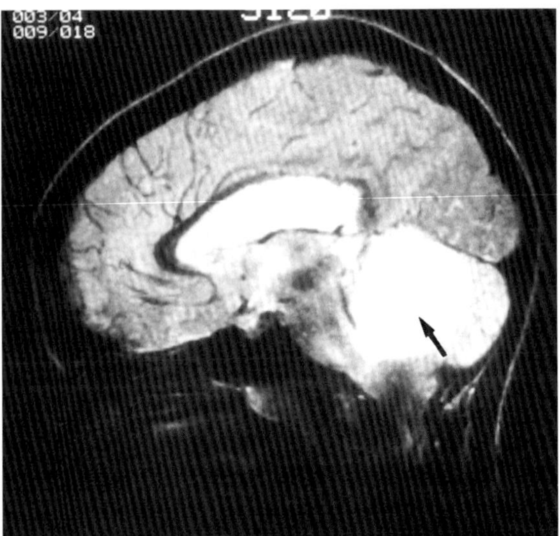

FIGURE 8-9. Cystic astrocytoma of the cerebellum in a 16-year-old presenting with esotropia and horizontal diplopia. The cystic portion of the tumor is identified by the *arrow*.

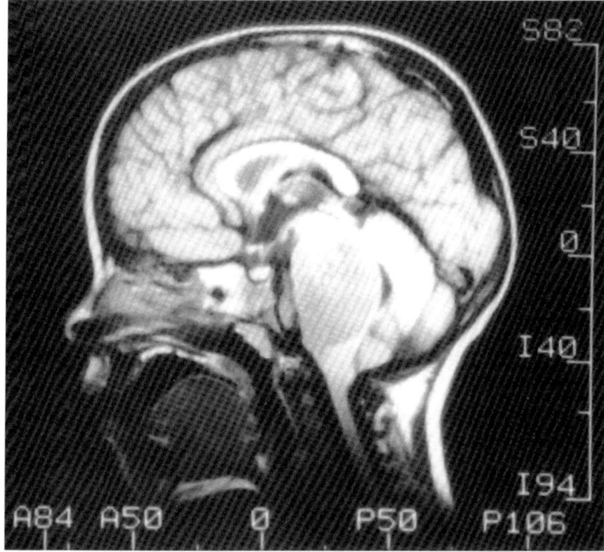

FIGURE 8-10. Sagittal MRI of a 4-year-old boy who presented with a left esotropia. Within 2 weeks, he began to have difficulty walking. Note the diffuse enlargement of the pons from a fibrillary astrocytoma. The tumor extends from the thalamus to the medulla.

radiation therapy of 8000 cGy consisting of divided doses delivered twice daily. Chemotherapy has been disappointing. The prognosis is usually quite poor, with a 5-year survival rate of only 20%.[39] Typical ophthalmologic signs and symptoms are a horizontal gaze paresis, horizontal nystagmus, trigeminal nerve paresis, and double vision, occurring in approximately 50% of the affected patients.

Astrocytoma of the cerebrum may arise in any portion of any hemisphere. These tumors are often infiltrative so that complete surgical resection is usually impossible. These patients are usually treated with surgical excision, followed in some cases by radiation therapy. Chemotherapy has generally been disappointing. Survival may vary from excellent for patients with benign pilocytic astrocytomas to poor for those patients with glioblastoma. Cerebral astrocytomas, although common in adults, are relatively rare in children. Ophthalmologic signs of these tumors may include visual field defects and increased intracranial pressure (Fig. 8-11). The most common non-ophthalmologic symptom is a seizure disorder.

Astrocytoma of the hypothalamus—in the region of the third ventricle—are quite common in childhood. These children present with hypothalamic dysfunction, visual loss, or both. Clinically, one suspects a primary origin in the hypothalamus when the visual loss is minimal compared to the level of hypothalamic or pituitary axis dysfunction. These tumors are usually of the juvenile pilocytic type. Treatment is usually radiation therapy unless the third ventricle is compromised. A ventricular peritoneal shunting or a surgical debulking of the tumor is needed. A biopsy has been desirable in the past, but modern imaging has made this test no longer mandatory.

Astrocytoma of the optic nerve is one of the most frequent tumors affecting children with ophthalmologic signs and symptoms. These tumors, whether they involve the optic nerve, the optic chiasm, or optic tract, are termed optic gliomas. These tumors are usually of very benign histological appearance (juvenile pilocytic astrocytoma).

Optic nerve gliomas may occur sporadically or be associated with neurofibromatosis type 1 (NF1). In a survey of patients with NF1, the incidence of optic pathway gliomas was found to be as high as 20%, with just less than half involving the optic nerve.[25] The ophthalmologic findings are generally decreased visual function, optic disc swelling or pallor, strabismus, and proptosis. Visual loss or optic nerve atrophy occurs in about one-third of children with NF1.[2,16,26] Visual loss is more common in the sporadic patients. Gayre and coworkers found visual loss in 63% of the children they have followed.[14]

A tumor involving the optic nerve usually causes a fusiform enlargement of the nerve. The tumor diffusely replaces the normal neural architecture. In a patient with neurofibromatosis type 1 and an optic nerve glioma, the nerve is enlarged, but much of the tumor is in the subarachnoid space, surrounding and compressing an apparently normal optic nerve. One of the commonly associated findings of optic nerve gliomas is meningeal vascular hyperplasia. The hyperplasia often extends well beyond the limit of the optic nerve involvement. This benign reaction makes it difficult on neuroimaging to accurately determine the true extent of nerve involvement.

Astrocytomas of the chiasm are similar to those of the optic nerve in appearance. Because they lack a meningeal covering,

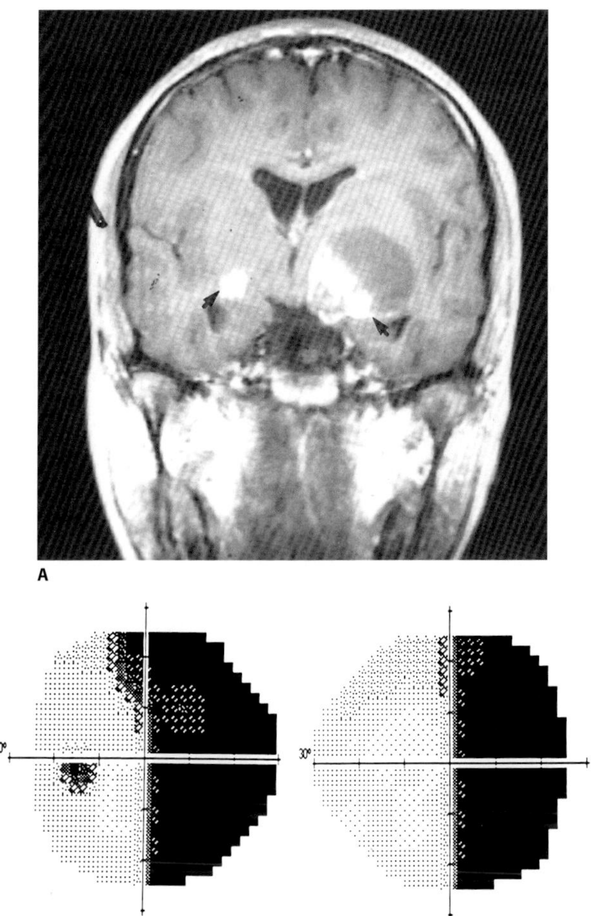

FIGURE 8-11A,B. A 16-year-old boy with no visual complaints presented for ophthalmologic evaluation. **(A)** A coronal MRI demonstrates bilateral astrocytomas infiltrating the lateral geniculate nuclei (*arrows*). The left lesion has a substantial cystic component. **(B)** Visual acuity and pupils were normal, but an automated visual field examination demonstrated a dense right homonymous hemianopsia.

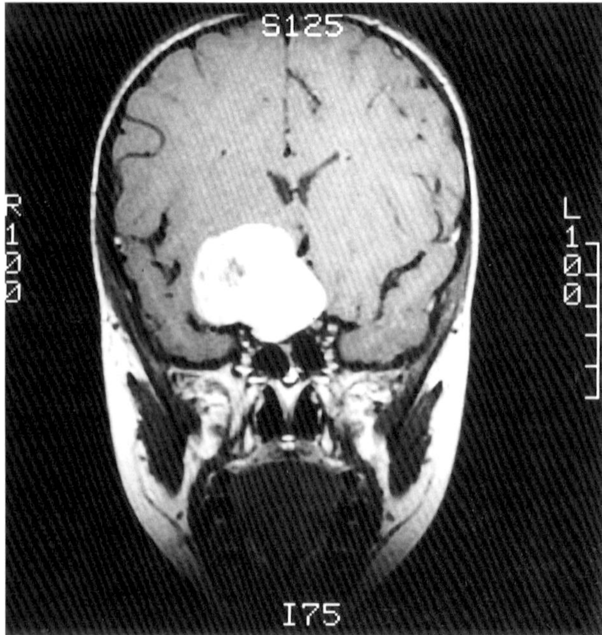

FIGURE 8-12. Coronal MRI of optic chiasmatic glioma in a 6-year-old boy. This patient was treated for 20/200 amblyopia for 1 year before his diagnosis. At that time, a right afferent pupillary defect and optic atrophy were noted. Note the compression of the midline third ventricle.

they may have a significant exophytic portion. That portion of the tumor may fill the suprasellar cistern compressing the hypothalamus and third ventricle (Fig. 8-12). These patients have optic atrophy, strabismus, and decreased vision. Six percent of patients with NF1 may harbor a chiasmatic glioma.[25] These patients may also develop endocrinopathies from upward extension into the hypothalamus or symptoms of increased intracranial pressure from extension into the third ventricle with compromise of CSF flow. Such extension portends a poorer prognosis.

The diagnosis of optic gliomas involves neuroimaging, particularly magnetic resonance imaging, of the visual pathways. In addition to the optic glioma, MRI may often demonstrate "hamartomatous" lesions of the basal ganglia in patients with neurofibromatosis. These lesions have disappeared during long-term follow-up.

The natural history of optic nerve and chiasmatic gliomas is uncertain. In some cases, the tumor remains static, in other cases there may be slow growth, while in rare cases there may be rapid growth with invasion of contiguous structures. Wright and colleagues followed 17 patients with optic nerve gliomas.[44] Nine of their patients demonstrated no growth of the tumor, while 8 showed enlargement. Patients with neurofibromatosis may have had a slightly more benign prognosis. Hoyt and Baghdassarian described 18 patients with chiasmatic gliomas.[16] Only eight eyes showed any deterioration of visual function, suggesting that these lesions do not grow, and may be hamartomas. Imes and Hoyt reported the long-term follow-up (median, 20 years) for 28 patients with chiasmatic glioma, including some from the initial study.[18] Five had died, but four deaths were from tumor before 1969, suggesting a static course for most optic gliomas. More troublesome in the Imes and Hoyt report was the high incidence of secondary intracranial tumors, which were responsible for death in a number of patients.[18] Perhaps these patients are more prone to tumor development, or did these tumors develop because of the radiotherapy they had received?

The visual prognosis is varied; some patients are unchanged whereas others show a slow loss of vision, even after an extended period of stability.[2,14] More striking is a report that has shown that these tumors may even regress spontaneously and the vision improve. Parsa and colleagues presented 13 cases of spontaneous regression with no treatment.[30] In many cases, the regression was associated with improvement in visual function.

As the natural history of optic glioma is unknown, the treatment remains controversial. It is impossible with the available tests to predict which tumor will progress. For optic nerve gliomas, appropriate management should be close serial examinations of the patient for evidence of progressive visual loss or tumor enlargement. Such examinations should include neuroimaging at least every 6 months, determination of visual acuity and fields at 3-month intervals for the first year, then at 6-month intervals thereafter. If there is deterioration in visual function or enlargement of the tumor, many authors advocate removal of the optic nerve, usually using a combined orbitotomy-craniotomy approach. However, surgical resection should be undertaken only when necessary, usually due to extreme proptosis, in light of the reports of spontaneous regression.[30] If both optic nerves or the chiasm are involved, radiation therapy is the most appropriate therapeutic approach.

For optic chiasm glioma, a biopsy is performed only when there is an atypical presentation or a need to debulk an exophytic portion of the tumor because of compression of normal structures (see Fig. 8-12). There does not seem to be a deleterious effect on visual function from removal of such an exophytic portion. These patients, like those with optic nerve tumors, are followed very carefully for radiologic enlargement or visual deterioration. If there is either radiologic expansion or visual deterioration, treatment usually consists of chemotherapy for children less than age 4 and radiotherapy for older children.[29] Vincristine and carboplatin are the agents typically used.

Ependymomas are the third most frequent childhood brain tumor, with a peak incidence occurring early in life. Ependymomas arise from the ependymal cells of the lining epithelium of the ventricles, cerebral aqueduct, and spinal canal. The most common location for such a tumor in childhood is the fourth ventricle. The tumor characteristically occludes the ventricle, producing increased intracranial pressure. It may infiltrate normal tissues or extend into the cerebellopontine angle. About 11% of patients have metastasis to other parts of the craniospinal axis at the time of their presentation.[31] The treatment is partial surgical resection, followed by radiation therapy to the tumor bed with additional treatment to the whole brain and spinal cord. The survival rate for this tumor is variable, depending on the histology and extent of surgical resection.

Colloid cysts of the third ventricle are also tumors of glial origin. These tumors produce symptoms of increased intracranial pressure including papilledema and abduction weakness. These tumors are benign. They may be diagnosed by MRI. The treatment is resection.

Choroid plexus tumors usually occur in the lateral ventricles of children, less frequently in the third or fourth ventricles. These tumors often secrete excess CSF, producing hydrocephalus and papilledema. Most tumors have a benign histological appearance. The mainstay of treatment is complete surgical resection. If the tumor is only partially resected, craniospinal irradiation is necessary.

Oligodendrogliomas are usually located in the cerebral hemispheres but may occur in any part of the brain. They are usually of benign histological appearance and often calcified. Due to their location in the hemispheres, the ophthalmologic signs are hemianopsia and papilledema. Seizures are a frequent symptom. The treatment of these tumors is surgical resection followed by adjuvant radiation therapy.

Tumors of Neural Origin

Only a small number of tumors affecting the child's brain are of neural origin: these are the medulloblastoma, by far the most common, neuroblastoma, ganglioglioma, and retinoblastoma. The last tumor is discussed elsewhere in this text.

Medulloblastoma is one of the most common tumors of childhood, representing about 25% of all brain tumors in this age group. It usually arises in the midline of the cerebellum, and is frequently associated with necrosis but only rarely with calcification (Fig. 8-13), unlike the cerebellar cystic astrocytoma,

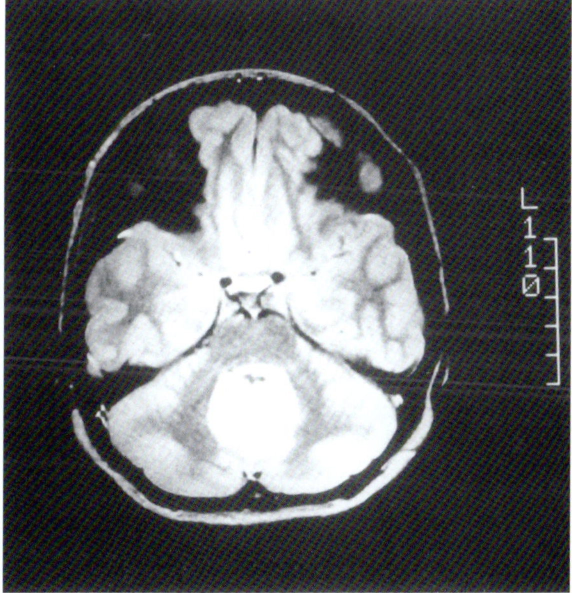

FIGURE 8-13. Axial MRI of an 8-year-old boy with a medulloblastoma enveloping the fourth ventricle, infiltrating the dorsal brainstem and cerebellum.

which is often calcified. A medulloblastoma may obliterate the fourth ventricle and infiltrate the cerebellum, the brainstem, and the meninges. It may also metastasize to any location bathed by CSF. There is usually a brief history of headache and vomiting from increased intracranial pressure. There may also be ocular motor signs from infiltration of the brainstem and disruption of ocular motor nuclei and their interconnections. Such signs include internuclear ophthalmoplegia, gaze palsy, and ocular motor neuropathy.

Medulloblastomas are highly malignant with a poor prognosis. Treatment consists of an aggressive resection followed by craniospinal irradiation. Chemotherapy is also employed, particularly in younger patients. The survival rate for 5 years is approximately 50%.[10]

Other tumors of neuronal origin include *neuroblastomas*, which may arise in the central nervous system but are quite rare. Most CNS neuroblastomas occur during childhood. They have a poor prognosis. Only approximately 30% of patients are alive at 5 years.[4]

Gangliogliomas are benign tumors, usually occurring in the third ventricle, which often present with hypothalamic dysfunction or noncommunicating hydrocephalus. Because of their location, they might be confused with optic glioma. The ophthalmologist may help in the diagnosis, because usually the visual function is better than with optic gliomas and there is little optic atrophy.

Tumors of Meningeal Origin

Tumors of the meninges are very rare in childhood and represent only a small percentage of tumors during childhood and the teenage years.[35] There is no sex predilection observed for the tumors presenting in childhood, in contrast to the female predilection in adulthood. Meningiomas may have a more aggressive behavior in childhood than they have in adulthood. The tumors arise from the arachnoid layer of the meninges and may have an intracranial, intraspinal, or intraventricular location. There is a striking association with NF1. A patient with neurofibromatosis often has multiple foci of meningioma as well as other intracranial tumors such as acoustic neuromas, neurofibromas, and gliomas.

Intracranial meningiomas may produce symptoms because of mass effect, direct compression of the tumor on brain tissue or cranial nerves, and obstruction of the venous sinuses. The precise symptoms developed by a patient depend on the location of the tumor. For example, a meningioma in the cerebellopontine angle produces nystagmus and ocular motor dysmetria as well as increased intracranial pressure.

The treatment of intracranial meningioma is complete surgical resection wherever possible. Radiation therapy has been attempted for tumors located in inoperable locations with varying degrees of success.

Meningiomas may also occur, primarily associated with the sheath of the optic nerve; they occur in this location about as often in children as in adults.[28] A patient with a primary orbital meningioma usually presents with unilateral visual loss. In childhood, the visual loss is usually quite advanced at the time of presentation. The optic disc may be swollen or atrophic, although it is most often atrophic. Optociliary shunt vessels may be present on the surface of the disc. The tumor is readily diagnosed with neuroimaging. Radiologic features include tubular enlargement of the optic nerve associated with calcification. The appearance is often described as a "train track," with enhancing parallel lines surrounding a lucent space in axial CT sections of the optic nerve.

The appropriate treatment for primary orbital meningiomas is controversial. Alper has said that many of these tumors behave malignantly in children and should be resected completely and immediately.[1] In general, resection of the affected optic nerve should be performed before the tumor spreads intracranially. Radiotherapy remains an alternative treatment. There are case reports of improvement after radiotherapy.[37]

In our center, we prefer to follow these tumors at 3-month intervals in a fashion analogous to that for optic nerve gliomas. Visual acuity is monitored as well as tumor volume and extent by neuroimaging. A patient who demonstrates increasing encroachment of the meningioma toward the intracranial space, tumor enlargement, or complete loss of vision should be considered for a combined craniotomy/orbitotomy resection.[1]

Tumors of Congenital Origin

Three distinct tumors of congenital origin present during childhood: germinoma, craniopharyngioma, and arachnoid cyst.

Germinomas are relatively rare tumors that arise from germ cells. They most often arise in the region of the pineal gland

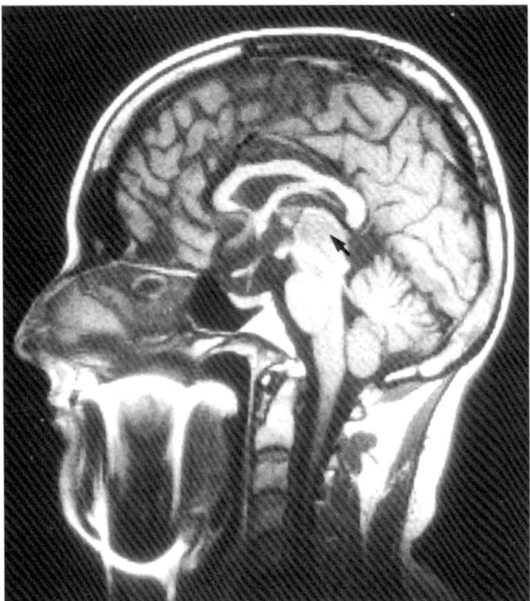

FIGURE 8-14. Midsagittal MRI of a 12-year-old boy with a germinoma. His symptoms were difficulty seeing the blackboard. He had bilateral pupillary light–near dissociation, anisocoria, and convergence-retraction nystagmus. The tumor (*arrow*) is seen compressing the tectal plate.

but contain no cells typical of the pineal gland. They may also appear in the hypothalamic or thalamic region. As in all brain tumors, the presenting signs of germinoma depend on their location. If the tumor arises in the region of the pineal gland, the patient will have signs of increased intracranial pressure from compression of the dorsal midbrain and of the cerebral aqueduct (Fig. 8-14). The ophthalmologic signs of the dorsal midbrain syndrome (Parinaud) are a skew deviation, fourth and sixth cranial nerve pareses, convergence-retraction nystagmus, impaired upgaze, anisocoria, and corectopia. The differential diagnosis of germinoma in the region of the pineal includes pinealoma and teratoma.

If the tumor is in the hypothalamic region, downward extension may cause visual loss and upward extension may cause papilledema from obstruction of the third ventricle. Germinomas in the region of the thalamus also cause visual loss from infiltration of the lateral geniculate body, optic tracts, or portions of the geniculocalcrine radiations. The diagnosis in each of these locations is made by biopsy. Treatment is radiation therapy. These tumors are extraordinarily sensitive to radiation therapy, with a 10-year survival rate of approximately 72%.[40]

Craniopharyngioma is the third most common brain tumor of children in some studies, representing about 10% of tumors.[20] It often presents to the ophthalmologist as visual loss of unknown etiology or as a sensory strabismus. The physician should be very wary of this tumor when diagnosing amblyopia or functional visual loss. For instance, we saw a 6-year-old with exotropia and 20/200 vision in one eye. Mild optic atrophy was present. An MRI demonstrated a large craniopharyngioma. In childhood, this tumor usually presents after visual symptoms are present because of the delay in diagnosis with children.

Craniopharyngiomas arise from embryonic rests of Rathke's pouch. The tumor is composed of a capsule, a cystic portion containing the classic "machine oil," and a solid mass. The tumor may compress the optic pathways, the hypothalamus, the third ventricle, and the pituitary gland (Fig. 8-15). The optic pathway may be compressed from above, below, or from the side, thus causing nearly any visual field defect. We previously reported on the clinical course of 12 children with craniopharyngiomas. Nearly all these children suffered severe visual loss and most presented with profound optic atrophy.[33] There was no recovery of function following treatment in children, unlike the improvement seen in adults.

The treatment of craniopharyngioma involves an attempt at total resection when accompanied by an acceptable minimal morbidity. If complete resection is impossible, as is often the case, a partial resection is performed. For older children, teenagers, and adults, postoperative radiotherapy is employed. For young children, radiotherapy is delayed, relying on clinical examination and repeat neuroimaging at 3-month intervals for the first year and at 6-month intervals thereafter to detect recurrences. These studies evaluate the suprasellar space for regrowth and consequent compromise of the visual system. If there is regrowth, repeat resection and/or drainage of the reaccumulated cystic material followed by radiotherapy is performed. In our experience, children with visual loss and especially those with

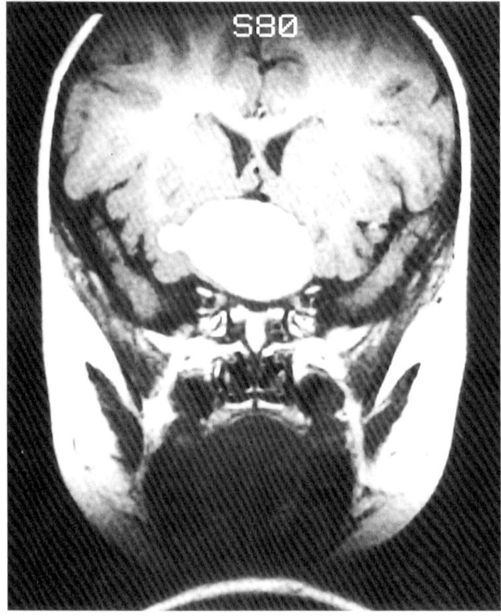

FIGURE 8-15. Coronal MRI of a craniopharyngioma in a 1-year-old patient that is obliterating the suprasellar cistern.

optic atrophy at the time of their presentation will not have significant visual improvement after decompression. However, they do not seem to suffer further visual loss.

The differential diagnosis of craniopharyngioma includes suprasellar epidermoid and dermoid cysts, Rathke pouch cysts, arachnoid cysts, and pituitary adenoma. Pituitary adenomas are uncommon in children but may present similarly to craniopharyngioma with endocrine dysfunction, hypopituitarism, and/or visual loss.

Arachnoid cysts are collections of CSF contained within a membrane of meningeal tissue. They may arise anywhere there are meninges. In some circumstances, arachnoid cysts may enlarge because of the active production of fluid. Enlargement may cause symptoms of mass effect, increased intracranial pressure, or, if there is a suprasellar cyst, an optic neuropathy. Suprasellar arachnoid cysts most often present in young patients

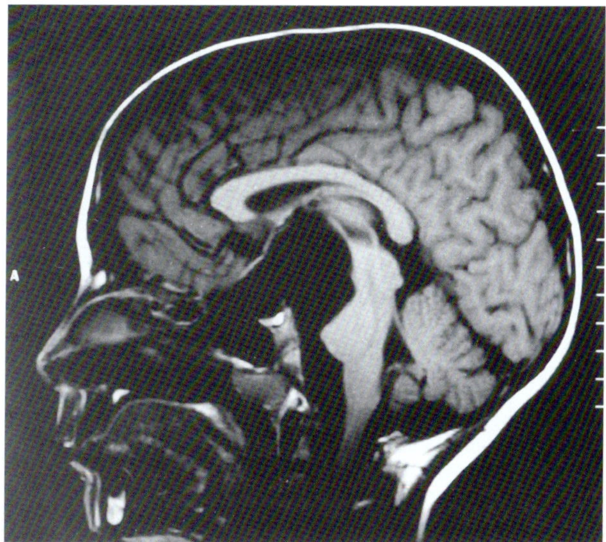

FIGURE 8-16. Sagittal MRI of a suprasellar arachnoid cyst in a 4-year-old patient. No ophthalmologic defect could be detected.

(Fig. 8-16).[15] Pituitary and hypothalamic signs as well as third ventricle compression may occur from expansion of a suprasellar or arachnoid cyst in addition to visual loss. Diagnosis of a cyst is usually incidental but is easily made by MRI. Treatment of symptomatic lesions is drainage with capsule removal. There is only a very low chance of recurrence, even when removal of the capsule is incomplete.

References

1. Alper MG. Management of primary optic nerve meningiomas: current status—therapy and controversy. J Clin Neuroophthalmol 1981;1:101–117.
2. Balcer LJ, Liu GT, Heller G, et al. Visual loss in children with neurofibromatosis type 1 and optic pathway gliomas: relation to tumor location by magnetic resonance imaging. Am J Ophthalmol 2001;131:442–445.
3. Barr M Jr, Hanson JW, Currey K, et al. Holoprosencephaly in infants of diabetic mothers. J Pediatr 1983;102:565–568.

4. Bennett JP Jr, Rubenstein LJ. The biological behavior of primary cerebral neuroblastoma: a reappraisal of the clinical course in a series of seventy cases. Ann Neurol 1984;16:21–27.
5. Britt RH. Brain abscess. In: Wilkins RH, Rengachary SS (eds) Neurosurgery. New York: McGraw-Hill, 1985:1928–1956.
6. Brown JK, Purvis RJ, Forfar JO, Cockburn F. Neurologic aspects of perinatal asphyxia. Dev Med Child Neurol 1974;16:567–580.
7. Burger PC. Malignant astrocytic neoplasms: classification, pathologic anatomy, and response to treatment. Semin Oncol 1986;13:16–26.
8. Conboy TJ, Pass RF, Stagno S, et al. Early clinical manifestations in intellectual outcome in children with symptomatic congenital cytomegalovirus infection. J Pediatr 1987;111:343–348.
9. De Morsier G. Etudes sur les dysgraphies cranioencephaliques et genesie du septum lucidum avec malformation du tractus optique. La dysplasie septo-optique. Schweiz Arch Neurol Psychiatr 1956;76:267.
10. Dhellemmes P, Demaille MC, Lejeune JP, Barazanelli MC, Combells G, Torrealbi G. Cerebellar medulloblastoma: results of multidisciplinary treatment. Surg Neurol 1986;25:290–294.
11. Fielder AR, Russell-Eggitt IR, Dodd KL, Mellor DH. Delayed visual maturation. Trans Ophthalmol Soc UK 1985;104:653–661.
12. Forrest JM, Menser MA. Congenital rubella in school children and adolescents. Arch Dis Child 1970;45:63–69.
13. Gaston H. Ophthalmic complication of spina bifida and hydrocephalus. Eye 1991;5:279–290.
14. Gayre GS, Scott IU, Feuer W, Saunders TG, Siatkowski RM. Long-term visual outcome in patients with anterior visual pathway gliomas. J Neuroophthalmol 2001;21:1–7.
15. Hoffman HJ, Hendrick EB, Humphries RP, Armstrong EA. Investigation and management of suprasellar arachnoid cysts. J Neurosurg 1982;57:597–602.
16. Hoyt WF, Baghdassarian SB. Optic glioma of childhood: natural history and rationale for conservative management. Br J Ophthalmol 1969;53:793–798.
17. Huber A. Eye signs and symptoms in brain tumors. St. Louis: Mosby, 1976.
18. Imes RK, Hoyt WF. Childhood chiasmal gliomas: update on the fate of patients in the 1969 San Francisco study. Br J Ophthalmol 1986;70:179–182.
19. Ingraham FD, Matson DD. Neurosurgery in infancy and childhood. Springfield: Thomas, 1954.
20. Ingraham FD, Scott HW Jr. Craniopharyngiomas in children. J Pediatr 1946;29:95–116.
21. Karp LA, Zimmerman LE, Borrett A, Spencer W. Primary intraorbital meningiomas. Arch Ophthalmol 1974;91:24–38.
22. Lambert SR, Hoyt CS, Nahara MH. Optic nerve hypoplasia. Surv Ophthalmol 1987;32:1–9.

23. Lambert SR, Kriss A, Gresty M, Banton S, Taylor D. Joubert syndrome. Arch Ophthalmol 1989;107:709–713.
24. Laurence KM. The pathology of hydrocephalus. Ann R Coll Surg Engl 1959;24:388–401.
25. Lewis RA, Gerson LP, Axelson KA, Riccardi VM, Whitford RP. von Recklinghausen neurofibromatosis. II. Incidence of optic gliomata. Ophthalmology 1984;91:929–935.
26. Listernick RA, Charrow J, Greenwald M, Mets M. Natural history of optic pathway tumors in children with neurofibromatosis type 1: a longitudinal study. J Pediatr 1994;125:63–66.
27. Menkes JH. Textbook of child neurology. Philadelphia: Lea & Febiger, 1990:197.
28. Menkes JH. Textbook of child neurology. Philadelphia: Lea & Febiger, 1990:254.
29. Packer RJ, Savino PJ, Bilaniuk LT, et al. Chiasmatic gliomas of childhood: a reappraisal of natural history and effectiveness of cranial irradiation. Child's Brain 1983;10:393–403.
30. Parsa CF, Hoyt CS, Lesser RL, et al. Spontaneous regression of optic gliomas: 13 cases documented with serial neuroimaging. Arch Ophthalmol 2001;119:516–529.
31. Pierre-Kahn A, Hirsch JF, Roux FX, Renier D, Sante-Rosa EC. Intracranial ependymomas of childhood: survival and functional results of 47 cases. Child's Brain 1983;10:145–156.
32. Repka MX, Miller NR. Optic atrophy in children. Am J Ophthalmol 1988;106:191–193.
33. Repka MX, Miller NR, Miller MJ. Visual outcome after surgical removal of craniopharyngiomas. Ophthalmology 1989;96:195–199.
34. Russell DC, Rubenstein LJ. Pathology of tumors of the nervous system. Baltimore: Williams & Wilkins, 1977.
35. Schulte FJ. Intracranial tumors in childhood: concepts of treatment and prognosis. Neuropediatrics 1984;15:3–12.
36. Skarf B, Hoyt CS. Optic nerve hypoplasia: association with anomalies of the endocrine and CNS. Arch Ophthalmol 1984;102: 62–67.
37. Smith JL, Vuksanovic MM, Yates BM, Bienfang DC. Radiation therapy for primary optic nerve meningiomas. J Clin Neuroophthalmol 1981;1:85–99.
38. Speer C, Pearlman J, Phillips PH, Cooney M, Repka MX. Fourth cranial nerve palsy in pediatric patients with pseudotumor cerebri. Am J Ophthalmol 1999;127:236–237.
39. Stroink AR, Hoffman HJ, Hendrick EB. Diagnosis and management of pediatric brain stem gliomas. J Neurosurg 1986;65:745–750.
40. Takakura K. Intracranial germ cell tumors. Clin Neurosurg 1985;32: 429–444.
41. Traboulsi EI, Maumenee IH. Ophthalmologic manifestation of X-linked childhood adrenoleukodystrophy. Ophthalmology 1987;94: 47–52.

TABLE 9-1. Nystagmus Types as Identified by History, Physical Examination, and Ocular Motility Recordings.

1. Acquired
2. Arthrokinetic
3. Associated
4. Audiokinetic
5. Bartel's
6. Bruns'
7. Centripetal
8. Cervical
9. Circular/elliptic/oblique
10. Congenital/infantile syndrome
11. Convergence
12. Dissociated
13. Downbeat
14. Drug-induced
15. Epileptic
16. Flash-induced
17. Gaze-evoked
18. Horizontal
19. Induced (provoked)
20. Intermittent vertical
21. Jerk
22. Latent/manifest latent
23. Lateral medullary
24. Lid
25. Miner's (occupational)
26. "Muscle-paretic"
27. Optokinetic
28. Optokinetic after (induced)
29. Pendular
30. Periodic/aperiodic alternating
31. Physiological (endpoint, fatigue)
32. Pursuit (after induced)
33. Rebound
34. Reflex (Baer's)
35. See-saw
36. Somatosensory induced
37. Spasmus nutans
38. Spontaneous ("voluntary")
39. Torsional
40. Uniocular
41. Upbeat
42. Vertical
43. Vestibular (central, peripheral, geotropic, ageotropic, galvanic, head shaking, positional, caloric, rotational)

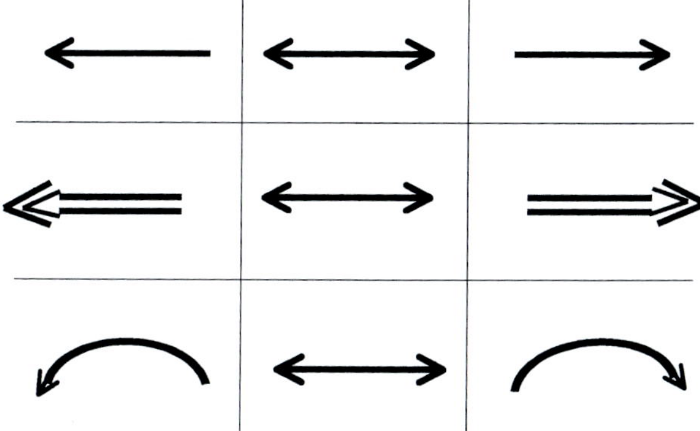

FIGURE 9-1. Diagram of nystagmus in nine positions of gaze. *Arrowheads* indicate direction of jerk: fast phase if on one end, pendular nystagmus if on both ends, and increasing frequency with *more arrowheads*. *Additional lines* indicate increased nystagmus amplitude. The *curved lines* indicate torsional nystagmus.

in synchrony. The nystagmus may be predominantly pendular or jerky, the former referring to equal velocity of the to-and-fro movement of the eyes, and the latter referring to the eyes moving faster in one direction and slower in the other. Involuntary ocular oscillations containing only fast phases are referred to as "saccadic oscillations and intrusions" and *not* nystagmus (Table 9-2). It is well documented that differentiating true nystagmus from saccadic oscillations and intrusions is sometimes

TABLE 9-2. Saccadic Intrusions and Oscillations Identified by History, Physical Examination, and Ocular Motility Recordings.

1. Bobbing/dipping
2. Double saccadic pulses
3. Dynamic overshoot
4. Dysmetria
5. Flutter
6. Flutter dysmetria
7. Macrosaccadic oscillations
8. Myoclonus
9. Opsoclonus
10. Psychogenic flutter (voluntary nystagmus)
11. Saccadic lateropulsion
12. Saccadic pulses/pulse trains ("abduction," ataxic, intrusions)
13. Square wave jerks/oscillations
14. Superior oblique myokymia

impossible clinically. Recent advances in eye movement recording technology have increased its application in infants and children who have disturbances of the ocular motor system.[1,4]

INCIDENCE

In 1991, Stang retrospectively reviewed the records of Group Health Inc. (White Bear Lake, Minnesota, U.S.A.) and in their pediatric population of 70,000 found a prevalence of clinical "nystagmus" of 1 in 2850.[66] Other estimates of its incidence range from 1 in 350 to 1 in 6550.[11,28,38,41,55] Up to 50% of the infantile strabismic population have some associated nystagmus.[9,20,39,42,44,45,54,60] If these cases are included in the prevalence estimates, then up to 0.5% of the population would be considered to have some form of nystagmus.

ETIOLOGY

The theoretical neuronal mechanisms of nystagmus continue to evolve and a single unifying explanation is still lacking. However, three major supranuclear inputs to the oculomotor system are clearly important in stabilizing eye movements; their dysfunction may lead to nystagmus. These inputs are the pursuit system, the vestibular system, and the neural integrator.

The pursuit system, previously thought to have only a dynamic function, provides a major input for fixation stability (e.g., pursuit at "0 velocity" is stable fixation).[37,57] The outputs of the right and left vestibular apparati are neural discharges, each of which tends to drive the eyes contralaterally. Normally the right and the left outputs are equal and cancel each other. Head rotation and unilateral vestibular damage alter this balance. For example, right vestibular damage causes the eyes to drift to the right side. A corrective saccade is then made toward the left. A distinguishing feature of vestibular nystagmus is that the slow phase of the nystagmus toward the affected side is of constant velocity as recorded by electronystagmography. It is important to realize that most forms of acquired nystagmus are caused by disease of the vestibular system (centrally or peripherally). Eye movement recordings show various combinations of slow phases including uniplanar or multiplanar, simple pendular, linear, and decelerating.[52]

The neutral integrator is a theoretical neuronal system that changes the resting firing rate to the extraocular muscles to (1) overcome the viscoelastic forces of the orbit and (2) maintain a position of eccentric gaze. The exact location of the neural integrator is unknown, but much of its function resides in the nucleus prepositus hypoglossi (NPH), located just caudal to the abducens nucleus.[53,57] Two types of dysfunction of the neural integrator are postulated: integrator leak and high-gain instability. With integrator leak, the firing rate of the extraocular muscles is inadequate to overcome the viscoelastic forces of the orbit and maintain the desired eccentric position of gaze; this results in a slow drift of the eyes toward the primary position of gaze and a corrective saccade back toward the desired eccentric position. The slow phase of the nystagmus as recorded by ocular motility recordings is linear (i.e., of constant velocity) or decelerating. Clinically, one observes gaze-evoked or gaze-paretic nystagmus.

High-gain instability is a term borrowed from engineering to try to explain the pathophysiology of infantile (congenital) nystagmus. In infantile nystagmus, the slow-phase velocity increases as the eyes move from the desired position of gaze; this is referred to as an accelerating slow phase. The ocular motor system (the "output") is improperly calibrated with the afferent visual system (the "input"). Gain is the ratio of output to input, and in the developing visual system, gain is properly calibrated in the first few weeks to months of life.[24,46,73] Faulty calibration of the gain may be a contributing factor in the etiology of infantile nystagmus. The pathophysiology of latent nystagmus and manifest/latent nystagmus (LN/MLN) (referred to by some as fusion maldevelopment nystagmus syndrome) is different from and less well understood than infantile nystagmus. Because it commonly is associated with the infantile strabismus syndrome, its cause may be related to the documented persistence of nasotemporal motion processing asymmetry that is also characteristic of the syndrome.

CLINICAL FEATURES OF NYSTAGMUS IN INFANCY AND CHILDHOOD

Neonatal and Early Infantile Nystagmus

Distinguishing acquired from the benign neonatal/infantile forms of nystagmus is important because of the implication for underlying neurological disease in acquired nystagmus (Table 9-3). A

TABLE 9-3. Types of Early-Onset Nystagmus.

Characteristic	*INS*	*LN/MLN*	*SN*
Onset first few months of life	Yes	Yes	Yes
May be only visual system deficit ("motor" only)	Yes	Yes	Yes
May be associated with sensory system disease	Yes; e.g., albinism, achromatopsia, aniridia, optic nerve hypoplasia	Yes; e.g., strabismic amblyopia	Yes, occasional chiasmal, hypothalamic, optic pathway gliomas and retinal dystrophy
Oscillation characteristics	Bilateral, conjugate, symmetrical, uniplanar, jerk/pendular	Bilateral, conjugate, symmetrical, uniplanar, jerk (can be worse in amblyopic eye)	Low amplitude, high frequency, dysconjugate, asymmetrical, pendular, multiplanar
Oscillopsia	No	No	No
Worsens with increased fixation effort and anxiety	Yes	No	No
Improves with convergence, fatigue, sleep	Yes	Yes	???
Anomalous head posture	Yes, ~20% by 1 year of age, due to "gaze-null"	Yes, ~5%–10%, due to an "adduction-null," fixation with the preferred eye	Yes, usually multiplanar (e.g., a tilt and turn)
Associated strabismus	~50%	Almost 100%	Yes, ~10%–20%
Associated head bobbing	No	No	Yes
A "latent" component (direction of jerk toward fixing eye)	~50%	100%	No
Natural history	Decreases but persists	Decreases but persists	"Disappears" by 2–3 years of age
Oculography	"Increasing" velocity slow phases	"Decreasing/linear" velocity slow phases	>10 Hz, dysconjugate, multiplanar, pendular slow phases

INS, infantile nystagmus syndrome; LN/MLN, latent nystagmus/manifest latent nystagmus; SN, spasmus nutans.

solid history of the onset of nystagmus in the first month of life is reassuring because such cases are usually neurologically benign. Efforts are being made to add precision and uniformity to nystagmus terminology. The terms congenital nystagmus (CN) infantile nystagmus, and idiopathic motor nystagmus have become synonymous with the most common form of neonatal nystagmus.[4,20,44,45,61] The term infantile nystagmus syndrome (INS) is a broader and more inclusive term that we prefer when referring to the broad range of neonatal nystagmus types, including those with identifiable causes. The distinguishing characteristic of INS is the presence of an accelerating slow phase. The major types of nystagmus waveforms are shown in Figure 9-2.

In general, a clearly documented history of onset of any form of nystagmus in the first months of life should put the exam-

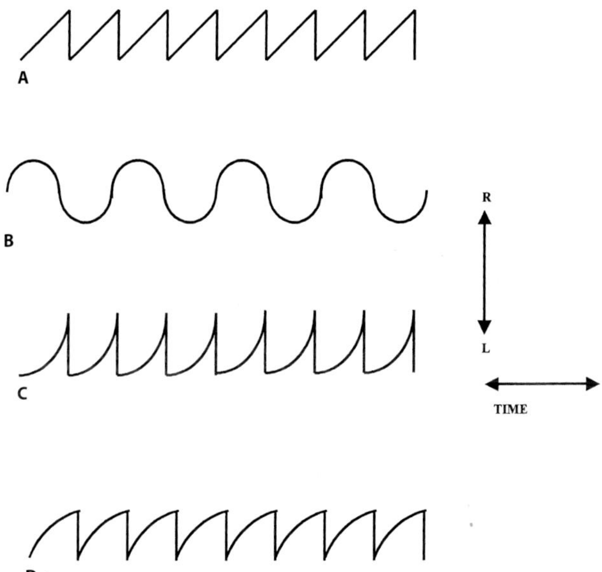

FIGURE 9-2A–D. Representation of major types of nystagmus waveforms. Continuous periods of time are depicted in each tracing. Rightward eye movements are up, and leftward eye movements are down. **(A)** Pure jerk left nystagmus. **(B)** Pendular nystagmus. **(C)** Jerk left with increasing velocity slow phases. **(D)** Jerk left with decreasing velocity slow phases.

iner at ease. Unfortunately, such history is not usually available because neonatal-onset nystagmus is frequently not noticed until later in life. However, the characteristics of INS and LN/MLN are so typical that when encountered in older patients the nystagmus can be assumed to have begun in the neonatal period. All other forms of nystagmus should be assumed to have been acquired, unless there is clear documentation of their neonatal onset.

Infantile Nystagmus Syndrome (Previously Congenital Motor Nystagmus, CN)

Familiarity with the clinical features of infantile nystagmus syndrome (INS) permits the examiner to avoid unnecessary testing. INS is an ocular motor disorder that presents at birth or early infancy and is clinically characterized by involuntary oscillations of the eyes. Estimations of the incidence of INS vary enormously, from 1 in 350 to 1 in 20,000, although the generally quoted estimated incidence is 1 in 6550 or 0.015%.[44,45] These movements most commonly have a slow and fast phase, although they may be purely pendular; they are usually horizontal with a small torsional component and may (rarely) have a vertical component. Other clinical characteristics, not always present, include increased intensity with fixation and decreased intensity with sleep or inattention; variable intensity in different positions of gaze (usually about a null position); changing direction in different positions of gaze (about a neutral position); decreased intensity (damping) with convergence; anomalous head posturing; strabismus; and an increased incidence of significant refractive errors. INS can occur in association with congenital or acquired defects in the visual sensory system (e.g., albinism, achromatopsia, and congenital cataracts). The cause or causes and pathophysiological mechanisms of INS have not been elucidated. Children with this condition frequently present with a head turn, which is used to maintain the eyes in the position of gaze of the null point (point of minimum nystagmus). This maneuver is particularly prominent when the child is concentrating on a distant object, as this form of nystagmus tends to worsen with attempted fixation. The head turn is an attempt to stabilize the image under these conditions. Head oscillations are common in INS and probably reflect underlying instability of cervical motor control. Hence, the head movements are pathological and not adaptive.

Oscillopsia, an illusory movement of the stationary world, is almost never present in INS. The reason for this is unclear, but may be explained by efference copy mechanisms, in which a copy of the motor output signal to the extraocular muscles (EOMs) is also sent to other sensory and motor areas in the brain.[2,8] Presumably this corollary discharge then permits suppression of oscillopsia. In those rare patients with intermittent oscillopsia, it tends to occur at gaze angles in which the nystagmus is maximal or if a new sensory system defect develops (e.g., retinal disease). Absence of oscillopsia is usually not helpful in distinguishing congenital from acquired nystagmus in children because, even with acquired nystagmus, small children rarely have this complaint.

Numerous studies of INS in infants and children confirm an age-dependent evolution of waveforms during infancy from pendular to jerk.[4,20,44,61] This concept is consistent with the theory that jerk waveforms reflect modification of the nystagmus by growth and development of the visual sensory system. Many forms of visual sensory system abnormalities are associated with the motor defects present in INS. Therefore, classification of INS as either "sensory" or "motor" is confusing and often inaccurate. Nevertheless, the practical task for the physician is to determine if an identifiable etiology or cause of the nystagmus is present. Accurate, uniform, and repeatable classification and diagnosis of nystagmus in infancy as INS is best accomplished by a combination of clinical and motility findings; in some cases, motility findings are indispensable for diagnosis (Fig. 9-3).

If an infant is diagnosed with INS, ocular motility analysis can also be helpful in determining visual status. Analysis of binocular or monocular differences in waveforms and foveation periods reflect development of the afferent visual system. Pure pendular or jerk waveforms *without foveation periods* are associated with poorer vision whereas waveforms of either type *with extended periods of foveation* are indicators of good vision. Significant interocular differences in a patient reflect similar differences in vision between the two eyes. Ocular motility analysis in infants also accurately determines nystagmus changes with gaze (null and neutral zones).

Although numerous studies have described INS pathophysiology and its effect on the visual system, its etiology remains elusive. Defects have been proposed involving the saccadic, optokinetic, smooth pursuit, and fixation systems as well as the

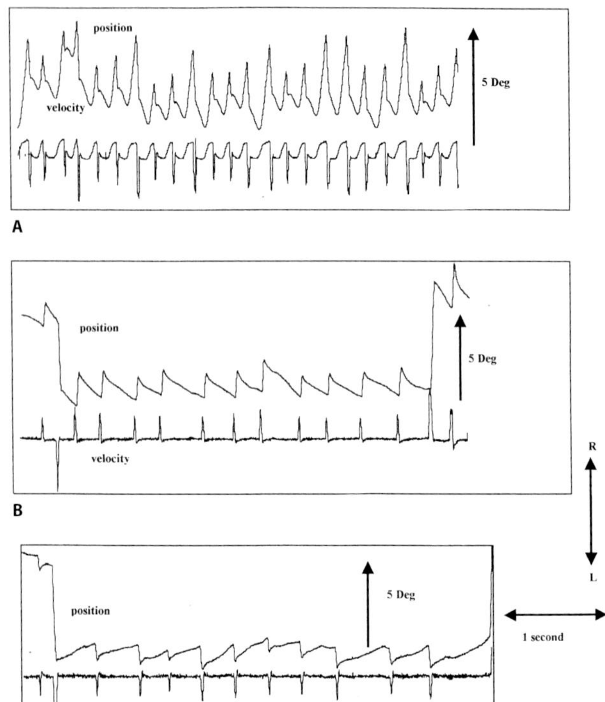

FIGURE 9-3A–C. (**A**) OU open-OD recording, jerk left INS. (**B**) OD viewing (OS cover), OD recording, jerk right LN/FDN. (**C**) OS viewing (OD cover), OS recording, jerk left LN/FDN. *INS*, infantile nystagmus syndrome; *FDN*, fusion maldevelopment nystagmus syndrome.

neural integrator for conjugate horizontal gaze. As mentioned previously, biomedical control system models have reproduced this oscillation, and it has been attributed to a "high-gain instability" in the ocular motor system. This term loosely translates as an error in "calibration" of the eye movement system during attempted fixation. Including genetic predisposition, many clinical conditions are associated with the INS oscillation. The immature ocular motor system is a required condition for the development of this ocular oscillation. The etiology may be multifactorial, with the final common pathway being interference with ocular motor calibration during a period of sensitivity, at which time an insult results in irreversible changes. Sensitive periods during development of other aspects of visual function are well recognized, including visual acuity and binocularity.

A model for the development of a stable ocular motor system is depicted in Figure 9-4. Motor system calibration is an active process that may start in utero and continues at least through early infancy. Sensory system development is a parallel visual process that has been more thoroughly studied and also continues to develop through the first decade of life. Previous studies have documented connections between parallel visual processes (cross-talk) that modify, instruct, and coordinate these systems, resulting in smooth and coordinated function. INS may result from a primary defect (e.g., familial X-linked) of ocular motor calibration. INS may also result from abnormal cross-talk from a defective sensory system to the developing motor system at any time during the motor system's sensitive period; this can

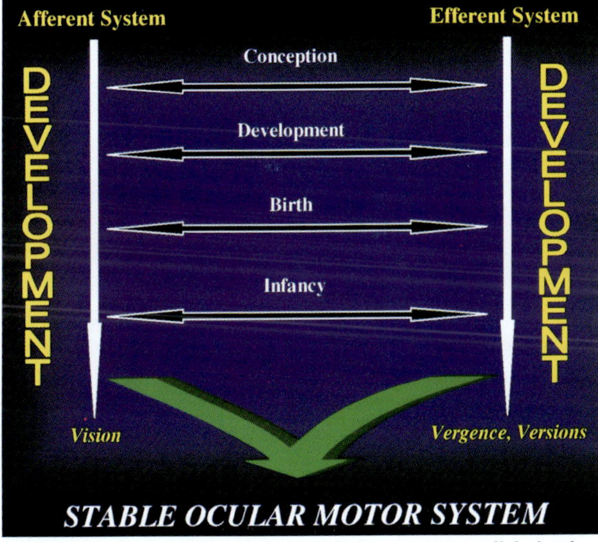

FIGURE 9-4. Diagram of model of interaction among parallel, developmental, visual processes, the interruption of which may result in infantile nystagmus syndrome (formerly termed CN).

occur from conception due to a primary defect (e.g., retinal dystrophy), during embryogenesis due to a developmental abnormality (e.g., optic nerve hypoplasia), or after birth during infancy (e.g., congenital cataracts). This theory of the genesis of INS incorporates a pathophysiological role for the sensory system in its genesis and modification. Although the set of physiological circumstances may differ, the final common pathway is abnormal calibration of the ocular motor system during its sensitive period. The primary ocular motor instability underlying INS is the same, but its clinical and oculographic expression is modified by both initial and final developmental integrity of all parallel afferent visual system processes. As the bidirectional arrows suggest (see Fig. 9-4), abnormal motor development would be expected to affect sensory development. As mentioned previously, this new knowledge forces us to abandon the classic "motor" and "sensory" classification introduced by Cogan more than 30 years ago.

Latent Nystagmus/Manifest Latent Nystagmus

Latent nystagmus/manifest latent nystagmus (LN/MLN) is a benign, jerk nystagmus that begins in early infancy and is easily observed under monocular viewing conditions. If the nystagmus is present under binocular viewing, then manifest latent nystagmus is said to be present. If monocular occlusion is needed to bring out the nystagmus, then latent nystagmus is present. LN/MLN is bilateral and conjugate with the slow phase toward the covered eye and the fast phase toward the viewing or suppressed eye. Strabismus, usually in the form of esotropia, is almost always present. It may be difficult to distinguish LN/MLN from INS with associated estropia without the aid of eye movement recordings. Latent nystagmus and manifest latent nystagmus have slow phases that are predominantly decreasing in velocity and linear (see Fig. 9-3).[20,22,35,75]

The term fusion maldevelopment nystagmus syndrome is preferred by some because all patients with this form of nystagmus have poor or absent fusion. Furthermore LN/MLN is an awkward and cumbersome term. However, it remains the most widely used term, and we continue to employ it in this text.

Patients with frank esotropia may demonstrate LN/MLN. Because these patients usually suppress one eye at a time, the nystagmus is often present even without covering an eye. The direction of the nystagmus depends on which eye is fixating.

LN/MLN can appear to be converted to "pure" latent nystagmus if the strabismus is repaired.

With electronystagmography, mild LN/MLN can usually be detected in those patients who appear to have only latent nystagmus clinically. The nystagmus simply becomes more prominent when one eye is occluded. True latent nystagmus is uncommon. LN/MLN tends to dampen on adduction, so patients with this condition may present with a head turn toward the side of the fixating eye. These patients have an adduction null with the fixing eye and not a true "gaze" null position. In addition to causing the anomalous head position, LN/MLN can cause the patient to have much worse monocular than binocular visual acuity.

Infantile Nystagmus Syndrome and Vision Loss (INS and Afferent System Defects)

Vision loss before 2 years of age is usually associated with a less well developed form of INS (previously Cogan's "sensory" nystagmus).[13,26,28–30,48,49] Visual loss should be highly suspected in any infant or toddler with onset of nystagmus after early infancy because mild to moderate visual loss may not be readily apparent in the preverbal years. It is never caused by pure cortical visual loss; consequently, careful evaluation of the eye is of utmost importance. The examiner should look for media opacities, high refractive errors, foveal hypoplasia, optic nerve hypoplasia, optic atrophy, and pigmentary retinopathy. Examination of the fundus with adequate magnification to assess the size and color of the optic disc is important. Foveal hypoplasia may be an isolated anomaly, or it may suggest albinism, aniridia, or rod monochromatism. A careful slit lamp examination for iris anomalies or transillumination defects and an electroretinogram (ERG) are necessary in such cases. Optic atrophy may be caused by tumors, hydrocephalus, and neurodegenerative disease. These possibilities need to be evaluated with good radiographic images of the brain and orbit, serum lactate and pyruvate levels, and leukocyte galactocerebrosidase levels.

A complete endocrinological evaluation is necessary in all cases of optic nerve hypoplasia because hypothalamic dysfunction is a commonly associated finding. Growth hormone deficiency in particular may be missed in the first few years of life. Lack of vigilance for this condition may result in unacceptable delays in treatment. We obtain brain MRI scans on young patients with optic nerve hypoplasia primarily to evaluate the structure of the infundiblum and pituitary gland. Finally, if a child with nystagmus has suspected visual loss but a normal ocular examination, an ERG is necessary because retinal dysfunction may be present even in the absence of pigmentary degeneration[17]; this may be caused by a primary photoreceptor dysgenesis such as Leber's congenital amaurosis or rod monochromatism. Alternatively, it may result from retinal degeneration associated with neuronal ceroid lipofuscinosis, or peroxisomal disease such as Refsum's disease, infantile adrenoleukodystrophy, or Zellweger's syndrome. Such cases should be evaluated with conjunctival biopsy to look for typical cytoplasmic inclusions by electron microscopy and with analysis of levels of serum very long chain fatty acid levels.

Spasmus Nutans

Spasmus nutans (SN) is the third most common oscillation beginning in infancy. The classic triad of findings includes high-frequency, small-amplitude, dys-conjugate oscillations; a head nodding oscillation; and a head tilt (Fig. 9-5). These findings usually become less noticeable as the infant becomes a toddler. Unlike ISN, the head nodding may result in improvement of vision and decrease in the nystagmus; the reason for this is unclear. The characteristic feature of spasmus nutans is the very fine, rapid pendular nature of the nystagmus. The eyes appear to have a shimmering appearance with horizontal, vertical, or

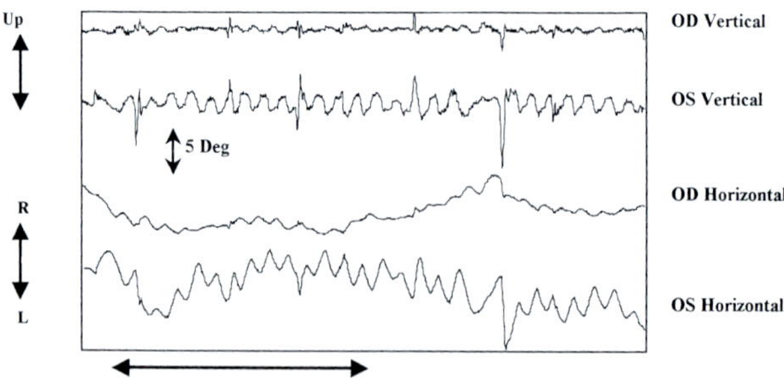

FIGURE 9-5. OU open. High-frequency (12–14 Hz), asymmetrical, dysconjugate, multiplanar, (torsional) pendular nystagmus typical of spasmus nutans.

TABLE 9-4. Extended Nystagmus Workup Is Not Necessary.

History
Onset of nystagmus in the first few 4–6 months of life
Family history of INS
No developmental or genetic diseases
Normal pregnancy, labor, delivery, growth, and developmental milestones
No exposure to toxins or drugs
Ophthalmic examination
Normal visual behavior in both eyes (e.g., F & F, C, US, M, normal Teller acuity card vision for age)
Normal structural examination of the eyes
Nystagmus pattern characteristic of INS or FDN
General pediatric examination
Normal growth and/or development.

INS, infantile nystagmus syndrome; LN/MLN, latent nystagmus/manifest latent nystagmus.

torsional movements. SN is usually asymmetrical to the point that it may appear unilateral. Pure unilateral forms are not uncommon. It may appear to switch eyes with changes in direction of gaze and frequently appears worse in the abducting eye. Large degrees of asymmetry are associated with amblyopia of the more involved eye.[5,31–33,36,71]

Spasmus nutans may be a completely benign condition with onset in infancy and resolution within 2 years. However, tumors of the anterior visual pathway and diencephalon can cause a condition indistinguishable from spasmus nutans. Consequently, neuroimaging or careful monitoring for visual, neurological, or endocrinological decline is essential. An intracranial tumor should be strongly suspected in any child who develops spasmus nutans after 3 years of age. Characteristics of infantile nystagmus syndrome, fusion maldevelopment nystagmus syndrome, and spasmus nutans are listed in Table 9-3.

Acquired Nystagmus

Toxins, drugs, and intracranial disease commonly cause acquired nystagmus. Consequently, further evaluation of acquired nystagmus is typically required (Tables 9-4, 9-5, 9-6).[18,25,40,51,52,62,63,70]

In general, the workup of nystagmus is directed toward identifying features that are not consistent with typical INS or LN/MLN. If these features are found and the etiology is not readily apparent by history or physical examination, neuroimaging studies are usually warranted. Atypical features

TABLE 9-5. Extended Nystagmus Workup Is Necessary.

- History
  - Onset of nystagmus after 6–9 months of age
  - History of severe prematurity or developmental or genetic diseases
  - Abnormal pregnancy, labor, or delivery
  - Abnormal and/or delayed growth
  - Exposure to toxins or drugs
- Ophthalmic examination
  - Abnormal vision of the eye(s) (e.g., photophobia, delayed visual behavior)
  - Abnormal structural examination of the eye(s) (e.g., foveal or optic nerve dysplasia)
  - Nystagmus pattern vertical, asymmetrical, dysconjugate, or associated with other ocular motor disorders, e.g., decreased pursuit, abnormal saccades, and paretic gaze
- General pediatric examination
  - Pediatrician is concerned with growth and development, or patient has manifest "hard" or "soft" focal or diffuse neurological signs

include vertical, circular, or elliptical components, dissociation of the nystagmus between the two eyes, the presence of oscillopsia, hearing loss, loss or reversal of developmental milestones, ataxia, and weakness. The rationale for specific neuroimaging studies can be derived from the following sections on various forms of acquired nystagmus.

TABLE 9-6. Components of Extended Nystagmus Workup.

- Ophthalmologic
  - Electroretinogram
  - Visual evoked response
  - Ocular motility recordings
- Neurological
  - Pediatric neurological examination
  - Neuroimaging (e.g., CAT Scan or MRI)
  - ±Brainstem auditory evoked potential
  - ±Electroencephalography
- Developmental/genetic
  - Genetic specialist evaluation (e.g., pedigree, specialized physical exam, chromosome analysis)
  - Pediatric developmental specialist evaluation (e.g., psychometric, fine and gross motor and cognitive evaluations)
- Serum and/or urine for metabolic diseases
  - Storage diseases (Neimann–Pick C, Gaucher, sialidosis types I and II, Pelizaeus–Merzbacher disease, GM_2 type III
  - Amino acidurias
  - Leukodystrophies and other degenerative neurological conditions
  - Lipid metabolism disorders
  - Amyloidosis

Periodic Alternating Nystagmus

Periodic alternating nystagmus (PAN) resembles INS except that the null point shifts position in a cyclic pattern, resulting in changes in the amplitude and direction of the nystagmus every few minutes. Adequate observation of the patient for several minutes should exclude this diagnosis. However, PAN should be considered any time a patient's head turn is different from one examination to the next. PAN is fairly common in patients with oculocutaneous albinism.

Periodic alternating nystagmus is usually congenital and benign. Acquired forms may be associated with vestibulocerebellar lesions, neurodegenerative conditions such as Friedreich's ataxia, visual loss, and hindbrain abnormalities such as Chiari type I malformation. Neuroimaging is warranted in all cases unless the nystagmus has been stable for a prolonged period of time. Acquired PAN responds to treatment with low-dose baclofen.

Gaze-Evoked Nystagmus

Gaze-evoked nystagmus is a jerk nystagmus that occurs in the direction of eccentric gaze. In contradistinction to INS, most forms of gaze-evoked nystagmus can be stabilized by, or improved with, visual fixation and are accentuated by darkness or image blur. Gaze-evoked nystagmus is called *gaze-paretic nystagmus* if it occurs in the direction of limited eye movement, as may be associated with a cranial nerve palsy or myasthenia gravis. Gaze-paretic nystagmus may appear dissociated if the limitation of eye movement is asymmetric between the two eyes.

One form of gaze-evoked nystagmus that is completely benign is endpoint nystagmus; this occurs in extreme positions of lateral or upward gaze. It can be distinguished from pathological forms of gaze-evoked nystagmus by its low amplitude, symmetry on right and left gaze, poor sustainability, and absence of associated neurological abnormalities.

Drugs, particularly anticonvulsants and sedatives, as well as posterior fossa disease are the most common causes of pathologic gaze-evoked nystagmus. Such etiologies can usually be elicited by a careful medical history and review of systems. Disease of the cerebellum or vestibular system usually results in asymmetry of gaze-evoked nystagmus. For example, tumors of the cerebellopontine angle may result in a special type of nystagmus called Bruns' nystagmus. In gaze toward the side of the lesion, there is a low-frequency, large-amplitude oscillation due to defective gaze-holding (gaze-evoked nystagmus). In gaze away from the side of the lesion, a high-frequency, small-amplitude oscillation caused by vestibular imbalance is seen. In patients with pathological gaze-evoked nystagmus, associated neurologic abnormalities such as ataxia, hearing loss, tremor, or hemiparesis should always be sought. Certain characteristics of vestibular nystagmus can localize the etiology to the peripheral or central neuronal pathways of the vestibular systems. Central vestibular nystagmus is frequently uniplanar in contrast to peripheral vestibular nystagmus, which is usually torsional or multiplanar. Visual fixation easily inhibits peripheral vestibular nystagmus but not central vestibular nystagmus. Vertigo and tinnitus are common in peripheral vestibular nystagmus and uncommon in central vestibular nystagmus.

Acquired Pendular Nystagmus

Acquired pendular nystagmus may be caused by tumors, infarction, inflammation, or degeneration of the brainstem or cerebellum. The nystagmus may be horizontal, vertical, or both. A single lesion in the brain results in horizontal and vertical components that oscillate at the same frequency of 2 to 7 cycles per second. If the horizontal and vertical components are in phase, the nystagmus will appear oblique; if they are out of phase, it will appear circular or elliptical. Circular or elliptical nystagmus that is constantly changing character is caused by horizontal and vertical components that are oscillating on different frequencies and implies more than one lesion in the brain.

Localizing Forms of Acquired Nystagmus

Certain forms of acquired nystagmus have features so distinct that neuroanatomic localization of the lesion can be determined by clinical examination alone (Fig. 9-6). *See-saw nystagmus* consists of an upward and incyclotorsional movement of one eye with a simultaneous downward and excyclotorsional movement of the other eye. Lesions of the diencephalon are the usual cause. Congenital see-saw nystagmus is a rare form of neonatal nystagmus with upelevation and excyclotorsion of one eye and concomitant depression and incyclotorsion of the other eye.[6]

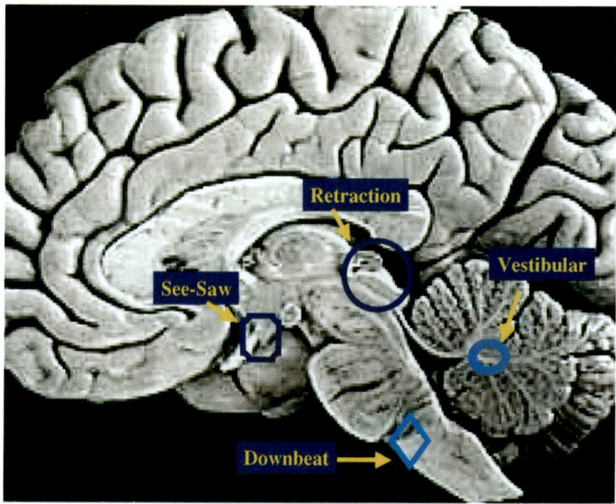

FIGURE 9-6. Sites within the brain responsible for the "localizing" forms of acquired nystagmus.

Isolated *downbeat nystagmus* is usually caused by drugs (particularly lithium or sedatives) or lesions at the cervicomedullary junction. In children, it is usually due to Arnold–Chiari malformation or syringo-myelia. Without a drug history, downbeat nystagmus should be evaluated in all patients with a sagittal MRI scan of the brainstem and cervical spinal cord.[12]

Convergence-retraction nystagmus is usually caused by lesions of the dorsal midbrain, especially those affecting the posterior commissure. It is not true nystagmus because there is no slow phase. A pinealoma is the most common etiology. Involvement of the pupillary light reflex pathway in the posterior commissure results in light–near dissociation of the pupils. The patients have a deficiency of upgaze, because supranuclear upgaze pathways also travel through the posterior commissure. The convergence-retraction nystagmus generally occurs when upgaze is attempted, and it is associated with lid retraction (Collier's sign). Unlike most forms of nystagmus, the pathological movement is the converging fast phase, which is associated with retraction of the globes into their orbits.[10,50] Convergence-retraction nystagmus is most easily elicited with a downward rotating OKN drum. Convergence-retraction nystagmus may be elicited with OKN stimulation long after other signs of dorsal midbrain involvement have resolved.

Saccadic Oscillations and Other Eye Movements

Saccadic oscillations may be mistaken for nystagmus on cursory examination. However, on closer inspection, or with eye movement recordings, their nonrhythmic nature and lack of slow phases make them distinguishable. As in nystagmus, recognizing those forms of saccadic oscillations that indicate intracranial or systemic disease is important (Fig. 9-7).[64,72]

Ocular dysmetria is a consistent undershooting or overshooting of a saccade toward a target. Saccades falling short of the target are hypometric; saccades that are too long are hypermetric. This event is usually followed by one or more correctional saccades toward the target. Ocular dysmetria usually is a sign of cerebellar disease, although it can occur with brainstem lesions it tends to have a stereotypical pattern in any given individual. Any patient with new-onset dysmetria requires neurological evaluation.

Ocular flutter consists of random conjugate, to-and-fro horizontal saccades that disrupt fixation. An additional pathological feature is the absence of the normal intersaccadic latency period. Ocular flutter also indicates cerebellar disease and is usually associated with ocular dysmetria.

Opsoclonus is multidirectional ocular flutter. It presents as conjugate, chaotic saccades sometimes described as "saccadomania" or "lightening eye movements." It is also a sign of cerebellar disease and frequently occurs as a manifestation of postviral encephalitis. When it is associated with ataxia and myoclonus, it is known as the *dancing eyes, dancing feet syndrome*. It may also occur as a paraneoplastic syndrome associated with neuroblastoma. Consequently, all children with opsoclonus should have a complete medical evaluation, CT scan of the abdomen and thorax, and urinary vanillylmandelic acid levels. Opsoclonus may respond to treatment with steroids or ACTH. It may convert to ocular flutter as it resolves. It can be elicited by forced eyelid closure long after it has otherwise resolved.

Square-wave jerks refer to small, conjugate, horizontal saccades away from fixation followed by a saccadic return to fixa-

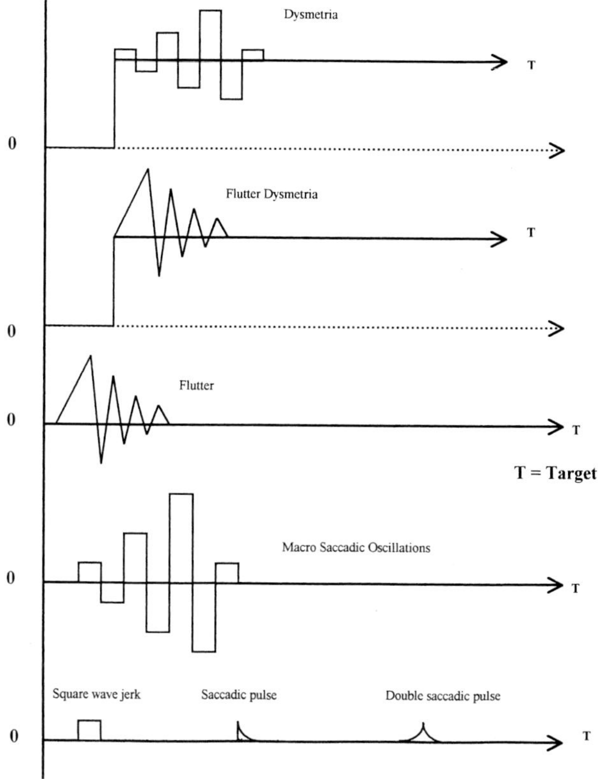

FIGURE 9-7. Saccadic oscillations and intrusions. Ocular motility recordings of major types of saccadic disorders. 0, the point of origin of eye.

tion after a 200-ms interval. These jerks may occur in normal individuals, particularly in the elderly. More than nine square-wave jerks per minute is considered abnormal in children. Such children should have a neurological evaluation and neuroimaging for a possible cerebellar disease.

Voluntary nystagmus (present in 7%–15% of the population) refers to a series of volitional, rapid alternating saccades with little to no intersaccadic interval (more like flutter). It is not a true nystagmus. The movements are usually horizontal but may be vertical or torsional and can only by sustained for a few seconds. Voluntary nystagmus is a popular party trick and is often seen in patients with functional visual complaints. It is frequently associated with convergence of the eyes or facial grimacing. Voluntary nystagmus warrants no laboratory or radiographic investigation.

CLINICAL ASSESSMENT

Examination Techniques: General

The first goal of the history and physical examination is to determine whether the nystagmus has been present from birth (the first few months of life) or acquired later. Information regarding a family history of neonatal eye disease, the pregnancy, labor, delivery, and growth and development since birth should be sought. Neonatal forms are generally benign, whereas acquired forms require further investigation. Patience is essential in the examination of childhood nystagmus. Because anxiety can affect nystagmus, the eye movements should be observed at a comfortable distance, in a nonthreatening manner, while talking to the child or the parent. The most important features of nystagmus can usually be ascertained while playing with the child. Head turns or tilts while the child is viewing distant or near objects should be noted. An adequate fundus examination is a necessary part of the evaluation of involuntary ocular oscillations in infants and children. Many of these patients have prechiasmal visual disorders.

The second goal of the history and physical examination is to assess the level of vision (see Techniques, following). This information may, in fact, be easier to determine than establishing the time of onset of the nystagmus. The types of nystagmus associated with decreased vision differ from nystagmus without visual loss, and this information, combined with the age of onset of the nystagmus, will aid in diagnosis. For example, in a child with acquired nystagmus and good vision, the finding of a conjugate, jerk, downbeat nystagmus points to a hindbrain abnormality and an MRI is indicated. As another example, if there is vision loss along with the nystagmus, the ocular examination is unremarkable and the child is neurologically normal, then an ERG is indicated to evaluate for possible retinal dystrophy. Figure 9-8 gives

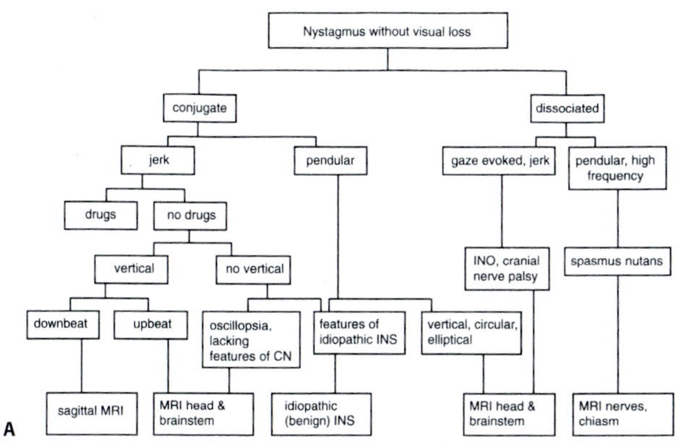

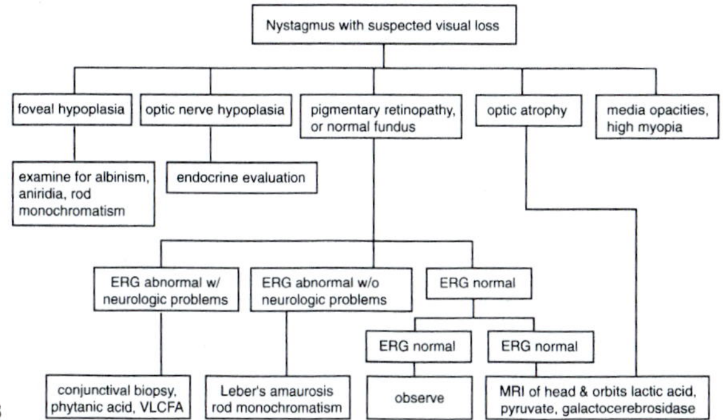

FIGURE 9-8A,B. (**A**) Algorithm for the evaluation of nystagmus without visual loss. Principal goal is to identify features that are not typical of idiopathic infantile nystagmus syndrome. (**B**) Algorithm for the evaluation of nystagmus with suspected visual loss.

algorithms for the evaluation and laboratory testing of children with nystagmus based upon the presence or absence of visual loss.

Examination Techniques: Vision

Vision testing procedures assume special importance and are dependent on the patient's ability to supply subjectively accurate data. Subjective accuracy depends on both the patient's age and neurological status. At this point it must be emphasized the patient's "*binocular acuity*" be tested first. If present, the patient must be allowed to assume their anomalous head posture (AHP) (which is often impossible if a phoropter is being used). During the examination of visual acuity in nystagmus patients with an AHP, it is imperative to observe the direction of the posture during a 5- to 7-min period. Up to 17% of patients with INS (with and without associated sensory system defects) have a periodicity to the direction of their fast phase.[25,65] This periodicity manifests clinically as a changing head posture in the direction of this fast phase.

It is important not to forget that binocular acuity is the "person's" acuity and monocular acuity is the "eye's" acuity. These two are often very different in patients with nystagmus. Legal documentation of a nystagmus patient's best acuity must take this into consideration. In a nonverbal child or adult, various tests can be used to help determine both binocular and monocular acuity; these include fixation behavior, the 10 prism diopter base-down test, Teller acuity cards, and matching of single, surrounded, HOTV optotypes, Lea symbols, or Wright Figures. The best test of visual acuity in an older child and cooperative adult is the ETDRS chart. The ETDRS chart provides LogMar evaluation of all acuities, especially those between 20/400 and 20/100. Simple testing of binocular function is always attempted, as the results are important if convergence is to be stimulated or fusion is to be aided by refractive therapy, for example, Worth 4-dot and near stereopsis.

Examination Techniques: Refraction

In older children a subjective refraction is the foundation for any type of refractive therapy. All "refractionists" develop their own method in this regard, and each of their idiosyncrasies assists them with rapid and accurate subjective refraction. Try to ignore the oscillation and start with the distance retinoscopy in a phoropter in those patients without an AHP or trial frame (in those patients who have a significant AHP). The next step is to do "binocular" refraction. Although this goes against the classic teaching for subjective refraction, it is the most important step in these patients because many (>50%) have significant changes in their nystagmus under complete monocular conditions (often decreasing their best possible acuity). The best way to do this is to fog the fellow eye with only enough extra plus to decrease the vision in that eye 1 to 3 lines. In many patients with coincidental strabismus (about 50% of the childhood nystagmus population), voluntary control of fixation is adequate, so no fogging is necessary.[20,44] Now, your usual routine for subjective refraction can be implemented.

In children a complete cycloplegic refraction (e.g., 40 min after 1% cyclogyl, 50 to 60 min after 1% atropine) provides additional and important data for treatment decisions. In many older children with nystagmus from infancy there are uncorrected (and now "latent") refractive errors. The error is usually mixed astigmatism or hyperopia and is not discovered with subjective refraction. In those patients in whom there is a different refraction under cycloplegia, record *both* subjective and objective refraction for decision making regarding spectacle prescription.

Examination Techniques: Motility

Complete clinical evaluation of the ocular oscillation also includes fast-phase direction, movement intensity, conjugacy, gaze effects, convergence effects, and effect of monocular cover. The amplitude, frequency, and direction of the nystagmus in all directions of gaze can be documented with a simple diagram (see Fig. 9-1). The clinician can also observe the nystagmus while moving the patient's head. Evaluation of associated motility systems (e.g., strabismus, pursuit, saccades, and vestibulo-ocular reflex) can be clinically evaluated and recorded separately from observations of the oscillation; this is most commonly accomplished with prism cover and/or alternate cover measurements in all gaze positions and near. In older children, fusional and accommodative amplitudes can be measured using prisms and a gradient technique, respectively. Changes in the character of the nystagmus with convergence or monocular viewing should be noted. If the nystagmus can be seen to increase beneath closed eyelids, vestibular or brainstem pathology should be suspected because visual fixation may suppress nystagmus from lesions in these regions. Conjugacy of eye movements should be observed. Nystagmus that is asymmetrical between the two eyes, especially in the primary position of gaze, frequently suggests anterior visual pathway disease. Conjugacy of nystagmus can be checked by holding a pair of stacked 40 diopter prisms placed

INHERITANCE

X-linked, autosomal dominant, and autosomal recessive modes of inheritance all have been reported in cases of INS. However, X-linked inheritance is probably the most common.[3,14,47,58,69] A survey of 40 individuals registered with the Canadian National Institute for the Blind (CNIB) as blind from INS revealed that an abnormal single gene was responsible for the disorder in 33 patients. Fifteen of these were caused by autosomal recessive conditions whereas X-linked disorders accounted for another 15 patients. In 3 cases, the pedigrees were consistent with both autosomal recessive and X-linked inheritance. A clearly defined environmental origin was present in 1 case while specific genetic or environmental factors were not detected in the remaining 6 patients. The albinism, achromatopsia, and Leber's congenital amaurosis groups of disorders were those most frequently detected.[3,14,47,58,69] Many systemic syndromes and genetic disorders are associated with both "acquired" and infantile types of nystagmus.[19,59,67,68]

TREATMENTS

There are a number of signs and symptoms due to nystagmus that are amenable to treatment.[43] The first and most obvious is *decreased vision* ("central visual acuity," "gaze-angle" acuity, near acuity). Correction of significant refractive errors in children with nystagmus is the single most powerful therapeutic intervention for improving vision and visual function in these patients. Refractive etiologies of decreased vision include either one or a combination of conditions, for example, myopia, hyperopia, astigmatism, and anisometropia. These refractive conditions can contribute significantly to already impaired vision in patients with other organic etiologies of decreased vision, such as amblyopia, optic nerve and/or retinal disease, oscillopsia, and the oscillation itself. The second is *anomalous head posturing (AHP)*. Etiologies of AHP include a "gaze-null" due to INS or acquired nystagmus (e.g., chin-down in downbeat nystagmus); an "adduction null" due to LN/MLN (manifest strabismus with the preferred eye fixing in adduction); convergence damping due to INS ("nystagmus blockage"); and a periodically changing head posture due to periodic alternating nystagmus. The third is *oscillopsia,* which is usually caused by either acquired nystagmus or a change in the sensory/motor status of patient with INS (e.g., "decompensated" strabismus, a change in the gaze null angle or decreasing acuity). Other less-common associated signs and symptoms include hypoaccommodation (can be associated with acquired nystagmus and/or INS) and photophobia (INS associated with the congenital cone dystrophies and albinism). General treatment medical and surgical indications and guidelines are outlined in Tables 9-7 and 9-8.

In patients with INS, after subjective refraction is completed two other optical maneuvers can be performed in some patients to try and improve their vision. If the patient has INS and is orthophoric, add 7 diopters of base-out prism in front of each eye with an additional −1.00 sphere (for the coincidental accommodation) to test the effect of "convergence damping" on acuity at distance. The improvements in acuity, nystagmus intensity, and AHP obtained by this maneuver can be quite impressive in this subset of INS patients *without strabismus*. The second maneuver is addition of prisms to correct the strabismic devia-

TABLE 9-7. Indications and Surgical Treatments of Nystagmus.

Anomalous head/face posture
"Anderson–Kestenbaum" resection-recession OU (horizontal gaze null)
Vertical rectus resection-recession OU (vertical gaze null)
Bilateral oblique muscle recession/transposition (vertical gaze null)
Horizontal transposition of vertical recti (torsional gaze null)
Bilateral oblique muscle transposition (torsional gaze null)
Resection/recession of fixing adducted eye (adduction null in FDN)
Bimedial rectus recession ("nystagmus blockage syndrome")
Strabismus
Recession/resection surgery as indicated (promotion of fusion)
Oscillopsia
Retroequatorial rectus recession[a]
Botulinus toxin injection[b]
INS and "convergence damping"
Bimedial rectus recession
Decreased vision[c]
Retroequatorial rectus recession[a]
Horizontal rectus tenotomy[d]

FDN, fusion defect nystagmus.

[a,d] These procedures have been reported to decrease the intensity of the ocular oscillations associated with INS, but their effect on vision is unpredictable.

[b] Botulinus injections slow the nystagmus and improve oscillopsia at the expense of a reduction or loss of the vestibulo-ocular reflex, causing other disturbing visual symptoms.

[c] Decreased vision due to the effect of the oscillation and not associated sensory system deficits, e.g., foveal hypoplasia.

TABLE 9-8. Indications and Medical Treatments of Nystagmus.

Anomalous head/face posture
Prism spectacles (base-out adducting eye and base-in abducting eye)
Strabismus
Prism spectacles (promotion of fusion)
Oscillopsia
Optical retinal image stabilization
Neurontin[a]
Baclofen[a]
Clonazepam[a]
INS and "convergence damping"
Prism spectacles (base-out prism both eyes)
Decreased vision
Complete manifest/cycloplegic refraction
Contact lens correction
Optical retinal image stabilization
Low-vision telescopes (bioptics)

[a] These and similar medicines have been used in both childhood and "acquired" nystagmus with varied effects on the nystagmus intensity, vision, and oscillopsia.

tion. If this approach assists with sensory fusion or any binocular cooperation, the patient's nystagmus is often reduced, potentially improving acuity and/or other visual functions. Binocular visual acuity is tested before and after these maneuvers, demonstrating whether they are effective; if so, they can be incorporated in a treatment approach.

PROGNOSIS

The prognosis of all these ocular oscillations depends on the type of underlying ocular and systemic disease. In general, infantile forms improve with time unless they are associated with a degenerative ocular or systemic disease. Acquired forms are more visually disturbing and follow the course of the underlying neurological disease.

FUTURE RESEARCH

Nystagmus is a common finding in patients with disease affecting the brainstem and cerebellum. Basic research into mechanisms that normally control eye movements will lead to a better understanding of the pathogenesis of different types of acquired nystagmus. Nystagmus is caused by disorders of the mechanisms that normally function to hold gaze steady: the vestibular system, the gaze-holding mechanism, the visual stabilization system, and the smooth pursuit system. Thus, evaluation of a patient's nystagmus requires a systematic examination of each functional class of eye movements. Measurement of the nystagmus waveform, using reliable methodology, is often helpful in securing a diagnosis. Such measurements help differentiate acquired nystagmus from congenital forms of nystagmus and from saccadic disorders that lead to instability of gaze.[52] There is evidence that both strabismus and LN/MLN are related to the nasotemporal optokinetic imbalance, which persists because of failure to develop binocular vision, and that LN/MLN and INS arise from a genetic or acquired embryologic disorder with various degrees and directions of expression.[38] The application of molecular genetics and biology in the study of patients with nystagmus will ultimately provide answers regarding etiology and future treatments.

References

1. Abadi RV, Dickinson CM. Waveform characteristics in INS. Doc Ophthalmol 1986;64(2):153–167.
2. Abadi RV, Worfolk R. Retinal slip velocities in INS. Vision Res 1989;29(2):195–205.
3. Abadi RV, et al. Congenital idiopathic nystagmus in identical twins. Br J Ophthalmol 1983;67(10):693–695.
4. Abel LA. Ocular oscillations. Congenital and acquired. Bull Soc Belge Ophthalmol 1989;237:163–189.
5. Antony JH, Ouvrier RA, Wise G. Spasmus nutans: a mistaken identity. Arch Neurol 1980;37(6):373–375.
6. Apkarian P, et al. Non-decussating retinal-fugal fibre syndrome. An inborn achiasmatic malformation associated with visuotopic misrouting, visual evoked potential ipsilateral asymmetry and nystagmus. Brain 1995;118(pt 5):1195–1216.
7. Baloh RW. Pathologic nystagmus: a classification based on electro-oculographic recordings. Bull Los Angel Neurol Soc 1976;41(3):120–141.
8. Bedell HE, Currie DC. Extraretinal signals for INS. Investig Ophthalmol Vis Sci 1993;34(7):2325–2332.
9. Berk AT, et al. Ocular findings in 55 patients with Down's syndrome. Ophthalmic Genet 1996;17(1):15–19.
10. Biedert S, Reuther R. Pathologic nystagmus and related phenomena. A review. Nervenarzt 1985;56(6):281–286.

11. Bothe N, Lieb B, Schafer WD. Development of impaired vision in mentally handicapped children. Klin Monatsbl Augenheilkd 1991; 198(6):509–514.
12. Brodsky MC. Congenital downbeat nystagmus. J Pediatr Ophthalmol Strabismus 1996;33(3):191–193.
13. Brodsky MC, et al. Ocular and systemic findings in the Aarskog (facial-digital-genital) syndrome. Am J Ophthalmol 1990;109(4): 450–456.
14. Cabot A, et al. A gene for X-linked idiopathic INS (NYS1) maps to chromosome Xp11.4–p11.3. Am J Hum Genet 1999;64(4):1141–1146.
15. Catalano RA, et al. Asymmetry in congenital ocular motor apraxia. Can J Ophthalmol 1988;23(7):318–321.
16. Ciancia AO. Early esotropia. Int Ophthalmol Clin 1971;11(4):81–87.
17. Cibis GW, Fitzgerald KM. Electroretinography in congenital idiopathic nystagmus. Pediatr Neurol 1993;9(5):369–371.
18. Cross SA, Smith JL, Norton EW. Periodic alternating nystagmus clearing after vitrectomy. J Clin Neuroophthalmol 1982;2(1):5–11.
19. Czeizel A, et al. An aetiological study on 6 to 14 years-old children with severe visual handicap in Hungary. Acta Paediatr Hung 1991; 31(3):365–377.
20. Dell'Osso LF. Congenital, latent and manifest latent nystagmus—similarities, differences and relation to strabismus. Jpn J Ophthalmol 1985;29(4):351–368.
21. Dell'Osso LF, Flynn JT. INS surgery. A quantitative evaluation of the effects. Arch Ophthalmol 1979;97(3):462–469.
22. Dell'Osso LF, Schmidt D, Daroff RB. Latent, manifest latent, and INS. Arch Ophthalmol 1979;97(10):1877–1885.
23. Dell'Osso L, et al. Eye movement recordings as a diagnostic tool in a case of INS. Am J Optom Arch Am Acad Optom 1972;49(1):3–13.
24. Dell'Osso LF, et al. Foveation dynamics in INS. II: Smooth pursuit. Doc Ophthalmol 1992;79(1):25–49.
25. DiBartolomeo JR, Yee RD. Periodic alternating nystagmus. Otolaryngol Head Neck Surg 1988;99(6):552–557.
26. Fielder AR, et al. Delayed visual maturation. Trans Ophthalmol Soc UK 1985;104(pt 6):653–661.
27. Flynn JT, Dell'Osso LF. The effects of INS surgery. Ophthalmology 1979;86(8):1414–1427.
28. Good PA, et al. Value of the ERG in INS. Br J Ophthalmol 1989; 73(7):512–515.
29. Gottlob I. Eye movement abnormalities in carriers of blue-cone monochromatism. Investig Ophthalmol Vis Sci 1994;35(9):3556–3560.
30. Gottlob I, Reinecke RD. Eye and head movements in patients with achromatopsia. Graefe's Arch Clin Exp Ophthalmol 1994;232(7):392–401.
31. Gottlob I, et al. Signs distinguishing spasmus nutans (with and without central nervous system lesions) from infantile nystagmus. Ophthalmology 1990;97(9):1166–1175.

32. Gottlob I, et al. Head nodding is compensatory in spasmus nutans. Ophthalmology 1992;99(7):1024–1031.
33. Gottlob I, Wizov SS, Reinecke RD. Spasmus nutans. A long-term follow-up. Investig Ophthalmol Vis Sci 1995;36(13):2768–2771.
34. Gottlob I, Wizov SS, Reinecke RD. Quantitative eye and head movement recordings of retinal disease mimicking spasmus nutans. Am J Ophthalmol 1995;119(3):374–376.
35. Gradstein L, et al. Relationships among visual acuity demands, convergence, and nystagmus in patients with manifest/latent nystagmus. J Am Assoc Pediatr Ophthalmol Strabismus 1998;2(4):218–229.
36. Gresty MA, Ell JJ. Spasmus nutans or INS? Classification according to objective criteria [Letter]. Br J Ophthalmol 1981;65(7):510–511.
37. Gresty MA, et al. Assessment of vestibulo-ocular reflexes in INS. Ann Neurol 1985;17(2):129–136.
38. Gresty MA, et al. Neurology of latent nystagmus. Brain 1992;115(pt 5):1303–1321.
39. Guo SQ, et al. Visual pathway abnormalities in albinism and infantile nystagmus: VECPs and stereoacuity measurements. J Pediatr Ophthalmol Strabismus 1989;26(2):97–104.
40. Halmagyi GM, et al. Treatment of periodic alternating nystagmus. Ann Neurol 1980;8(6):609–611.
41. Helveston EM. Dissociated vertical deviation—a clinical and laboratory study. Trans Am Ophthalmol Soc 1980;78:734–779.
42. Helveston EM. 19th annual Frank Costenbader Lecture—the origins of congenital esotropia [see comments]. J Pediatr Ophthalmol Strabismus 1993;30(4):215–232.
43. Hertle RW. Examination and refractive management of patients with nystagmus. Surv Ophthalmol 2000;45(3):215–222.
44. Hertle RW, Dell'Osso LF. Clinical and ocular motor analysis of INS in infancy [see comments]. J Am Assoc Pediatr Ophthalmol Strabismus 1999;3(2):70–79.
45. Hertle RW, Zhu X. Oculographic and clinical characterization of thirty-seven children with anomalous head postures, nystagmus, and strabismus: the basis of a clinical algorithm. J Am Assoc Pediatr Ophthalmol Strabismus 2000;4(1):25–32.
46. Hoffmann KP, Distler C, Markner C. Optokinetic nystagmus in cats with congenital strabismus. J Neurophysiol 1996;75(4):1495–1502.
47. Hu DN. Prevalence and mode of inheritance of major genetic eye diseases in China. J Med Genet 1987;24(10):584–588.
48. Jacobson SG, Mohindra I, Held R. Visual acuity of infants with ocular diseases. Am J Ophthalmol 1982;93(2):198–209.
49. Jan JE, et al. Visually impaired children with sensory defect nystagmus, normal appearing fundi and normal ERGS. Dev Med Child Neurol 1996;38(1):74–80.
50. Keltner JL. Neuro-ophthalmology for the pediatrician. Pediatr Ann 1983;12(8):586, 590–598, 600–602.
51. Kori AA, et al. Pendular nystagmus in patients with peroxisomal assembly disorder. Arch Neurol 1998;55(4):554–558.

52. Leigh RJ. Clinical features and pathogenesis of acquired forms of nystagmus. Baillieres Clin Neurol 1992;1(2):393–416.
53. Leigh RJ, et al. Effect of monocular visual loss upon stability of gaze. Investig Ophthalmol Vis Sci 1989;30(2):288–292.
54. Nelson LB, et al. Congenital esotropia. Surv Ophthalmol 1987;31(6): 363–383.
55. Norn MS. Congenital idiopathic nystagmus. Incidence and occupational prognosis. Acta Ophthalmol 1964;42(4):889–896.
56. Ong E, Ciuffreda KJ, Tannen B. Static accommodation in INS. Investig Ophthalmol Vis Sci 1993;34(1):194–204.
57. Optican LM, Zee DS. A hypothetical explanation of INS. Biol Cybern 1984;50(2):119–134.
58. Pearce WG. INS—genetic and environmental causes. Can J Ophthalmol 1978;13(1):1–9.
59. Pike MG, Jan JE, Wong PK. Neurological and developmental findings in children with cataracts. Am J Dis Child 1989;143(6):706–710.
60. Pratt-Johnson JA. 18th annual Frank Costenbader Lecture. Fusion and suppression: development and loss. J Pediatr Ophthalmol Strabismus 1992;29(1):4–11.
61. Reinecke RD. Costenbader Lecture. Idiopathic infantile nystagmus: diagnosis and treatment. J Am Assoc Pediatr Ophthalmol Strabismus 1997;1(2):67–82.
62. Sakata E, et al. Recent development of the study on clinical significance of abnormal eye movement. Auris Nasus Larynx 1985;12(3): 169–182.
63. Selz PA, et al. Vestibular deficits in deaf children. Otolaryngol Head Neck Surg 1996;115(1):70–77.
64. Shallo-Hoffmann J, Petersen J, Muhlendyck H. How normal are "normal" square wave jerks? Investig Ophthalmol Vis Sci 1989;30(5): 1009–1011.
65. Shallo-Hoffmann J, Faldon M, Tusa RJ. The incidence and waveform characteristics of periodic alternating nystagmus in INS. Investig Ophthalmol Vis Sci 1999;40(11):2546–2553.
66. Stang HJ. Developmental disabilities associated with INS. J Dev Behav Pediatr 1991;12(5):322–323.
67. Silengo MC, et al. A new syndrome with cerebro-oculo-skeletal-renal involvement. Pediatr Radiol 1990;20(8):612–614.
68. Steinlin M, Zangger B, Boltshauser E. Non-progressive congenital ataxia with or without cerebellar hypoplasia: a review of 34 subjects. Dev Med Child Neurol 1998;40(3):148–154.
69. Summers CG, King RA. Ophthalmic features of minimal pigment oculocutaneous albinism. Ophthalmology 1994;101(5):906–914.
70. Troost BT. Nystagmus: a clinical review. Rev Neurol 1989;145(6-7):417–428.
71. Weissman BM, et al. Spasmus nutans. A quantitative prospective study. Arch Ophthalmol 1987;105(4):525–528.
72. Yee RD, et al. A study of INS: waveforms. Neurology 1976;26(4): 326–333.

73. Yee RD, Baloh RW, Honrubia V. Study of INS: optokinetic nystagmus. Br J Ophthalmol 1980;64(12):926–932.
74. Zubcov AA, Reinecke RD, Calhoun JH. Asymmetric horizontal tropias, DVD, and manifest latent nystagmus: an explanation of dissociated horizontal deviation. J Pediatr Ophthalmol Strabismus 1990;27(2):59–64; discussion 65.
75. Zubcov AA, et al. Treatment of manifest latent nystagmus. Am J Ophthalmol 1990;110(2):160–167.

10

Neurodegenerative Conditions of Ophthalmic Importance

Mark S. Borchert and Sarah Ying

The pediatric ophthalmologist is frequently asked to evaluate children with multiple neurological impairments for ophthalmic manifestations of heritable neurological diseases. Occasionally these are diseases with specific ocular findings such as Kayser–Fleischer rings in Wilson's disease or cherry-red spots in Tay–Sachs disease. More typically, they are diseases with nonspecific findings such as optic atrophy or nystagmus. Such findings can be used to help direct the neurological workup. Less commonly, these children present to the ophthalmologist with ocular complaints primarily. The ophthalmologist must recognize those signs and symptoms that may be associated with neurodegenerative conditions and institute an appropriate workup. Although all these conditions are rare, a general ophthalmologist is likely to encounter several of them in their career.

Most of the neurodegenerative conditions are metabolic and represent dysfunction of specific enzymes or enzyme systems. Many of these enzyme systems are associated with particular cellular organelles, allowing for the classification of these diseases according to the organelle that is disrupted. Examples of these are the lysosomal storage diseases, the mitochondrial disorders, and the peroxisomal diseases. Other neurodegenerative diseases have characteristic clinical and pathological findings without known enzyme defects. Clinically, these diseases each have their own stereotypical time and mode of onset, which allows for easy division of the neurodegenerative conditions into groups that present in infancy, early childhood, or late childhood (Tables 10-1 through 10-3).

LYSOSOMAL STORAGE DISEASES AND LEUKODYSTROPHIES

The lysosomal storage diseases are caused by dysfunction of lysosomal enzymes involved in the catabolism of complex lipids and sugars normally present in tissues, resulting in accumulation of intracellular storage products. Substances that may accumulate in nerve cell bodies and ultimately cause neuronal degeneration include sphingolipids, mucopolysaccharides, mucolipids, and oligosaccharides.[81]

When the catabolic defect affects primarily myelin constituents, it results in white matter fibrosis known as leukodystrophy. The leukodystrophies typically have visual loss as a primary manifestation of the disease. Those that are caused by lysosomal enzyme defects include metachromatic leukodystrophy and globoid cell leukodystrophy (Krabbe's disease). Adrenoleukodystrophy is now recognized to result from defects of peroxisomal function. Spongiform leukodystrophy (Canavan disease) and sudanophilic leukodystrophy (Pelizaeus–Merzbacher disease) are disorders of myelin production. The metabolic defect in other leukodystrophies remains obscure. Other lysosomal diseases with ophthalmic manifestations, including secondary visual loss, are covered elsewhere.

Krabbe's Disease

Krabbe's disease (globoid cell leukodystrophy, galactosylceramide lipidosis) is an autosomal recessive condition characterized by the accumulation of periodic acid–Schiff- (PAS-) positive material within microglial cells in the brain imparting a typical "globoid cell" appearance histologically. It is caused by a deficiency of the lysosomal enzyme galactocebroside β-galactosidase (*galactocerebrosidase*), which is encoded on chromosome 14. The accumulation of galactocerebroside results in central nervous system and peripheral nervous system demyelination.

Typical infantile-onset Krabbe's disease presents at age 4 to 5 months with irritability and muscular hypertonicity. Loss of vision or failure to develop vision is noted soon thereafter, as are recurrent low-grade fevers. Spasticity and opisthotonos rapidly supervene. Death usually occurs by age 2 years.[186] The principal ophthalmoscopic finding is primary optic atrophy. Rarely, macular cherry red spots are seen.[115]

TABLE 10-2. Neurodegenerative Conditions with Onset in Late Infancy or Early Childhood.

Defective organelle	*Condition*	*Principal ophthalmic manifestation*	*Principal systemic manifestations*	*Biochemical defect*
Lysosome sphingolipidoses	Metachromatic leukodystrophy	Optic atrophy, nystagmus	Weakness, ataxia, dementia	Arylsulfatase A
	Gaucher disease type 3	Abducens palsy, ocular motor apraxia	Dysphagia, spasticity, dementia, myoclonus organomegaly, osseous lesions	Glucocerebrosidase
	Niemannn–Pick type IS (formerly type B)	Pigmentary maculopathy	Organomegaly, mental retardation	Sphingomyelinase
	Niemann–Pick type IIS (formerly type C)	Vertical gaze palsy	Organomegaly, psychomotor retardation	NPC1 or HE1/NPC2 product
Lysosome oligosaccharidoses	Aspartylglycosaminuia	Crystalline cataracts	Coarse facies, mental retardation, diarrhea, recurrent infections	Aspartylglycosaminadase
	Fucosidosis	Tortuous conjunctival vessels	Coarse facies, psychomotor deterioration, dysostosis multiplex, angiokeratoma	α-L-Fucosidase
	Mannosidosis type II	Spokelike cataracts, corneal opacities	Coarse facies, psychomotor deterioration, dysostosis, multiplex, deafness, recurrent infections	α-Mannosidase
	Schindler's neuroaxonal dystrophy	Optic atrophy, nystagmus	Weakness, peripheral neuropathy, psychomotor retardation	α-*N*-Acetylogalactosaminidase
Lysosome mucolipidoses	Mucolipidosis III (pseudo–Hurler polydystrophy)	Corneal clouding, pigmentary retinopathy, hyperoptic astigmatism	Dysostosis multiplex, mental retardation, coarse facies (mild)	UPD-*N*-Acetylglucosamine: lysosomal enzyme *N*-acetylglu-cosaminyl-1-phosphotransferase
Lysosome mucopolysaccharidoses	MPS 1H (Hurler)	Corneal clouding, pigmentary retinopathy	Dysostosis multiplex, organomegaly, coarse facies, mental retardation	α-L-Iduronidase
	MPS II (Hunter)	Pigmentary retinopathy, corneal clouding (rare)	Dysostosis multiplex, organomegaly coarse facies, psychomotor retardation	Iduronate sulfatase

	MPS III (Sanfilippo)	Pigmentary retinopathy	Severe mental retardation, mild dysostosis multiplex, deafness	Heparan *N*-sulfatase (MPS IIIA) α-L-Acetylglucosaminidase (MPS IIIB) Acetyl-Co-A:α-glucosaminide acetyltransferase (MPS IIIC) *N*-Acetylglucosamine 6-sulfatase (MPS IIID)
Lysosome ceroidoses	Late infantile NCL (Jansky–Bielschowsky)	Pigmentary retinopathy, optic atrophy	Seizures, ataxia, spasticity, loss of speech	Pepstatin-insensitive lysosomal peptidase
Mitochondria	MELAS syndrome	Hemianopsia, cortical visual loss	Seizures, lactic acidosis, hemiparesis	Mitochondrial $tRNA^{leu}$
Peroxisome	Adrenoleukodystrophy	Cortical blindness, optic atrophy	Quadriparesis, dysarrthria, cognitive decline, Addison's disease	Lignoceroyl CoA ligase
Unknown	Riley–Day syndrome (familial dysautonomia)	Dry eyes, corneal hypoesthesia, band keratopathy, optic atrophy	Vomiting, motor delay, poor temperature control, postural hypotension, emotional lability	IKAP protein
	Chediak–Higashi syndrome	Iris transillumination, foveal hypoplasia, nystagmus	Oculocutaneous albinism, recurrent infections, ataxia, polyneuropathy	Unknown
	Neuroaxonal dystrophy	Optic atrophy, cortical blindness, nystagmus, esotropia	Weakness, peripheral neuropathy, spasticity	Unknown
	Ataxia telangiectasia (Louis–Bar syndrome)	Conjunctival telangiectasia, dysmetric saccades, nystagmus, optic atrophy	Ataxia, polyneuropathy, immunologic impairment	ATM protein kinase

TABLE 10-3. Neurodegenerative Conditions with Onset in Late Childhood or Adolescence.

Defective organelle	*Condition*	*Principal ophthalmic manifestation*	*Principal systemic manifestations*	*Biochemical defect*
Lysosome sphingolipidoses	Metachromatic leukodystrophy (late onset)	Optic atrophy	Personality changes, ataxia, incontinence, gallstones	Arylsulfatase A
Lysosome oligosaccharidoses	Sialidosis (type I)	Cherry-red spots, nyctalopia, cataracts	Myoclonus, ataxia	Neuroaminidase (oligosaccharide sialidase)
Lysosome ceroidosis	Juvenile NCL (Spielmeyer–Vogt)	Pigmentary maculopathy	Behavioral problems, cognitive decline, seizures, spasticity	Palmitoyl protein thioesterase and others
Peroxisome (presumed)	Refsum's disease	Pigmentary retinopathy, nyctalopia, cataracts	Ataxia, hearing loss, cardiac arrhythmia	Phytanic acid α-hydroxylase
Mitochondria	Fukuhara's disease (MERRF)	Optic atrophy	Myoclonus, ataxia, weakness	Mitochondrial $tRNA^{lys}$
	Chronic progressive external ophthalmoplegia CPEO/Kearns–Sayre	Ptosis, ophthalmoplegia, pigmentary retinopathy, nystagmus	Weakness, heart block, ataxia, hearing loss, endocrine problems	Mitochondrial $tRNA^{leu}$; multiple mitochondrial enzymes
None	SSPE	Macular chorioretinitis, optic atrophy, papilledema	Cognitive decline, myoclonus, epilepsy, rigidity	Immune response to measles virus
	Hallervorden–Spatz disease	Vertical gaze palsy, saccadic pursuit, eyelid apraxia, pigmentary retinopathy	Rigidity, choreoathetosis, dysarthria, dysphagia, dementia	Pantothenate kinase
	Wilson disease	Kayser–Fleischer rings, sunflower cataracts, saccadic pursuit	Liver failure, choreoathetosis, renal stones, cardiomyopathy	Copper-transporting ATPase
	Myotonic dystrophy	Ptosis, blepharospasm, cataracts, pigmentary retinopathy	Myotonia, muscle atrophy	Myotonic dystrophy protein kinase (DMPK)
	Friedreich's ataxia	Optic atrophy, nystagmus	Ataxia, dysarthria, pes cavus, kyphoscoliosis, proprioceptive loss, hyporeflexive joints, hearing loss	Frataxin

Late-onset forms of Krabbe's disease exist with symptoms beginning as late as 15 years of age; these usually present with rapid visual loss due to a combination of optic atrophy and cortical blindness. Ataxia, spasticity, polyneuropathy, and psychosis usually follow visual loss. Late-onset forms are often associated with prolonged survival and are believed to be manifestations of allelic variants in the defective galactocerebrosidase gene.[92,186]

Diagnosis of Krabbe's disease is made by assay of galactocerebrosidase activity in peripheral blood leukocytes or in cultured skin fibroblasts. However, the clinical measurements of residual activity do not necessarily correlate with clinical type or severity. Intermediate levels of activity can also be detected in the carrier state, but do not constitute a reliable screen in the general population. Prenatal diagnosis can be made by assay of galactocerebrosidase activity in cultured chorionic villus or amniotic fluid cells.[2,58,186]

Laboratory studies reflect the central and peripheral demyelination. Nerve conduction velocities may be slowed. Visual evoked potentials (VEPs), brainstem auditory evoked potentials (BAEPs), and somatosensory evoked potentials (SSEPs) are all delayed or absent.[85] Cerebrospinal fluid (CSF) protein may be elevated, particularly in early-onset disease. T_2- or proton density-weighted magnetic resonance images of the brain typically show high signal intensity white matter lesions sparing the subcortical U fibers,[32] which are nonspecific findings of any leukodystrophy.

As with any lysosomal storage disease, treatment with bone marrow transplantation to replace the defective enzyme is theoretically possible; this has resulted in remarkable reversal of neurological abnormalities and laboratory studies in several examples of late-onset disease. Early-onset disease has been successfully engrafted, with promising initial results in one patient so far. Intrauterine engraftment has not yet been successfully accomplished, but studies continue.[84] Other avenues of research include the use of umbilical cord blood, neuronal stem cells, or viral gene therapy.[186]

Metachromatic Leukodystrophy

Metachromatic leukodystrophy (MLD), or sulfatide lipidosis, is an autosomal recessive condition with a defect in either the lysosomal enzyme *arylsulfatase-A* (chromosome 22q)[47] or its sphingolipid activator protein (chromosome 10),[66] which together comprise *cerebroside sulfatase*; it results in the accumulation of cerebroside sulfate, a metachromatic material in the urinary sediment and viscera. Cerebroside sulfate is a major lipid component of myelin, and its accumulation in white matter results in demyelination of the central and peripheral nervous systems.

There are many forms of the disease, characterized by age of onset and clinical course, but they can generally be divided into three categories: late infantile, juvenile, and adult. The later onset forms have slower progression, but all three forms are lethal.[32] More than 70 mutations have been identified,[71] with a direct genotype–phenotype correlation between the different mutant alleles, residual enzyme activity, and severity of the disease form.[47]

The most common form of metachromatic leukodystrophy, late infantile, begins in the second or third year of life, and is preceded by normal development. Subsequently, there is developmental delay followed by progressive weakness, ataxia, spasticity, dementia, and optic atrophy. Death usually occurs within 2 to 4 years. Optic atrophy is rarely appreciated before the onset of other symptoms.

The juvenile-onset form arbitrarily begins between 4 and 16 years of age. It is intermediate in severity and duration between the adult and the late infantile varieties. Some cases may be compound heterozygotes of the adult and late infantile alleles. Patients may present initially with either neurological or psychological deterioration. Seizures occur in 80% of patients.

The adult form of MLD begins after 16 years of age and accounts for 10% of cases. Personality changes and inattention are usually the first signs. Patients with this condition are frequently misdiagnosed as schizophrenic. Eventually, ataxia, incontinence, and vision loss due to optic atrophy supervene. Biliary tract dysfunction caused by metachromatic gallstones is common. In contrast to the late infantile form, peripheral neuropathy is not a prominent feature. Deterioration occurs over years to decades.[32]

Diagnosis is based on finding decreased arylsulfatase-A activity in peripheral leukocytes or fibroblasts. Other laboratory studies reflect central and peripheral demyelination. As in Krabbe's disease, visual, auditory, brainstem, and somatosensory evoked responses show abnormal prolongation, and nerve conduction velocities are slowed. CSF protein may be markedly elevated.

Brain MRI scanning shows diffuse high signal on T_2 or proton density sequences. MLD is classically associated with diffuse symmetrical anterior leukoencephalopathy that spares the subcortical arcuate *U fibers*. However, it may have a focal asymmetrical, leopard skin, or even a tigroid appearance (previously believed to be pathognomonic of Pelizaeus–Merzbacher disease). The disease eventually progresses to involve the subcortical U fibers, cerebellum, and cortical gray matter.[33,195]

The MLD allele is present in approximately 1 in 100 normal people. Given recent advances in treatment options, efforts are currently underway to establish general population screening, using sulfatide levels from urine-soaked filter paper. Assaying arylsulfatase-A activities in chorionic villus homogenates permits prenatal diagnosis.

Genetic counseling in affected families has been confounded by the measurement of low arylsulfatase-A activities in otherwise healthy individuals; this is known as arylsulfatase-A pseudodeficiency. The frequency of the pseudodeficiency (PD) allele in the general population is estimated to be as high as 15%.[59] Presumably individuals with arylsulfatase-A pseudodeficiency have sufficient arylsulfatase-A activity to avoid disease. It is particularly important to screen for the PD allele in families with MLD, as compound heterozygotes with both the MLD and the PD alleles would have abnormal arylsulfatase-A activity but a clinically normal prognosis.[86]

The only available treatment for MLD is bone marrow transplantation, which has been shown to slow or even arrest the progress of the disease, although reversal of neurological damage has not been demonstrated. Prognosis is best for later-onset forms, before significant progression of the disease. In fact, presymptomatic individuals treated with transplantation may remain asymptomatic.[84] Thus, early diagnosis and treatment is critical.

Neuronal Ceroid-Lipofuscinosis (Batten Disease)

Neuronal ceroid lipofuscinosis (NCL) refers to a group of four clinically related diseases that are characterized by severe brain atrophy and by accumulation of the autofluorescent lipopigments, ceroid and lipofuscin, within neurons. It is the most common neurodegenerative condition in children,[16] with an estimated annual incidence of 300 to 350 cases in the United States and a collective incidence of 1 in 12,500 live births globally.[136,185]

F.E. Batten in 1906 provided the first pathological description of NCL, but the four diseases carry eponyms recognizing those who first described them.[135] Traditionally, these diseases have been classified by their age of onset, although recent discoveries have enabled further classification on a molecular genetic basis. The infantile variety (*Santavouri–Haltia* or *Hagberg–Santavouri disease*) presents in the first 2 years of life, the late variety infantile (*Jansky–Bielschowsky disease*) at age 2 to 4 years, and the juvenile variety (*Spielmeyer–Vogt–Sjogren* or *Batten–Mayou disease*) at age 5 to 10 years. These disorders all exhibit an autosomal recessive mode of inheritance. The adult variety (*Kufs' disease*), inherited in either a dominant or recessive fashion, presents in the third decade of life, and follows a more benign course. Kufs' disease is not discussed further in this text, as there are no ophthalmic manifestations.

The late infantile and juvenile varieties are the most common, together accounting for 70% to 85% of cases. The infantile variety accounts for an additional 10% to 20% of cases.[16,189,190] All childhood varieties of NCL develop cognitive impairment and loss of vision early in their course. In infantile NCL, regression occurs after about 8 months of normal development. Psychomotor deterioration is rapid, with hypotonia, ataxia, choreoathetosis, and seizures. Microcephaly as a manifestation of cerebral atrophy is common. Blindness from optic atrophy occurs by age 2 years. The electroretinogram becomes isoelectric by age 3 years, and death occurs in the first decade.

Late infantile NCL generally presents with a major motor seizure between 2.5 and 3 years of age.[15] Falls due to ataxia and hypotonia become commonplace, as do myoclonic jerks. Speech output gradually declines. Eventually spasticity develops, leading to flexion contractures. Retinal degeneration develops by age 3 years. By age 5 years, these children are reduced to a blind, cachectic, drooling state. They become prone to dehydration and infection. Death mercifully supervenes by age 10 years.

Declining vision due to pigmentary retinopathy is usually the first sign of juvenile NCL. Behavioral problems and cognitive decline insidiously follow. A more rapid deterioration is heralded by the onset of seizures at around 8 to 10 years of age. Myoclonic jerks become difficult to control, as does extrapyramidal rigidity. Dysarthria and echolalia characterize speech. Further decline to spasticity and mutism does not usually occur until the third decade of life. Death occurs by 40 years of age.

All three childhood forms of NCL may demonstrate a bull's-eye pigmentary maculopathy. There may also be a diffuse salt-

and-pepper appearance to the ophthalmic fundus. Bone spicule pigmentation is uncommon. By the time blindness develops, the electroretinogram is flat.

NCL has long been classified as a lysosomal storage disease because of the characteristic autofluorescent inclusion bodies within lysosomes, but only recently have the mutant lysosomal gene products been identified. At least eight NCL genetic loci (CLN1–CLN8) have been identified. So far, four have been found to encode for soluble or membrane-bound lysosomal proteins.[9] The protein product of CLN1, palmitoyl protein thioesterase 1 (PPT1), may be involved in intracellular regulation, whereas the product of CLN2, pepinase, appears to be involved in degradation of the membrane-bound mitochondrial subunit c of ATP synthase.[24] It is possible that the absence of cell division makes neurons particularly dependent on lysosomal protein degradation. The exact pathogenesis of the disease remains unclear, although apoptosis has been established as the final common pathway of neurodegeneration.[87]

The intracellular inclusions seen by electron microscopy have a characteristic appearance for each of the three childhood varieties of NCL. In infantile NCL they appear as granular osmiophilic deposits; they are curvilinear in late infantile NCL, and they have a fingerprint pattern in juvenile NCL. The inclusions can be identified within neurons, pericytes, macrophages, smooth muscle cells, lymphocytes, and capillary endothelial cells. The most popular tissue for biopsy is skin and rectum. We have found biopsy of the conjunctiva to be very productive in most cases. If the first biopsy is negative, biopsy of a different tissue should be considered in clinically suspicious cases.[16,49] Prenatal and carrier diagnosis is complicated by the extensive allelic diversity, but electron microscopic analysis provides additional information.[125]

Currently, genetic counseling, in conjunction with in vitro fertilization of high-risk individuals, is the only means of preventing the disease.[136] However, with advances in bone marrow transplantation and gene therapy for other diseases, presymptomatic treatment may become available for NCL as well.

Neuroaxonal Dystrophy

The neuroaxonal dystrophies are rare, heterogenous disorders that share a common histopathological finding. Histologically, there are accumulations of dense eosinophilic aggregates or "spheroids" in the axon terminals throughout the central nervous system, the peripheral nervous system, and the autonomic nervous system. These aggregates are free within the cytoplasm of the axon terminals and are thought to represent a manifestation of abnormal retrograde axonal transport.[154] The neuronal perikarya are normal, and there is no obvious loss of neurons. The white matter, glial cells, endothelial cells, and arachnoid cells are normal.

Seitelberger first described the classical clinical characteristics of neuroaxonal dystrophies in 1952. It generally presents in the second year of life with progressive weakness and difficulty in walking. A peripheral neuropathy is manifested by decreased sensitivity to pain and loss of tendon reflexes. Subsequently, the corticospinal tracts are involved, causing hyperactive reflexes and Babinski signs. At about the same time, loss of vision may bring the child to an ophthalmologist. The loss of vision can be due to optic atrophy, cortical damage, or both. Nystagmus and esotropia, along with the loss of vision, are common. Psychomotor deterioration soon gives way to dementia. The children are reduced to a decorticate state within the first decade of life. Seizures and extrapyramidal signs are rare.[36,116]

There are several notable variants to the clinical course of neuroaxonal dystrophy just described. A rare neonatal form has a preponderance of hypothalamic and autonomic manifestations including keratitis sicca, constipation, urinary retention, hypothyroidism, diabetes insipidus, and dysfunctional temperature regulation.[114] A more protracted course into late childhood with a predominance of cerebellar symptoms has also been described.[116]

Schindler's disease is one form of neuroaxonal dystrophy that is associated with a defect in the activity of the lysosomal enzyme alpha-*N*-acetylgalactosamin-idase. This loss results in accumulation of glycopeptides in the urine, which contain alpha-*N*-acetylgalactosaminyl residues.[147] The clinical spectrum ranges from the classical presentation of neuroaxonal dystrophy to angiokeratomata with vacuolization but without neurological manifestations.

Schindler's disease is transmitted in an autosomal recessive fashion and results from a single point mutation on chromosome 22q13-ter.[180,181] Other subjects with neuroaxonal dystrophies have not been found to have this enzyme defect.[25] The mechanism by which this defect causes the observed spectrum of neuropathology is unknown.

Marked cerebellar atrophy and diffuse hyperintensity of the cerebellar cortex on T_2-weighted MRI distinguish neuroaxonal dystrophy from other degenerative diseases with a similar age of onset. There are reports of hypointensity of the globus pallidus and substantia nigra (similar to those seen in Hallervorden–Spatz disease), which may represent progression of disease.[34,116,164]

Electromyography consistent with atrophy of motor neurons may be one of the earliest objective findings. A later but more suggestive finding includes fast rhythms on electroencephalography. As predicted by pathological findings, visual evoked responses are reduced or absent, whereas the electroretinogram is relatively preserved. Conjunctival biopsy may demonstrate spheroid inclusion in the unmyelinated axons.[38] Otherwise, the diagnosis of neuraxonal dystrophy remains largely dependent on clinical and eventual neuropathological findings.

Treatment is supportive.

PEROXISOMAL DISEASES

Peroxisomes are small cytosolic vesicles that are found in all cells except for mature erythrocytes. Peroxisomes are bounded by a single membrane and are not part of the cellular endomembrane system. They contain enzymes responsible for metabolism of very long chain fatty acids. This process consumes molecular oxygen and generates hydrogen peroxide. Continued beta-oxidation of the shortened fatty acid product is then carried out in the mitochondria. Peroxisomes are also partially responsible for the metabolism of steroids as well as synthesis of plasmalogens and bile acids. Biochemical markers of peroxisomal dysfunction include deficiency of plasmalogens or accumulation of pipecolic acid, phytanic acid, or very long chain fatty acids (VLCFA).

Some peroxisomal diseases are associated with normal peroxisomal structure; these are usually associated with defects in a single peroxisomal enzyme. X-linked adrenoleukodystrophy and Refsum's disease have the most ophthalmic significance and are detailed next. Other single enzyme defects of plasmalogen synthesis or beta-oxidation are also associated with normal peroxisomal structure. However, as they clinically mimic the peroxisomal biogenesis disorders, they are not discussed separately.

Peroxisomal biogenesis disorders (*PBD*) result from abnormalities of peroxins (PEX), which are required for import of proteins into the peroxisome. In turn, the activities of multiple peroxisomal enzymes are affected. The PBDs are currently categorized according to 12 complementation groups. For 11 of these groups, the mutated PEX gene has already been identified. Clinical severity is determined by functional differences of the mutant alleles. This continuum of disease was previously separated into four clinical presentations, here listed in decreasing order of severity: *Zellweger's syndrome*, *neonatal adrenoleukodystrophy*, *infantile Refsum's disease*, and *rhizomelic chondrodysplasia punctata*. We continue to describe this group of diseases according to clinical presentation for initial diagnostic categorization. Rhizomelic chondrodysplasia punctata is predominantly characterized by skeletal abnormalities and is not discussed here. Benign variants of other PBD syndromes without ophthalmologic involvement have also been reported.[52,94,108,109]

Adrenoleukodystrophy

Historically, adrenoleukodystrophy has referred to the X-linked disease first described by Siemerling and Creutzfeldt in 1923. It presents in 4- to 8-year-old boys with bronzing of the skin secondary to adrenal insufficiency. Personality changes and intellectual decline soon follow. Quadriparesis, dysarthria, dysphagia, and death supervene over a period of 2 to 4 years. The adrenal insufficiency is usually not clinically recognized until the neurological decline. Cortical visual loss presents at any time during the disease and may be associated with the development of exotropia. Eventually, optic atrophy is evident, further contributing to vision loss. As with any leukodystrophy, the neurological signs and symptoms correspond to massive degeneration of white matter.

A phenotypic variant of X-linked adrenoleukodystrophy known as adrenomyeloneuropathy occurs in men over 21 years of age.[106] This disorder presents mainly with a spinal neuropathy and peripheral neuropathy. Isolated cases are frequently mistaken for multiple sclerosis. Addisonian symptoms occur in many of these patients, but cerebral involvement is not common. These patients may have a normal lifespan. They may present in pedigrees containing persons with classical childhood onset X-linked adrenoleukodystrophy. A similar condition occurs in 20% of female carriers of the gene in their fifth or sixth decade of life.

In X-linked adrenoleukodystrophy (XALD), histologically normal peroxisomes are present, although lignoceroyl-Co-A ligase activation of *very long chain fatty acids (VLCFA)* for metabolism is impaired. The defective gene, found on chromosome Xq28, actually encodes for ALD protein (ALDP), an ATP-binding cassette (ABC) half-transporter that localizes to the peroxisomal membrane. The exact mechanism is unclear, but in vitro addition of ALDP to fibroblasts from XALD patients can restore VLCFA metabolism. It has been postulated that ALDP is required for the transfer of lignoceroyl-Co-A ligase into the peroxisome.[109,110]

The downstream pathogenesis of neurodegeneration also requires elucidation. It has been postulated that an increased proportion of VLCFAs may help to trigger a cytokine-mediated inflammatory cascade, particularly tumor necrosis factor (TNF). Pathologically, there is evidence of perivascular infiltrates by macrophages and lymphocytes. Absence of ALDP protein may be confirmed by immunohistochemistry but does not correlate with phenotype severity.[107]

Diagnosis in males may be made on the basis of elevated plasma levels of VLCFA. However, up to 15% to 20% of carrier females may demonstrate normal levels.[111] Measurement of VLCFA levels in chorionic villus or amniocyte samples is the most commonly used procedure for prenatal diagnosis, but the assay must be carefully regulated to avoid false-negative results.[105]

Although DNA analysis has been limited by the heterogeneity of mutations, recently an exon sequence-based identification of XALD heterozygotes was developed that may be applicable to any mutation. This analysis may be used for genetic counseling, prenatal diagnosis, and disease prevention.[11,105]

The characteristic radiographic finding is a symmetrical, posterior to anterior progression of white matter hyperintensity on T_2-weighted MRI. The leading edge of the abnormality may enhance with gadolinium-based contrast. As in most demyelinating disorders, the subcortical *U fibers* are typically spared. Involvement of the pontomedullary corticospinal tracts may help to distinguish X-linked ALD from other demyelinating disorders.[4] MR spectroscopy may show evidence of axonal injury before the appearance of any MRI changes.

Elevated very long chain fatty acid levels are now recognized as a biochemical anomaly of many peroxisomal disorders. The demonstration of lipid inclusions containing VLCFAs in adreno-cortical cells and skin fibroblasts of patients with X-linked adrenoleukodystrophy led to a plasma assay for VLCFAs considered to be specific for the disease.[104,132] Subsequently, elevation of plasma VLCFAs with a slightly different pattern was noted in an autosomal recessive neurodegenerative condition known as neonatal adrenoleukodystrophy.

Neonatal adrenoleukodystrophy is a disorder of peroxisomal biogenesis that is clinically and pathologically distinct from X-linked adrenoleukodystrophy. It occurs with equal frequency in boys and girls. The patients are markedly hypotonic at birth; they develop uncontrollable seizures early in infancy. Tanning of the skin due to adrenal insufficiency occurs late in the disease. Respiratory death usually occurs by age 3 years. Visual loss occurs early as a result of retinal photoreceptor degeneration, which can be confirmed by a flat electroretinogram. Pigmentary clumping may occur in the retina late in the disease. Pathologically, there is degeneration of the retinal photoreceptors and ganglion cells. Macrophages with cytoplasmic inclusions can be seen throughout the retina, histologically.[20,48,172] No normal peroxisomes are identifiable by electron microscopy.

A variant of adrenoleukodystrophy that looks clinically like neonatal adrenoleukodystrophy, but biochemically like X-linked adrenoleukodystrophy, has been reported.[127] These patients have enlarged peroxisomes and an isolated deficiency of peroxisomal fatty acyl-CoA oxidase.

Treatment for adrenoleukodystrophy requires careful consideration. Bone marrow transplantation in several cases has been associated with some reversal of neurological disability. It is not recommended for patients with rapidly advancing or severe neurological disease, as they cannot tolerate the transient exacerbation associated with the procedure itself. Given the considerable morbidity and mortality, it is also not recommended for patients without neurological deficit because less than 50% will progress to severe neurological disease.[111,158]

There are some noteworthy potential therapies currently under investigation. In a mouse model of XALD, administration of 4-phenylbutyrate increased expression of an ALD-related protein and normalized levels of VLCFA in the brain.[109] Anecdotal evidence suggests temporary improvement of neurological symptoms with intravenous gammaglobulin therapy. Therapeutic trials of thalidomide, interferon, and lovastatin are currently underway.[107] The use of gene therapy or transplantation of marrow-derived mesenchymal cells also warrant further investigation before entering human trials.[111]

Other treatment options have been less encouraging. Steroid replacement is quite effective for adrenal insufficiency but has no effect on neurological impairment. Dietary restriction of VLCFA with dietary administration of erucic acid (major component of Lorenzo's oil) does reduce plasma levels of VLCFA, although it has failed to affect disease progression in the childhood X-linked variety once symptoms have started.[107,176] Plasma exchange, carnitine therapy, and clofibrate have exerted no appreciable effect.[111]

Refsum's Disease

In 1946, Sigvald Refsum first described a unique hereditary ataxic syndrome in two Norwegian families that he termed heredopathia atactica polyneuritiformis. Many additional cases of this autosomal recessive condition have since been described, which usually presents in the first or second decade with progressive night blindness associated with ataxia and distal muscle weakness. Symptoms are generally progressive but infection, pregnancy, or other stress may trigger exacerbation. Many cases develop progressive neurosensory hearing loss and somatosensory loss associated with dorsal column degeneration and peripheral neuropathy. Nearly all have elevated protein levels in cerebrospinal fluid. Death from cardiac arrhythmia is common.

Ocular features of Refsum's disease are myriad, but the outstanding feature is a pigmentary retinopathy with progressive field loss and a flat ERG. Other findings include nystagmus, miosis, posterior subcapsular cataracts, and glaucoma.[171]

An unusual branched chain 20-carbon fatty acid, *phytanic acid*, was discovered in the tissues of patients with Refsum's disease. Phytanic acid is a breakdown product of phytol, a component of plant chlorophyll, and comes exclusively from dietary sources. Elevated plasma phytanic acid levels were once thought to be diagnostic of Refsum's disease but are now recognized in other diseases with peroxisomal dysgenesis. Phytanoyl CoA alphahydroxylase, the enzyme deficient in Refsum's disease, has been localized to chromosome 10.[113]

The pathophysiology is not clearly understood. Phytanic acid may accumulate more than 100 fold when peroxisomal phytanoyl-CoA hydroxylase is absent. One hypothesis suggests that incorporation of phytanic acid into tissue lipids may cause dysfunction by molecular distortion of myelin or membrane lipids. Another possible mechanism is via interference with normal prenylation, thus preventing posttranslational targeting of proteins to the membrane.[32,184]

In 1982, Scota et al. described a condition in young children with dysmorphism, hepatomegaly, anosmia, deafness, and pigmentary retinopathy. The discovery of intracellular lamellar structures resembling plant chloroplasts in the liver led the authors to check plasma phytanic acid levels. These were markedly elevated, which led to the title of infantile Refsum's disease. Subsequent studies of this disorder led to the discovery of generalized peroxisomal dysfunction as well as absence of peroxisomes histologically.[128,141,150] The disorder is therefore, much more analogous histologically and biochemically to neonatal adrenoleukodystrophy and Zellweger syndrome than to "adult" Refsum's disease.

Prenatal diagnosis of infantile Refsum's disease is possible by checking for the absence of peroxisomes in chorionic villus samples in the first or second trimester of gestation.[150] These can normally be detected with indirect immunofluorescence techniques using anticatalase antiserum. As yet, prenatal diagnosis of classical Refsum's disease is not possible.

Treatment is directed toward management of phytanic acid levels. Progression of Refsum's disease can be slowed with a diet free of chlorophyll and phytol.[30] Phytanic acid itself is commonly found in butter, cheese, lamb, beef, and certain fish. Failure of dietary restriction to reduce plasma phytanic acid levels or worsening of the clinical condition warrants treatment with plasma exchange. Lipapheresis may be equally effective.[57,184]

Zellweger Syndrome (Cerebrohepatorenal Syndrome)

Similar to infantile Refsum's disease and neonatal adrenoleukodystrophy, Zellweger syndrome is in the spectrum of autosomal recessive disorders of peroxisome biogenesis. The Zellweger phenotype is the most severe and has the most extensive systemic involvement. Peroxisomal enzymes are synthesized normally, but are rapidly degraded due to the deficiency of formed peroxisomes.[149] Some empty membranous structures may remain, known as peroxisome ghosts.[32]

Patients with Zellweger syndrome are born with significant dysmorphic features including prominent forehead, micrognathia, hypertelorism with epicanthal folds, hypoplastic supraorbital ridge, and high arched palate. Neuronal migration defects lead to seizures and severe retardation. Other neurological features include deafness and contractures of the limbs and digits. Organ dysgenesis problems include polycystic kidneys, intrahepatic biliary dysgenesis, and cardiac ventricular septal defects. Death from multiple factors usually occurs in the first year of life.

The ocular findings are also more severe than in other peroxisomal disorders; they include blindness from pigmentary retinopathy and optic atrophy. Corneal clouding, cataract, and glaucoma are common features, but need not be present to make the diagnosis.[40]

Treatment for Zellweger syndrome remains symptomatic, including antiepileptic medications or vitamin K for hemorrhage from cirrhosis. With the identification of a genetic defect, genetic counseling may soon become feasible. The development of mouse models may help to elucidate the pathogenesis and eventually provide a rational basis for definitive therapy.[35]

MITOCHONDRIAL DISEASES

Our understanding of mitochondrial diseases has been rapidly changing. It has been well established that mitochondria are organelles with a double membrane and are not part of the cellular endomembrane system. Their major function is the transfer of electrons from reduced nucleotides (e.g., NADH) to oxygen. This energy transfer is coupled to the generation of ATP, the chemical currency for all cellular anabolic processes. This oxidative respiration utilizes up to 65 protein components aggregated in five respiratory chain complexes.

It has been generally assumed that the clinical phenotype results from direct disruption of bioenergetics. Cellular demand for ATP frequently results in increased glycolysis and lactic acidosis. Other clinical features depend on the specific needs of different organ systems and the overall distribution of the defective mitochondria. The most common manifestations include seizures, strokes, optic atrophy, neuropathy, myopathy, cardiomyopathy, sensorineural hearing loss, or diabetes mellitus. Defects in different components of the respiratory chain can result in varied clinical presentation as well as considerable overlap among syndromes.

Recently, other pathogenetic mechanisms have been explored that implicate mitochondrially localized superoxide. One study showed that several pathogenic mitochondrial mutations confer cellular sensitivity to oxidant stress, which is in turn modulated by calcium ion (Ca^{2+}) levels. Indeed, in MERRF cytoplasmic Ca^{2+} is abnormally high, while ATP levels are not low. Oxidative stress and a rise in intracellular Ca^{2+} may induce a mitochondrial permeability transition, which may initiate apoptosis.[21]

The mitochondrion is the only organelle with its own genome and protein manufacturing system. Thirteen of the respiratory chain components are coded by *mitochondrial DNA* and translated within the mitochondrion itself. The majority of respiratory protein components are coded by nuclear DNA, translated by cytosolic ribosomes, and transported into the mitochondria where they undergo modification and aggregation into the respiratory chain complexes.

Most of the mitochondrial diseases show morphological disruption of the mitochondria on muscle biopsy. When stained with modified Gomori trichrome stain, accumulations of abnormal mitochondria within myofibers may cause an irregular appearance described as *ragged-red fibers*. Ultrastructurally, the mitochondria may be of abnormal size or shape or contain crystalline or globular inclusions. On the other hand, any of these diseases may present without cellular morphological abnormalities.

Mitochondrial DNA is transmitted almost exclusively by the mother via the ovum. Because many copies of mitochondrial DNA may be transmitted to the offspring and mitochondrial DNA replicates many times more frequently than nuclear DNA, the relative proportion of mutant and wild-type mitochondrial DNA may vary from cell to cell and from individual to individual (*heteroplasmy*). The varying mutational burden may result in considerable phenotypic variability, both within and across clinically distinct entities.

Nuclear DNA may have a far more complex interaction with mitochondrial DNA than previously suspected. Not only does nuclear DNA encode for mitochondrial proteins, but susceptibility to identified mitochondrial mutations may be inherited in Mendelian fashion, whether X-linked, autosomal dominant, or autosomal recessive[103]; this further complicates our approach to genetic counseling for mitochondrially encoded mutations. Oocyte donation or preimplantation diagnosis with in vitro fertilization are reliable, but difficult, means of preventing the disease in susceptible families. Oocyte nuclear transplantation is well described in other mammalian species but has not been attempted in humans.[139]

Prenatal diagnosis can be made with chorionic villus sampling or blood analysis of mitochondrial DNA mutations. These tests are most reliable when the mutant mitochondrial DNA load is closely correlated with disease severity, uniformly distributed throughout all tissues, and stable over time.[131] As already mentioned, these requirements are rarely met in mitochondrial diseases.

Five clinical syndromes transmitted via mitochondrial DNA are of ophthalmic importance (Table 10-4); these are chronic progressive external ophthalmoplegia (CPEO) or Kearns–Sayre syndrome; myoclonic epilepsy with ragged-red fibers (MERRF) or Fukuhara's disease; mitochondrial encephalopathy, lactic acidosis, and strokelike episodes (MELAS); neuropathy, ataxia, and retinitis pigmentosa (NARP); and Leber's hereditary optic neuropathy (LHON). This classification of disease is complicated by the lack of explicit genotype–phenotype correlation and by phenotypic overlap among syndromes.[103] The future may well see a reclassification of mitochondrial diseases according to genetic mutation, as in the case of the disorders of peroxisomal biogenesis.

Among diseases of Mendelian inheritance, Leigh syndrome is the most common pediatric disorder of mitochondrial function. Leigh syndrome itself is probably the common clinopatho-

TABLE 10-4. Features of the Mitochondrial Cytopathies.

Manifestation	*CPEO+*	*MERRF*	*MELAS*	*Leber's*	*NARP*
Ophthalmoplegia	+				
Retinal degeneration	+				+
Optic atrophy		+		+	
Cortical blindness			+		
Ataxia	+	+			+
Seizures		+	+		
Cardiac dysrhythmia	+			+	
Short stature	+	+	+		
Lactic acidosis	+	+	+		
Sensorineural deafness	+	+	+		
Ragged-red fibers	+	+	+		
Peripheral neuropathy					+

logic manifestation of a number of different mutations and respiratory chain defects. Although Leigh syndrome is usually transmitted in an autosomal dominant fashion, it has also been associated with autosomal dominant, X-linked, or maternal inheritance patterns.[23]

Leigh Syndrome (Subacute Necrotizing Encephalopathy)

In 1951, Denis Leigh described a child with lactic acidosis of the serum and cerebrospinal fluid and focal necrosis of gray matter in the brainstem. To this day, Leigh syndrome remains a postmortem diagnosis made by characteristic histopathological findings. These findings include spongiform lesions of the basal ganglia, thalamus, cerebellum, and brainstem formed by vacuoles representing intramyelin splitting.[76] There have been case reports of spongiform lesions in the white matter as well.[169] Capillary proliferation, demyelination, and gliosis are common.[23] The putamen has a reddish hue in fresh tissue.

Clinical, laboratory, and radiologic findings can be used to make a presumptive diagnosis. Patients with this disease usually present in the first 2 years of life with feeding difficulties, seizures, and ataxia. Severe psychomotor regression ensues with hypotonia, involuntary movements, and respiratory dysfunction. Ocular signs include nystagmus, ophthalmoplegia and optic atrophy. Lactate and pyruvate are almost always elevated in the serum and CSF. Magnetic resonance imaging classically demonstrates symmetrical spongiform basal ganglia lesions, although lesions of the white matter or gray matter nuclei may also be seen.[53,112,169] Death usually occurs within a couple of years.

Deficiencies of various mitochondrial enzymes including pyruvate dehydrogenase chain complex, pyruvate dehydrogenase activator, ATPase 6 subunit, and electron transport complexes I, II, and IV, as well as tRNA mutations, have been described in Leigh syndrome.[26] Pyruvate carboxylase deficiency in some patients suggests that the pathological changes may be secondary to the lactic acidemia. Similar histopathological findings in cases of hypoxia, carbon monoxide poisoning, Wilson's disease, and Wernicke's disease raise further questions about their specificity. Nonetheless, when linked to its distinctive clinical characteristics, Leigh syndrome can be considered as a group of similar nosological entities with defective mitochondria.

Treatment options are still anecdotal. Sodium dicholoracetate has been used to decrease lactic acidosis by disinhibition of pyruvate dehydrogenase complex, with clinical and radiologic improvement.[75] Thiamine has also been reported to improve lactic acidosis and neurological symptoms.[27]

Leber's Hereditary Optic Neuropathy

In 1871, Theodor Leber described a maternally inherited loss of central vision afflicting otherwise healthy young individuals, particularly young males. It is now known that the age of onset ranges from 1 to 80 years. More than 80% of clinically affected individuals are male. Patients typically experience acute or subacute progressive central or cecocentral scotomas, with involvement of the second eye within a couple months. Visual acuity usually stabilizes at 20/200 or worse within a few months. A minority of individuals has some recovery of vision. Color vision is lost early, and Uhthoff's phenomenon may be observed. Patients may report pain with eye movements, leading to confusion with optic neuritis.[19,64,161] Ataxia, dystonia, spasticity, peripheral neuropathy, or cardiac conduction abnormalities may also be present. Symptoms may cluster in families.[6,32]

Presymptomatically and during the acute phase of visual loss, the pathognomonic fundoscopic finding is a circumpapillary telangiectatic microangiopathy with swelling of the peripapillary retinal nerve fiber layer, without staining or leakage on fluorescein angiography. Within 6 months, optic atrophy supervenes, particularly affecting the temporal optic disc. Although visual evoked potentials may be normal early in the course, these too become undetectable.[19]

Three pathogenic mutations have been discovered so far, all affecting components of complex I of the respiratory chain. There is no apparent genotype–phenotype correlation. There are several other "secondary mutations" that have been found with increased frequency in affected individuals. It is possible that these represent nonpathogenic polymorphisms or haplotypic associations.[19] The search continues for a possible X-linked factor that renders males more susceptible to the disease.[64]

No specific treatment is available at this time.

Other Mitochondrial Cytopathies

MELAS syndrome (mitochondrial myopathy, encephalopathy, lactic acidosis, and strokelike episodes) is characterized by seizures, vomiting, and lactic acidosis in the first few years of life. Intermittent hemiparesis, hemianopsia, and cortical visual loss are prominent features. These episodes are believed to be caused by respiratory dysfunction of cortical neurons. A problem with autoregulation of blood flow at the level of pial arterioles has also been suggested.[120] Persons with this condition usually recover from the strokelike episodes, but are subject to multiple recurrences. Unlike other mitochondrial cytopathies, muscle weakness is not a prominent feature of this syndrome.

Patients with MELAS syndrome have ragged-red fibers of skeletal and cardiac muscle seen in many mitochondrial cytopathies.[119] The genetic defect in MELAS syndrome has been identified as a point mutation in the gene for mitochondrial $tRNA_{leu}$ in 85% of patients.[51,143] A mutation in tRNAphe has also been reported.[56] NADH-Co Q reductase deficiency has been reported in several patients with this condition.[77,119,194]

Fukuhara's disease, otherwise known as myoclonic epilepsy and ragged-red fiber disease (*MERRF*), usually presents with myoclonus in the second decade of life; this progresses to generalized seizures followed by ataxia and weakness. Patients with this disease become severely debilitated and blind from progressive optic atrophy. Pure maternal transmission and defects of oxidative phosphorylation have been confirmed, and a mitochondrial DNA point mutation has been identified in the gene for mitochondrial tRNAlys in most cases.[159]

NARP (neuropathy, ataxia, and retinitis pigmentosa) generally presents in the first decade of life with neurogenic weakness and pigmentary retinopathy. The retinopathy is typically similar to retinitis pigmentosa, with poor dark adaptation and progressive peripheral bone spicule formation on ophthalmoscopic examination, although other patterns have been reported.[122] These effects are followed by the development of progressive ataxia. NARP is caused by a T to G point mutation at position 8993 in the mitochondrial DNA affecting an ATPase subunit of complex V in the respiratory chain.[61]

Treatment of MELAS syndrome, MERRF, and NARP remain largely symptomatic.

DISORDERS OF MYELIN PRODUCTION

Canavan's Disease

Canavan's disease, also known as spongiform leukoencephalopathy, is an autosomal recessive, rapidly progressive leukodystrophy that most commonly affects Ashkenazi Jews. It usually presents in the first few months of life with diffuse hypotonia and head lag. Profound visual loss due to optic atrophy is an early feature. Soon thereafter, nystagmus and seizures develop. The hypotonia is replaced by spasticity, but nuchal hypotonia frequently persists. Death usually occurs by 5 years of age.

Enlarged head size is a characteristic early feature of the disease, a result of diffuse disruption of the white matter with cystic spaces, which have a characteristic spongiform appearance on histopathological section. The cystic spaces actually represent coalescence of vacuoles within swollen astrocytes. The mitochondria within the astrocytes have a pathognomonic elongated appearance on electron microscopy with short cristae and a dense matrix.[1] Other glial cells and neurons appear normal. There is a paucity of myelin, but no evidence of demyelination. Despite the abnormal appearance of the mitochondria in astrocytes, oxidative phosphorylation appears normal.[24a]

The finding of excessive urinary excretion of *N*-acetylaspartic acid (NAA) in patients with Canavan's disease led to the discovery of *aspartoacylase* deficiency as the primary enzyme defect. The mechanism by which this defect leads to the characteristic spongiform degeneration of the brain is unknown. It has been suggested that NAA plays a unique role in myelinogenesis as a transporter of acetyl groups for lipogenesis.[55] Elevated levels of this amino acid could disrupt this process. Alternatively, spongy degeneration may result from NAA accumulation and secondary edema.[97]

The gene encoding for aspartoacylase has been localized to the short arm of chromosome 17 (17p13-ter). Although mutations have been identified on all six exons, there are two specific mutations that account for 98% of mutations in Ashkenazi Jews.[32,97]

Diagnosis is made on the basis of massive elevations in urine NAA. Serum and CSF levels of NAA may also be elevated but are not required for diagnosis. Lesser elevations of NAA

macrophages, particularly in the perivascular region. Electron microscopy demonstrates defective lamellation and compaction of myelin. Although clinical characteristics may strongly suggest this disorder, absolute diagnosis can only be made by histologic evaluation of brain tissue.[42,155]

Patients with PMD have been found to have mutations in the gene for proteolipid apoprotein, PLP (lipophilin).[79] This protein represents approximately half the protein content of normal CNS white matter and is not present in peripheral nervous system myelin. It is believed to be important in forming the tight concentric apposition of oligodendrocyte membranes that make up CNS myelin.[166]

The PLP gene has been localized to the Xq22 chromosome. The nucleotide sequence is highly conserved among humans, rats, cows, mice, and dogs, which would indicate little room for error in the structure of the protein. Indeed, more than 60 different mutations in the PLP gene have been identified in different patients with Pelizaeus–Merzbacher disease, and similar point mutations have been found in animal models of the disease.[42,126]

Three different genetic mechanisms have been identified: deletion, duplication, or point mutation; these are associated with a range of overlapping phenotypes that do not specifically correlate with the clinical presentations described earlier. Deletions produce a loss of PLP function but result in a relatively mild phenotype. Duplication of the PLP sequence is the most common mechanism of mutation. It is postulated that variation in the disruption or inclusion of the flanking genes may determine phenotype with duplication mutations. Point mutations lead to amino acid substitutions and a gain of toxic function. Normal PLP folding is disrupted, resulting in accumulation of the abnormal protein in the endoplasmic reticulum and eventual oligodendrocyte apoptosis; this, too, results in a wide range of phenotypes. Of note, PMD is also allelic with X-linked spastic paraplegia type 2.[42,192]

A number of cases of PMD have had no identifiable mutations within the coding region of the PLP gene. Whether there are other genes that affect PLP translation or function is unknown, which could explain the autosomal recessive inheritance pattern in some cases.

The existence of numerous mutations and modes of inheritance makes genetic counseling very difficult in this condition. Furthermore, it makes prenatal diagnosis impractical. Prenatal diagnosis may be possible in affected families by tracking DNA polymorphisms linked to the PLP gene in chorionic villus samples.[17]

Currently, treatment is symptomatic only. Intraventricular transplantation of glial cell progenitors into a rat model PMD resulted in diffusely increased myelination, providing some hope for therapy in the not so distant future.[89]

DISORDERS OF UNKNOWN ETIOLOGY

Subacute Sclerosing Pancencephalities

Subacute sclerosing pancencephalities (SSPE) is a term developed to link two diseases, subacute inclusion body encephalitis and subacute sclerosing leukoencephalitis, with a common nosologic entity, persistent measles virus infection of the CNS.[54] This disease is a rare consequence of measles virus infection in infancy or early childhood. The incidence of the disease in the United States has dropped dramatically with the advent of effective vaccination programs.

Typically the victim of SSPE does well for 5 to 10 years following an otherwise uneventful measles infection. Thereafter, insidiously progressive neurological problems supervene, usually beginning with abnormal behavior and intellectual decline. Eventually most patients develop myoclonic seizures, spasticity, and extrapyramidal dyskinesia. This condition ultimately evolves to decerebrate rigidity, coma, and death over a period of months to years.

Up to 50% of patients with SSPE develop visual loss, typically due to a chorioretinitis in the macular region[138] that generally presents as subretinal pigmentary changes with overlying retinal edema, folds, and occasionally hemorrhages. Vitreous cells are rare. Occasionally, chorioretinitis is the presenting manifestation of the disease.[196] Other ocular findings include papilledema, optic atrophy, and nystagmus. A characteristic EEG abnormality termed a suppression burst occurs in about 80% of patients[193] and may precede the onset of clinical myoclonus. CSF IgG is usually elevated, although total CSF protein levels may be normal. Antibodies against measles virus are disproportionately elevated in the CSF.[170]

Pathologically, mutant measles virus can be demonstrated nearly anywhere in the brain, although the cerebellum is characteristically spared.[63,168] White matter lesions appear to be immunomediated rather than caused by direct viral infection.[130] These lesions are pathologically indistinguishable from those of other viral infections such as subacute AIDS encephalomyelitis, progressive rubella encephalitis, and postinfectious encephalomyelitis.

There is no definitely effective treatment of SSPE. Preliminary studies in the use of alpha interferon have been promising, however.[44,102]

Familial Dysautonomia

Familial dysautonomia (*Riley–Day syndrome*) is a rare autosomal recessive condition that mainly afflicts Ashkenazi Jews. Most cases are associated with a tissue-specific splicing mutation in the IKBKAP gene on chromosome 9q31.[161a] It generally presents in early childhood with vomiting, failure to thrive, delayed motor development, and emotional lability. Autonomic dysfunction manifests as orthostatic hypotension, failure to produce tears, excessive sweating, and irregular temperature control.

In addition to autonomic dysfunction patients with this condition have sensory impairment manifested by hyporeflexia, and absence of pain and temperature sensation. Sensation to pressure and light touch is generally preserved. A characteristic finding is absence of fungiform papillae on the tongue and deficiencies in the sensation of taste.[124]

Most of the ocular problems are a consequence of dry eyes and corneal hypesthesia. Patients with this condition are prone to corneal ulceration and band keratopathy. The pupils show supersensitivity to methacholine, suggesting parasympathetic denervation.[50] Others have questioned this interpretation.[82]

Patients who escape corneal scarring tend to develop mild to moderate vision loss due to optic atrophy in the second or third decade of life.[28,137]

Hallervorden–Spatz Disease

Hallervorden–Spatz disease (neurodegeneration with brain iron accumulation type 1, or NBIA1) is a rare autosomal recessive condition with varied age of onset and rate of neurodegeneration. It usually presents in the first or second decade with progressive rigidity of the legs. Choreoathetosis is common.

Extrapyramidal involvement of the bulbar muscles may manifest as difficulty with speech and swallowing. Progressive dementia eventually supervenes, and death occurs within 15 years of diagnosis.

Generally, the ophthalmic manifestations of Hallervorden–Spatz disease are nonspecific supranuclear gaze disorders typical of extrapyramidal disease that include defective smooth pursuit, downgaze paralysis, and apraxia of eyelid movements.[67,188] A pigmentary retinopathy with bull's-eye maculopathy and yellow-white flecks in the retinal periphery is estimated to occur in one-fourth of cases.[93,118]

Pathologically, iron deposits within the globus pallidus, substantia nigra, and red nuclei give these structures a distinctive brown pigmentation.[29] The ferromagnetic material causes a characteristic hypointensity of these structures on T_2 and gradient echo magnetic resonance images that may prove to be diagnostic.[144] Additionally, affected regions develop swollen axon terminals suggestive of neuroaxonal dystrophy. However, other features of the disease are so distinctive as to make grouping of Hallervorden–Spatz disease with neuroaxonal dystrophy untenable.

Recently, it has been shown that cortical and brainstem-type Lewy bodies are immunoreactive for alpha, beta, and gamma synuclein.[41,117] No metabolic or genetic defect has ever been found for Hallervorden–Spatz disease. Tests of serum iron and iron metabolism have been normal thus far.

There is no treatment. Chelating agents and L-dopa have been ineffective.

HEREDITARY ATAXIA SYNDROMES

The hereditary ataxia syndromes are a heterogeneous group of disorders that are frequently associated with oculomotor abnormalities or retinal degeneration. The nosologic classification of hereditary ataxias has undergone multiple metamorphoses over the past century. Greenfield attempted to use an anatomic basis for separation: predominantly spinal, spinocerebellar, and predominantly cerebellar. The more familiar Harding classification of autosomal dominant cerebellar ataxias (ADCA) emphasized clinical and pathogenic categories, further subdividing the autosomal dominant cerebellar ataxias into those with systemic features, those including retinal degeneration, and purely cerebellar syndromes. Olivopontocerebellar atrophy (OPCA) is a pathological description that may be associated with many different clinical presentations. However, recent advances have permitted a new classification of the autosomal dominant spinocerebellar ataxias on a genetic basis.[10,78] The most notable ataxia syndrome inherited in a recessive fashion is ataxia-telangiectasia.

Spinocerebellar Ataxias

The spinocerebellar ataxias (SCA) are now classified by a sequential numbering system according to their gene mutations. They typically present later in life with progressive cerebellar degeneration, which may also variously involve visual, oculomotor, pyramidal, extrapyramidal, cerebral cortical, or peripheral nervous system features. They are important to recognize because of *genetic anticipation*, the predisposition to more severe disease with succeeding generations. All SCA demonstrate an autosomal dominant pattern of inheritance, and all mutations identified thus far are associated with microsatellite expansions in different genes. Most expansions consist of CAG triplet repeats, except for an ATTCT pentanucleotide expansion that was recently discovered in SCA10. Like other triplet repeat diseases such as Huntington's disease or myo-tonic dystrophy, most SCAs show evidence of anticipation, particularly with paternal transmission. In general, infantile- or juvenile-onset diseases are associated with larger microsatellite expansions as well as more extensive neuropathology.[99,146]

Because a given mutation may have various clinical manifestations, the ADCA classification of Harding remains a useful independent clinical guide to diagnosis. In all types of SCA, patients typically present with slowly progressive gait ataxia, followed by a cerebellar dysarthria.

In the "pure cerebellar ataxias" (ADCA III), most notably SCA6, oculomotor signs referable to the midline cerebellum predominate, including gaze-evoked and downbeat nystagmus, disruption of the visual pursuit system, and impaired visual–vestibular interaction.

In the group of cerebellar ataxias with extracerebellar manifestations (ADCA I), patients exhibit a spectrum of symptoms. In SCA2, prominent slowing of saccades and optic atrophy is observed. Tremor and appendicular dysmetria and hyporeflexia may also be evident. In SCA3 (Machado–Joseph disease), oculomotor findings resemble those of the pure cerebellar ataxias, with the addition of ophthalmoplegia. Patients frequently also complain of diplopia due to asymmetrical ophthalmoplegia as well as impaired divergence.[121] Symptoms of SCA1 overlap with those of both SCA2 and SCA3.

In SCA7, the only genetically defined cerebellar ataxia with retinal degeneration (ADCA II), severity is strongly correlated to the number of repeats, and there is a strong anticipation, especially through paternal transmission. In addition to cerebellar ataxia and dysarthria, variable pyramidal tract signs, posterior column dysfunction, and dysphagia may also be observed. Progressive bilateral symmetrical pigmentary maculopathy is seen, with early blue-yellow dyschromatopsia. Oculomotor abnormalities include supranuclear palsy and slowing of saccades.[165]

The pathophysiological mechanisms involved in SCAs are still unclear.

Treatment is supportive, although there is some anecdotal use of antioxidant therapy.

Ataxia Telangiectasia

Ataxia telangiectasia is a rare autosomal recessive disease that presents in early childhood with progressive ataxia associated with disruption of the cytoarchitecture of *Purkinje cells* in the cerebellum; this leads to gross motor delay and frequent misdiagnosis as "cerebral palsy." Also in early childhood, telangiectatic vessels appear on the conjunctivae. Children with this finding are often treated for "chronic conjunctivitis" before accurate diagnosis is made. Cutaneous telangiectasias also develop in most patients.

Neurological impairment is slowly progressive, with eventual involvement of basal ganglia, spinal cord, and peripheral nerves. Most patients are confined to a wheelchair by their second decade. Mental deterioration occurs in some patients, but most have good cognitive function.

Eye movement abnormalities begin with delayed initiation of saccades followed by dysmetria, impaired pursuit, and eventually nystagmus. An optic neuropathy leading to mild visual impairment develops in older patients.[13] The amplitude of the visual evoked potential is diminished out of proportion with the visual loss.[13,22]

Immunological impairment is characterized by diminished circulating IgA.[101] However, the susceptibility to infection is greater than expected from absence of IgA alone, and most patients succumb to recurrent pulmonary infections in early adulthood. In addition, cancer susceptibility is high for patients with ataxia telangiectasia. This increased susceptibility to cancer also affects heterozygous carriers of the mutated ataxia-telangiectasia allele,[69,167] because of a hypersensitivity to ionizing radiation among affected individuals and carriers.

The defective protein (ATM) in ataxia telangiectasia is a protein kinase that plays a role in the repair of double-strand breaks in DNA caused by ionizing radiation. It is thought to be important in activation of the tumor suppressor gene p53.[162] The genetic defect has been mapped to chromosome 11q22.[175] Mutations that cause truncation of ATM result in significantly shorter survival than mutations that do not alter protein length.[91] However, others have questioned genotype–phenotype correlation.[7]

It remains uncertain what role ATM protein may have in affecting the function of nonmitotic cells, such as Purkinje cells, that are not considered very susceptible to ionizing radiation. It has been hypothesized that the ATM protein is also protective of oxidative damage and that cerebellar Purkinje cells are particularly affected by oxidative damage.[5]

References

1. Adachi M, Wallace BJ, Schneck L, et al. Fine structure of spongy degeneration of the central nervous system (van Bogaert and Bertrand type). J Neuropathol Exp Neurol 1966;25(4):598–616.
2. Baker RH, Trautmann JC, Younge BR, et al. Late juvenile-onset Krabbe's disease. Ophthalmology 1990;97(9):1176–1180.
3. Barkovich AJ. Concepts of myelin and myelination in neuroradiology. AJNR (Am J Neuroradiol) 2000;21(6):1099–1109.
4. Barkovich AJ, Ferriero DM, et al. Involvement of the pontomedullary corticospinal tracts: a useful finding in the diagnosis of X-linked adrenoleukodystrophy. AJNR (Am J Neuroradiol) 1997;18(1):95–100.
5. Barlow C, Dennery PA, et al. Loss of the ataxia-telangiectasia gene product causes oxidative damage in target organs. Proc Natl Acad Sci USA 1999;96:9915–9919.
6. Beal MF. Energetics in the pathogenesis of neurodegenerative diseases. Trends Neurosci 2000;23(7):298–304.
7. Becker-Catania SG, Chen G, et al. Ataxia-telangiectasia: phenotype/genotype studies of ATM protein expression, mutations, and radiosensitivity. Mol Genet Metab 2000;70:122–133.
8. Begleiter ML, Harris DJ. Autosomal recessive form of connatal Pelizaeus–Merzbacher disease. Am J Med Genet 1989;33(3):311–313.

9. Bennett MJ, Hofmann SL. The neuronal ceroid-lipofuscinoses (Batten disease): a new class of lysosomal storage diseases. J Inherit Metab Dis 1999;22(4):535–544.
10. Berciano J, Pascual J, et al. History of ataxia research. Handbook of ataxia disorders, vol 50. New York: Dekker, 2000:77–100.
11. Boehm CD, Cutting GR, et al. Accurate DNA-based diagnostic and carrier testing for X-linked adrenoleukodystrophy. Mol Genet Metab 1999;66(2):128–136.
12. Bohne W, von Figura K, Gieselmann V. An 11-bp deletion in the arylsulfatase A gene of a patient with late infantile metachromatic leukodystrophy. Hum Genet 1991;87:155–158.
13. Borchert MS, McCulloch D, Kaleita T. VEPs and visual pathway function in ataxia telangiectasia. Investig Ophthalmol Vis Sci 1991;32(suppl):952.
14. Boustany RN, Aprille JR, Halperin J, Levy H, DeLong GR. Mitochondrial cytochrome deficiency presenting as a myopathy with hypotonia, external ophthalmoplegia, and lactic acidosis in an infant and as fatal hepatopathy in a second cousin. Ann Neurol 1983;14:462–470.
15. Boustany RM. Neurology of the neuronal ceroid-lipofuscinoses: late infantile and juvenile types. Am J Med Genet 1992;42(4):533–535.
16. Boustany RM, Ahoy J, Kolodny EH, et al. Clinical classification of neuronal ceroid-lipofuscinosis subtypes. Am J Med Genet Suppl 1988;5:47–58.
17. Bridge PJ, MacLeod PM, Lillicrap DP, et al. Carrier detection and prenatal diagnosis of Pelizaeus–Merzbacher disease using a combination of anonymous DNA polymorphisms and the proteolipid protein (PLP) gene cDNA. Am J Med Genet 1991;38(4):616–621.
18. Caro PA, Marks HG. Magnetic resonance imaging and computed tomography in Pelizaeus–Merzbacher disease. Magn Reson Imaging 1990;8:791–796.
19. Chalmers RM, Schapira AH. Clinical, biochemical and molecular genetic features of Leber's hereditary optic neuropathy. Biochim Biophys Acta 1999;1410(2):147–158.
20. Cohen SM, Green WR, et al. Ocular histopathologic studies of neonatal and childhood adrenoleukodystrophy. Am J Ophthalmol 1983;95(1):82–96.
21. Cortopassi GA, Wong A. Mitochondria in organismal aging and degeneration. Biochim Biophys Acta 1999;1410(2):183–193.
22. Cruz Martinez A, Barrio M, Gutierrez AM, Lopez E. Abnormalities in sensory and mixed evoked potentials in ataxia-telangiectasia. J Neurol Neurosurg Psychiatry 1977;40:44–49.
23. Dahl HH. Getting to the nucleus of mitochondrial disorders: identification of respiratory chain-enzyme genes causing Leigh syndrome. Am J Hum Genet 1998;63(6):1594–1597.
24. Dawson G, Cho S. Batten's disease: clues to neuronal protein catabolism in lysosomes. J Neurosci Res 2000;60(2):133–140.

24a. de Coo IF, Gabreels FJ, Renier WO, et al. Canavan disease: neuromorphological and biochemical analysis of a brain biopsy specimen. Clin Neuropathol 1991;10(2):73–78.
25. Desnick RJ, Wang AM. Schindler disease: an inherited neuroaxonal dystrophy due to alpha-*N*-acetylgalactosaminidase deficiency. J Inherit Metab Dis 1990;13(4):549–559.
26. Di Donato S. Disorders related to mitochondrial membranes: pathology of the respiratory chain and neurodegeneration. J Inherit Metab Dis 2000;23(3):247–263.
27. Di Rocco M, Lamba LD, et al. Outcome of thiamine treatment in a child with Leigh disease due to thiamine-responsive pyruvate dehydrogenase deficiency. Eur J Paediatr Neurol 2000;4(3):115–117.
28. Diamond GA, D'Amico RA, Axelrod FB. Optic nerve dysfunction in familial dysautonomia. Am J Ophthalmol 1987;104:645–648.
29. Dooling EC, Schoene WC, Richardson EP. Hallervorden–Spatz syndrome. Arch Neurol 1974;30:70–83.
30. Elbaz A, Vale-Santos J, et al. Hypokalemic periodic paralysis and the dihydropyridine receptor (CACNL1A3): genotype/phenotype correlations for two predominant mutations and evidence for the absence of a founder effect in 16 caucasian families. Am J Hum Genet 1995;56(2):374–380.
31. Eldjarn L, Try K, Stokke O, et al. Dietary effects on serum phytanic acid levels and on clinical manifestations in heredopathia atactica polyneuritiformis. Lancet 1966;1:691–693.
32. Evans OB, Parker C, et al. Inborn errors of metabolism of the nervous system. In: Bradley W, Daroff R, Fenichel G, Marsden C (eds) Neurology in clinical practice, vol 2. Boston: Butterworth-Heinemann, 2000:1595–1664.
33. Faerber EN, Melvin J, et al. MRI appearances of metachromatic leukodystrophy. Pediatr Radiol 1999;29(9):669–672.
34. Farina L, Nardocci N, et al. Infantile neuroaxonal dystrophy: neuroradiological studies in 11 patients. Neuroradiology 1999;41(5):376–380.
35. Faust PL, Hatten ME. Targeted deletion of the PEX2 peroxisome assembly gene in mice provides a model for Zellweger syndrome, a human neuronal migration disorder. J Cell Biol 1997;139(5):1293–1305.
36. Fenichel G. Psychomotor retardation and regression. In: Clinical pediatric neurology. Philadelphia: Saunders, 2001:117–148.
37. Fensom AH, Marsh J, Jackson M, et al. First-trimester diagnosis of metachromatic leukocystrophy. Clin Genet 1988;34:122–125.
38. Ferreira RC, Mierau GW, et al. Conjunctival biopsy in infantile neuroaxonal dystrophy. Am J Ophthalmol 1997;123(2):264–266.
39. Fischer G, Jatzkewitz H. The activator of cerebroside sulfatase. Binding studies with enzyme and substrate demonstrating the detergent function of the activator protein. Biochem Biophys Acta 1977;481:561–572.

40. Folz SJ, Trobe JD. The peroxisome and the eye. Surv Ophthalmol 1991;35(5):353–368.
41. Galvin JE, Giasson B, et al. Neurodegeneration with brain iron accumulation, type 1 is characterized by alpha-, beta-, and gamma-synuclein neuropathology. Am J Pathol 2000;157(2):361–368.
42. Garbern J, Cambi F, et al. The molecular pathogenesis of Pelizaeus–Merzbacher disease. Arch Neurol 1999;56(10):1210–1214.
43. Gardiner RM. Mapping the gene for juvenile onset neuronal ceroid lipofuscinosis to chromosome 16 by linkage analysis. Am J Med Genet 1992;42:539–541.
44. Gascon GG, Yamani S, Cafege A, et al. Treatment of subacute sclerosing panencephalitis with alpha interferon. Ann Neurol 1991;30: 227–228.
45. Gencic S, Abuelo D, Ambler M, Hudson LD. Pelizaeus–Merzbacher disease: an X-linked neurologic disorder of myelin metabolism with a novel mutation in the gene encoding proteolipid protein. Am J Hum Genet 1989;45:435–442.
46. Gieselmann V, von Figura K. Advances in molecular genetics of metachromatic leukodystrophy. J Inherit Metab Dis 1990;13:560–571.
47. Gieselmann V, Matzner U, et al. Metachromatic leukodystrophy: molecular genetics and an animal model. J Inherit Metab Dis 1998; 21(5):564–574.
48. Glasgow BJ, Brown HH, et al. Ocular pathologic findings in neonatal adrenoleukodystrophy. Ophthalmology 1987;94(8):1054–1060.
49. Goebel HH, Schochet SS, et al. Progress in neuropathology of the neuronal ceroid lipofuscinoses. Mol Genet Metab 1999;66(4):367–372.
50. Goldberg MF, Payne JW, Brunt SPW. Ophthalmologic studies of familial dysautonomia. Arch Ophthalmol 1968;80:732–743.
51. Goto Y, Nonaka I, Horai S, et al. A mutation in the tRNA(Leu) (UUR) gene associated with the MELAS subgroup of mitochondrial encephalomyopathies. Nature (Lond) 1990;348(6302):651–653.
52. Gould SJ, Valle D. Peroxisome biogenesis disorders: genetics and cell biology. Trends Genet 2000;16(8):340–345.
53. Greenberg SB, Faerber EN, Riviello JJ, et al. Subacute necrotizing encephalomyelopathy (Leigh disease): CT and MRI appearances. Pediatr Radiol 1990;21(1):5–8.
54. Greenfield J. Encephalitis and encephalomyelitis in England and Wales during the last decade. Brain 1950;73:141.
55. Hagenfeldt L, Bollgren I, Venizelos N, et al. *N*-Acetylaspartic aciduria due to aspartoacylase deficiency—a new aetiology of childhood leukodystrophy. J Inherit Metab Dis 1987;10(2):135–141.
56. Hanna MG, Nelson IP, et al. MELAS: a new disease associated mitochondrial DNA mutation and evidence for further genetic heterogeneity. J Neurol Neurosurg Psychiatry 1998;65(4):512–517.
57. Harari D, Gibberd FB, Dick JPR, et al. Plasma exchange in the treatment of Refsum's disease (heredopathia atactica polyneuritiformis). J Neurol Neurosurg Psychiatry 1991;54(7):614–617.

58. Harzer K, Schuster I. Prenatal enzymatic diagnosis of Krabbe disease (globoid-cell leukodystrophy) using chorionic villi. Pitfalls in the use of uncultured villi. Hum Genet 1989;84(1):83–85.
59. Herz B, Bach G. Arylsulfatase A in pseudodeficiency. Hum Genet 1984;66(2–3):147–150.
60. Hofman KJ, Naidu S, Moser HW, Maumenee IH, Wenger DA. Cherry red spot in association with galactosylceramide-beta-galactosidase deficiency. J Inherit Metab Dis 1987;10:273–274.
61. Holt IJ, Harding AE, Petty RKH, et al. A new mitochondrial disease associated with mitochondrial DNA heteroplasmy. Am J Hum Genet 1990;46:428–433.
62. Hoogerbrugge PM, Poorthuis BJHM, Romme AE, van de Kamp JJP, Wagemaker G, van Bekhum PW. Effect of bone marrow transplantation on enzyme levels and clinical course in the neurologically affected twitcher mouse. J Clin Invest 1988;81:1790–1794.
63. Horta-Barbosa L, Fuccillo DA, Sever JL, Zeman W. Subacute sclerosing pancephalitis: isolation of measles from brain biopsy. Nature (Lond) 1969;221:974.
64. Howell N. Leber hereditary optic neuropathy: mitochondrial mutations and degeneration of the optic nerve. Vision Res 1997;37(24):3495–3507.
65. Hudson LD, Puckett C, Berndt J, Chan J, Gencic S. Mutation of the proteolipid protein gene PLP in a human X chromosome-linked myelin disorder. Proc Natl Acad Sci USA 1989;86:8128–8131.
66. Inui K, Kao FT, et al. The gene coding for a sphingolipid activator protein, SAP-1, is on human chromosome 10. Hum Genet 1985;69(3):197–200.
67. Jankovic J, Kirkpatrick JB, Blomquist KA, et al. Late-onset Hallervorden–Spatz disease presenting as familial parkinsonism. Neurology 1985;35(2):227–234.
68. Järvelä I, Vesa J, Santavuori P, Hellsten E, Peltonen L. Molecular genetics of neuronal ceroid lipofuscinoses. Pediatr Res 1992;32:645–648.
69. Janin N, Andrieu N, et al. Breast cancer risk in ataxia-telangiectasia (AT) heterozygotes: haplotype study in French AT families. Br J Cancer 1999;80:1042–1045.
70. Kappler J, Leinekugel P, Conzelmann E, et al. Genotype-phenotype relationship in various degrees of arylsulfatase A deficiency. Hum Genet 1991;86:463–470.
71. Kaye EM. Update on genetic disorders affecting white matter. Pediatr Neurol 2001;24(1):11–24.
72. Kelley RI, Datta NS, Dobyns WB, et al. Neonatal adrenoleukodystrophy: new cases, biochemical studies, and differentiation from Zellweger and related peroxisomal polydystrophy syndromes. Am J Med Genet 1986;23:869–901.
74. Kelley RI, Moser HW. Hyperpipecolic acidemia in neonatal adrenoleukodystrophy. Am J Med Genet 1984;19:791–795.

75. Kimura S, Ohtuki N, et al. Clinical and radiologic improvements in mitochondrial encephalomyelopathy following sodium dichloroacetate therapy. Brain Dev 1997;19(8):535–540.
76. Kimura S, Kobayashi T, Amemiya F, et al. Myelin splitting in the spongy lesion in Leigh encephalopathy. Pediatr Neurol 1991;7(1): 56–58.
77. Kobayashi M, Morishita H, Sugiyama N, et al. Two cases of NADH-coenzyme Q reductase deficiency: relationship to MELAS syndrome. J Pediatr 1987;110:223.
78. Koeppen AH. The hereditary ataxias. J Neuropathol Exp Neurol 1998;57(6):531–543.
79. Koeppen AH, Ronca NA, Greenfield EA, et al. Defective biosynthesis of proteolipid protein in Pelizaeus–Merzbacher disease. Ann Neurol 1987;21(2):159–170.
80. Kolodny EL. Sulfatide lipidosis: metachromatic leukodystrophy. In: Scriver CR, Beaudet AL, Sly WS, Valle D (eds) The metabolic basis of inherited diseases. New York: McGraw-Hill, 1989:1721–1749.
81. Kolodny EH, Cable WJ. Inborn errors of metabolism. Ann Neurol 1982;11(3):221–232.
82. Korczyn AD, Rubenstein AE, Yahr MD, Axelrod FB. The pupil in familial dysautonomia. Neurology 1981;31:628.
83. Krivit W, Shapiro E, Kennedy W, et al. Treatment of late infantile metachromatic leukodystrophy by bone marrow transplantation. N Engl J Med 1990;322:28–31.
84. Krivit W, Peters C, et al. Bone marrow transplantation as effective treatment of central nervous system disease in globoid cell leukodystrophy, metachromatic leukodystrophy, adreno-leukodystrophy, mannosidosis, fucosidosis, aspartylglucosaminuria, Hurler, Maroteaux–Lamy, and Sly syndromes, and Gaucher disease type III. Curr Opin Neurol 1999;12(2):167–176.
85. Kurokawa T, Chen YJ, Nagates M, et al. Late infantile Krabbe leukodystrophy: MRI and evoked potentials in a Japanese girl. Neuropediatrics 1987;18(3):182–183.
86. Lake BD, Young EP, et al. Prenatal diagnosis of lysosomal storage diseases. Brain Pathol 1998;8(1):133–149.
87. Lane SC, Jolly RD, et al. Apoptosis as the mechanism of neurodegeneration in Batten's disease. J Neurochem 1996;67(2):677–683.
88. Lazo O, Contreras M, Hashnil M, Stanley W, Irazu C, Singh T. Peroxisomal lignoceroyl-CoA ligase deficiency in childhood adrenoleukodystrophy and adrenoneuropathy. Proc Natl Acad Sci USA 1988;85:7647–7651.
89. Learish RD, Brustle O, et al. Intraventricular transplantation of oligodendrocyte progenitors into a fetal myelin mutant results in widespread formation of myelin. Ann Neurol 1999;46(5):716–722.
90. Leigh D. Subacute necrotizing encephalomyelopathy in an infant. J Neurol Neurosurg Psychiatry 1951;14:216–221.
91. Li A, Swift M. Mutations at the ataxia-telangiectasia locus and clinical phenotypes of A-T patients. Am J Med Genet 2000;92:170–177.

92. Loonen MC, Van Diggelen OP, Janse HC, et al. Late-onset globoid cell leucodystrophy (Krabbe's disease). Clinical and genetic delineation of two forms and their relation to the early-infantile form. Neuropediatrics 1985;16(3):137–142.
93. Luckenbach MW, Green WR, Miller NR, Moser WH, Clark AW, Tennekoon G. Ocular clinicopathologic correlation of Hallervorden–Spatz syndrome with acanthocytosis and pigmentary retinopathy. Am J Ophthalmol 1983;95:369–382.
94. MacCollin M, De Vivo CD, et al. Ataxia and peripheral neuropathy: a benign variant of peroxisome dysgenesis. Ann Neurol 1990;28(6):833–836.
95. Manz HJ, Schvelein M, McCullough DC, Kishimoto Y, Eiben RM. New phenotypic variant of adrenoleukodystrophy: pathologic, ultrastructural, and biochemical study in two brothers. J Neurol Sci 1980;45:245–260.
96. Matalon R, Kaul R, Casanova J, et al. Aspartoacylase deficiency: the enzyme defect in Canavan disease. J Inherit Metab Dis 1989; 12(suppl 2):329–331.
97. Matalon R, Michals-Matalon K. Prenatal diagnosis of Canavan disease. Prenat Diagn 1999;19(7):669–670.
98. Matalon R, Michals-Matalon K. Recent advances in Canavan disease. Adv Pediatr 1999;46:493–506.
99. Matsuura T, Yamagata T, et al. Large expansion of the ATTCT pentanucleotide repeat in spinocerebellar ataxia type 10. Nat Genet 2000;26(2):191–194.
100. Mattei MG, Alliel PM, Dautigny A, et al. The gene encoding for the major brain proteolipid (PLP) maps on the q-22 band of the human X chromosome. Hum Genet 1986;72:352–353.
101. McFarlin DE, Strober W, Barlow M, et al. The immunological deficiency state in ataxia-telangiectasia. Res Publ Assoc Res Nerv Ment Dis 1971;49:275.
102. Miyazaki M, Hashimoto T, Fujino K, Goda T, Tayama M, Kuroda Y. Apparent response of subacute sclerosing pancephalitis to intrathecal interferon alpha. Ann Neurol 1991;29:97–99.
103. Morgan-Hughes JA, Hanna MG. Mitochondrial encephalomyopathies: the enigma of genotype versus phenotype. Biochim Biophys Acta 1999;1410(2):125–145.
104. Moser HW, Moser AB, Frayer KK, et al. Adrenoleukodystrophy: increased plasma content of saturated very long chain fatty acids. Neurology 1981;31:1241–1249.
105. Moser AB, Moser HW. The prenatal diagnosis of X-linked adrenoleukodystrophy. Prenat Diagn 1999;19(1):46–48.
106. Moser HW. The peroxisome: nervous system role of a previously underrated organelle. The 1987 Robert Wartenberg lecture. Neurology 1988;38(10):1617–1627.
107. Moser HW. Adrenoleukodystrophy: phenotype, genetics, pathogenesis and therapy. Brain 1997;120(pt 8):1485–1508.

108. Moser HW. Genotype-phenotype correlations in disorders of peroxisome biogenesis. Mol Genet Metab 1999;68(2):316–327.
109. Moser HW. Molecular genetics of peroxisomal disorders. Front Biosci 2000;5:D298–D306.
110. Moser HW, Kemp S, et al. Mutational analysis and the pathogenesis of variant X-linked adrenoleukodystrophy phenotypes. Arch Neurol 1999;56(3):273–275.
111. Moser H, Smith K, et al. X-linked adrenoleukodystrophy. In: Scriver C, Kinzler K, Vogelstein B, et al. (eds) The metabolic and molecular bases of inherited disease. New York: McGraw-Hill, 2000: 3257–3301.
112. Munoz A, Mateos F, et al. Mitochondrial diseases in children: neuroradiological and clinical features in 17 patients. Neuroradiology 1999;41(12):920–928.
113. Nadal N, Rolland MO, et al. Localization of Refsum disease with increased pipecolic acidaemia to chromosome 10p by homozygosity mapping and carrier testing in a single nuclear family. Hum Mol Genet 1995;4(10):1963–1969.
114. Nagashima K, Suzuki S, Ichikawa E, et al. Infantile neuroaxonal dystrophy: perinatal onset with symptoms of diencephalic syndrome. Neurology 1985;35(5):735–738.
115. Naidu S, Hofmann KJ, et al. Galactosylceramide-beta-galactosidase deficiency in association with cherry red spot. Neuropediatrics 1988;19(1):46–48.
116. Nardocci N, Zorzi G, et al. Infantile neuroaxonal dystrophy: clinical spectrum and diagnostic criteria. Neurology 1999;52(7):1472–1478.
117. Neumann M, Adler S, et al. Alpha-synuclein accumulation in a case of neurodegeneration with brain iron accumulation type 1 (NBIA-1, formerly Hallervorden–Spatz syndrome) with widespread cortical and brainstem-type Lewy bodies. Acta Neuropathol (Berl) 2000;100(5):568–574.
118. Newell FW, Johnson RO, Huttenlocker PR. Pigmentary degeneration of the retina in the Hallervorden–Spatz syndrome. Am J Ophthalmol 1979;88:467–471.
119. Nishizawa M, Tanaka K, Shinozawa K, et al. A mitochondrial encephalomyopathy with cardiomyopathy: a case revealing a defect of complex I in the respiratory chain. J Neurol Sci 1987;78:189.
120. Ohama E, Ohara S, Ikuta F, et al. Mitochondrial angiopathy in cerebral blood vessels of mitochondrial encephalomyopathy. Acta Neuropathol (Berl) 1987;74:226.
121. Ohyagi Y, Yamada T, et al. Vergence disorders in patients with spinocerebellar ataxia 3/Machado–Joseph disease: a synoptophore study. J Neurol Sci 2000;173(2):120–123.
122. Ortiz R, Newman NJ, Shoffner JM, et al. Variable retinal and neurologic manifestations in patients harboring the mitochondrial DNA 8993 mutation. Arch Ophthalmol 1993;111:1525–1530.

123. Ozand PT, Gascon GG, Al Ageel A, et al. Prenatal detection of Canavan disease. Lancet 1991;337:735–736.
124. Pearson JF, Finegold MJ, Budzilovich G. The tongue and taste in familial dysautonomia. Pediatrics 1970;45:739–745.
125. Peltonen L, Savukoski M, et al. Genetics of the neuronal ceroid lipofuscinoses. Curr Opin Genet Dev 2000;10(3):299–305.
126. Pham-Dinh D, Popot JL, Boespflug-Tanguy O, et al. Pelizaeus–Merzbacher disease: a valine to phenylalanine point mutation in a putative extracellular loop of myelin proteolipid. Proc Natl Acad Sci USA 1991;88(17):7562–7566.
127. Poll-The BT, Roels F, Ogien H, et al. A new peroxisomal disorder with enlarged peroxisomes and a specific deficiency of acyl-Co-A oxidase (pseudo-neonatal adrenoleukodystrophy). Am J Hum Genet 1988;42:422–434.
128. Poll-The BT, Saudubray JM, Ogier H, et al. Infantile Refsum's disease: biochemical findings suggesting multiple peroxisomal dysfunction. J Inherit Metab Dis 1986;9(2):169–174.
129. Polten A, Fluharty AL, Fluharty CB, von Figura K, Gieselmann V. Molecular basis of different forms of metachromatic leukodystrophy. N Engl J Med 1991;324:18–22.
130. Poser CM. Notes on pathogenesis of subacute sclerosing panencephalitis. J Neurol Sci 1990;95:219–224.
131. Poulton J, Marchington DR. Progress in genetic counselling and prenatal diagnosis of maternally inherited mtDNA diseases. Neuromusc Disord 2000;10(7):484–487.
132. Powers JM, Schaumburg HH, Johnson AB, et al. A correlative study of the adrenal cortex in adrenoleukodystrophy: evidence for a fatal intoxication with very long chain fatty acids. Investig Cell Pathol 1980;3:353–376.
133. Pratt VM, Trofatter JA, Schinzel A, Dlouhy SR, Conneally PM, Hodes ME. A new mutation in the proteolipid protein (PLP) gene in a German family with Pelizaeus–Merzbacher disease. Am J Med Genet 1991;38:136–139.
134. Refsum S. Heredopathia atactica polyneuritiformis. Acta Psychiatr Scand (Suppl) 1946;38:9.
135. Rider JA, Rider DL. Batten disease: past, present, and future. Am J Med Genet 1988;5(suppl):21–26.
136. Rider JA, Rider DL. Thirty years of Batten disease research: present status and future goals. Mol Genet Metab 1999;66(4):231–233.
137. Rizzo JF, Lessell S, Liebman SD. Optic atrophy in familial dysautonomia. Am J Ophthalmol 1986;102:463–467.
138. Robb RM, Watters GV. Ophthalmic manifestations of subacute sclerosing panencephalitis. Arch Ophthalmol 1970;83:426–435.
139. Roberts RM. Prevention of human mitochondrial (mtDNA) disease by nucleus transplantation into an enucleated donor oocyte. Am J Med Genet 1999;87(3):265–266.

140. Roels F, Cornelis A, Poll-The BT, et al. Hepatic peroxisomes are deficient in infantile Refsum disease: a cytochemical study of 4 cases. Am J Med Genet 1986;25:257–271.
141. Roels F, Cornelis A, et al. Hepatic peroxisomes are deficient in infantile Refsum disease: a cytochemical study of 4 cases. Am J Med Genet 1986;25(2):257–271.
142. Rushton AR, Shaywitz BA, Duncan CC, et al. Computed tomography in the diagnosis of Canavan's disease. Ann Neurol 1981;10(1): 57–60.
143. Sakuta R, Goto Y-I, Horai S, Nonaka I. Mitochondrial DNA mutations at nucleotide positions 3243 and 3271 in mitochondrial myopathy, encephalopathy, lactic acidosis, and stroke-like episodes: a comparative study. J Neurol Sci 1993;115:158–160.
144. Schaffert DA, Johnsen SD, Johnson PC, Drayer BP. Magnetic resonance imaging in pathologically proven Hallervorden–Spatz disease. Neurology 1989;39:440–442.
145. Scheffer IE, Boraitser M, Wilson J, et al. Pelizaeus–Merzbacher disease: classical or connatal? Neuropediatrics 1991;22(2):71–78.
146. Schelhaas HJ, Ippel PF, et al. Similarities and differences in the phenotype, genotype and pathogenesis of different spino-cerebellar ataxias. Eur J Neurol 2000;7(3):309–314.
147. Schindler D, Bishop DF, Wolfe DE, et al. Neuroaxonal dystrophy due to lysosomal alpha-*N*-acetylgalactosaminidase deficiency. N Engl J Med 1989;320(26):1735–1740.
148. Schram AW, Strijland A, Hashimoto RJA, Schutgens RBH, van den Bosch H, Tager JM. Biosynthesis and maturation of peroxisomal β-oxidation enzymes in fibroblasts in relation to the Zellweger syndrome and infantile Refsum disease. Proc Natl Acad Sci USA 1986;83:6156–6158.
149. Schram AW, Strijland A, et al. Biosynthesis and maturation of peroxisomal beta-oxidation enzymes in fibroblasts in relation to the Zellweger syndrome and infantile Refsum disease. Proc Natl Acad Sci USA 1986;83(16):6156–6158.
150. Schutgens RBH, Schrakamp G, Wanders RJA, Heymans HSA, Tager JM, van den Bosch H. Prenatal and perinatal diagnosis of peroxisomal disorders. J Inherit Metab Dis 1989;12(1):118–134.
151. Scotto JM, Hadchouel M, Odievre M, et al. Infantile phytanic acid storage disease, a possible variant of Refsum's disease: three cases, including ultrastructural studies of the liver. J Inherit Metab Dis 1982;5:83–90.
152. Seitelberger F. Eine unbekannte form von infantiler lipoid-specherkrankhect des gehirns. Proc First Int Cong Neuropathol, vol 3. Turin: Rosenberg and Sellier, 1952.
153. Seitelberger F. In: Vinken P, Bruyn G (eds) Peliazeus–Merzbacher disease. Leucodystrophies and poliodystrophies, vol 10. Amsterdam: North Holland, 1970:150–201.
154. Seitelberger F. Neuroaxonal dystrophy: its relation to aging and neurologic disease. In: Vinken P, Bruyn G, Klawans H (eds) Hand-

book of clinical neurology, vol 49. Amsterdam: Elsevier, 1986:391–415.

155. Seitelberger F. Neuropathology and genetics of Pelizaeus–Merzbacher disease. Brain Pathol 1995;5(3):267–273.
156. Shapiro LJ, Aleck KA, Kaback MM, et al. Metachromatic leukodystrophy without arylsulfatase A deficiency. Pediatr Res 1979;13: 1179–1181.
158. Shapiro E, Krivit W, et al. Long-term effect of bone-marrow transplantation for childhood-onset cerebral X-linked adrenoleukodystrophy. Lancet 2000;356(9231):713–718.
159. Shoffner JM, Lott MJ, Lezza AMS, et al. Myoclonic epilepsy and ragged-red fiber disease (MERRF) is associated with a mitochondrial DNA tRNAlys mutation. Cell 1990;61:931–937.
160. Siemerling E, Creutzfeldt HG. Bronzekrankheit und sklerosierende encephalomyelitis. Arch Psychiatr Nervenski 1923;68: 217–244.
161. Simon DK, Johns DR. Mitochondrial disorders: clinical and genetic features. Annu Rev Med 1999;50:111–127.
161a. Slaugenhaupt SA, Blumenfeld A, Gill SP, et al. Tissue-specific expression of a splicing mutation in the IKBKAP gene causes familial dysautonomia. Am J Hum Genet 2001;68(3):598–605.
162. Smith GC, Cary RB, et al. Purification and DNA binding properties of the ataxia-telangiectasia gene product ATM. Proc Natl Acad Sci USA 1999;96:11134–11139.
163. Steinberg D. Refsum's disease. In: Scriver CT, et al. (eds) The metabolic basis of inherited disease. New York: McGraw-Hill, 1989: 1533–1550.
164. Steinlin M, Blaser S, et al. Cerebellar involvement in metabolic disorders: a pattern-recognition approach. Neuroradiology 1998;40(6): 347–354.
165. Stevanin G, Durr A, et al. Spinocerebellar ataxia type 7. Handbook of ataxia disorders. New York: Dekker, 2000;50:469–486.
166. Stoffel W, Hillen H, Giersiefen H. Structure and molecular arrangement of proteolipid protein of central nervous system myelin. Proc Natl Acad Sci USA 1984;81:5012–5016.
167. Su Y, Swift M. Mortality rates among carriers of ataxia-telangiectasia mutant alleles. Ann Intern Med 2000;133:770–778.
168. Swoveland PT. Molecular events in measles virus infection of the central nervous system. Int Rev Exp Pathol 1991;32:355–375.
169. Topcu M, Saatci I, et al. Leigh syndrome in a 3-year-old boy with unusual brain MR imaging and pathologic findings. AJNR (Am J Neuroradiol) 2000;21(1):224–227.
170. Tourtellotte WW, Ma BI, Brandes DB, Walsh MJ, Potvin AR. Quantification of denovo central nervous system IgG measles antibody synthesis in SSPE. Ann Neurol 1981;9:551–556.
171. Toussaint D, Danis P. An ocular pathologic study of Refsum's syndrome. Am J Ophthalmol 1971;72(2):342–347.

172. Traboulsi EI, Maumenee IH. Ophthalmologic manifestations of X-linked childhood adrenoleukodystrophy. Ophthalmology 1987; 94(1):47–52.
173. Trobe JD, Sharpe JA, Hirsh DK, et al. Nystagmus of Pelizaeus–Merzbacher disease. A magnetic search-coil study. Arch Neurol 1991;48(1):87–91.
174. Trofatter JA, Dlouhy SR, De Myer W, Conneally PM, Hodes ME. Pelizaeus–Merzbacher disease: tight linkage to proteolipid protein gene axon variant. Proc Natl Acad Sci USA 1989;86:9427–9430.
175. Udar NS, Xu S, et al. Physical map of the region surrounding the ataxia-telangiectasia gene on human chromosome 11q22-23. Neuropediatrics 1999;30:176–180.
176. Uziel G, Bertini E, Rimoldi M, et al. Experience on therapy of adreno-leukodystrophy and adrenomyeloneuropathy. Dev Neurosci 1991;13(4–5):274–279.
177. Wallace DC, Zheng X, Lott MT, et al. Familial mitochondrial encephalomyopathy (MERRF): genetic, pathophysiological, and biochemical characterization of a mitochondrial DNA disease. Cell 1988;55:601.
178. Wanders RJ, Schutgens RB, et al. Infantile Refsum disease: deficiency of catalase-containing particles (peroxisomes), alkyldihydroxyacetone phosphate synthase and peroxisomal beta-oxidation enzyme proteins. Eur J Pediatr 1986;145(3):172–175.
179. Wang AM, Schindler D, Desnick RJ. Schindler disease: the molecular lesion in the α-*N*-acetylgalactosaminidase gene that causes an infantile neuroaxonal dystrophy. J Clin Investig 1990;86:1752–1756.
180. Wang AM, Desnick RJ. Structural organization and complete sequence of the human alpha-*N*-acetylgalactosaminidase gene: homology with the alpha-galactosidase A gene provides evidence for evolution from a common ancestral gene. Genomics 1991;10(1): 133–142.
181. Wang AM, Bishop DF, et al. Human alpha-*N*-acetylgalactosaminidase-molecular cloning, nucleotide sequence, and expression of a full-length cDNA. Homology with human alpha-galactosidase A suggests evolution from a common ancestral gene. J Biol Chem 1990;265(35):21859–21866.
182. Weimbs T, Dick T, Stoffel W, Bolthauser E. A point mutation at the X-chromosomal proteolipid protein locus in Pelizaeus–Merzbacher disease leads to disruption of myelinogenesis. Biol Chem Hoppe Seyler 1990;371:1175–1183.
183. Weinberg K, Moser A, Watkins P, et al. Bone marrow transplantation for adrenoleukodystrophy. Pediatr Res 1988;23:334A.
184. Weinstein R. Phytanic acid storage disease (Refsum's disease): clinical characteristics, pathophysiology and the role of therapeutic apheresis in its management. J Clin Apheresis 1999;14(4):181–184.

185. Weleber RG. The dystrophic retina in multisystem disorders: the electroretinogram in neuronal ceroid lipofuscinoses. Eye 1998; 12(pt 3b):580–590.
186. Wenger DA, Rafi MA, et al. Krabbe disease: genetic aspects and progress toward therapy. Mol Genet Metab 2000;70(1):1–9.
187. Willard HF, Riordan JR. Assignment of the gene for myelin proteolipid protein to the X chromosome: implications for X-linked myelin disorders. Science 1985;230:940–942.
188. Winkelman AC, Gray LG. Paralysis of down-gazed in familial progressive encephalopathy. Frank B. Walsh Society Annual Meeting, Salt Lake City, Utah, February 1991.
189. Wisniewski KE, Kida E, et al. Variability in the clinical and pathological findings in the neuronal ceroid lipofuscinoses: review of data and observations. Am J Med Genet 1992;42(4):525–532.
190. Wisniewski KE, Kida E, Patxot OF, et al. Neuronal ceroid lipofuscinoses: research update. Neurol Sci 2000;21(3):S49–S56.
191. Wolfe LS, Palo J, Santavouri P, et al. Urinary sediment dolichols in the diagnosis of neuronal ceroid-lipofuscinosis. Ann Neurol 1986; 19:270–274.
192. Woodward K, Malcolm S. Proteolipid protein gene: Pelizaeus–Merzbacher disease in humans and neurodegeneration in mice. Trends Genet 1999;15(4):125–128.
193. Wulff CH. Subacute sclerosing panencephalitis: serial electroencephalographic studies. J Neurol Neurosurg Psychiatry 1982;45: 418.
194. Yamanaka R, Nomura Y, Segawa M, et al. MELAS, myoclonus, ataxia and deficiencies of complexes I and IV in muscle mitochondria. Acta Paediatr Jpn 1987;29:761.
195. Zafeiriou DI, Kontopoulos EE, et al. Neurophysiology and MRI in late-infantile metachromatic leukodystrophy. Pediatr Neurol 1999; 21(5):843–846.
196. Zagami AS, Lethlean AK. Chorioretinitis as a possible very early manifestation of subacute sclerosing panencephalitis. Aust NZ J Med 1991;21:350–352.
197. Zhang X, Rafi MA, DeGala G, Wenger DA. The mechanism for a 33-nucleotide insertion in an RNA causing sphingolipid activator protein (SAP-1)-deficient metachromatic leukodystrophy. Hum Genet 1991;87:211–215.

11

Neurocranial Defects with Neuro-Ophthalmic Significance

Ronald M. Minzter and Edward G. Buckley

Patients with cranial/skeletal defects often exhibit neuro-ophthalmic abnormalities, which may be caused by specific anomalies within the spectrum of a given condition, or by an associated malformation of the nervous system, or be secondary to mechanical forces such as hydrocephalus. This chapter reviews the ophthalmic abnormalities found in progressive hemifacial atrophy, which are primarily due to structural defects, as well as ophthalmic abnormalities in Arnold–Chiari malformations, meningomyelocele, platybasia, and the Klippel–Feil syndrome, which are related to both structural and secondary neurological mechanisms.

PROGRESSIVE HEMIFACIAL ATROPHY (PARRY–ROMBERG DISEASE)

Progressive hemifacial atrophy (PHA), described by Parry in 1825, and by Romberg in 1846 as "trophoneurosis facialis," is a progressive variable hemiatrophy of facial fat and subcutaneous tissues.[102,111] Eulenburg[34] later named this condition "progressive facial hemiatrophy." The atrophy begins in childhood, progresses intermittently and rapidly over the next 2 to 10 years, and usually decelerates by young adulthood.[48,49,99] If onset is early enough, bone and cartilage may be affected because the facial structures have not yet fully matured[104] (Fig. 11-1, top). In addition to facial atrophy, there can be dental/oral changes, migraine headaches, and neurological disturbances such as

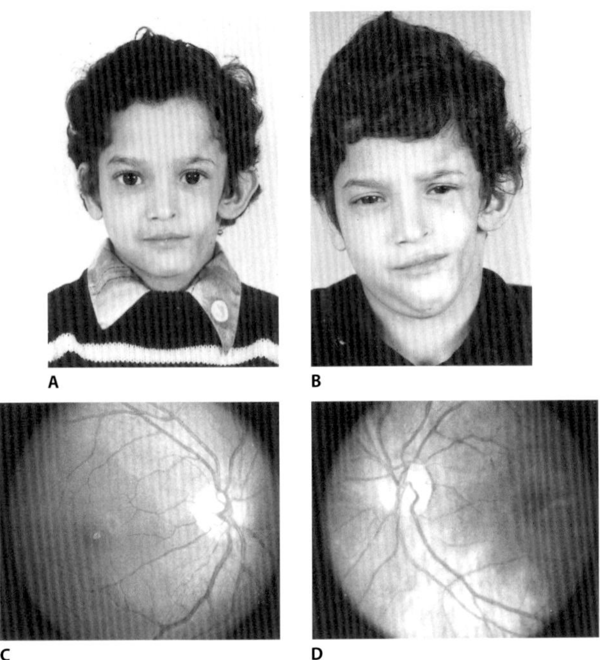

FIGURE 11-1A–D. Progressive nature of progressive hemifacial atrophy (PHA) in a patient at 8 years old (**A**) and again at 15 years (**B**), showing left-sided atrophy. Fundus photos of the normal contralateral side (**C**) and the ipsilateral affected side with hypopigmentary disturbances (**D**), particularly along the inferior arcade.

trigeminal neuralgia and seizures.[60,84] Unilateral trunk, limb, and even visceral changes have been associated in rare cases.[91,108,110]

Genetic patterns are unclear but, in a review by Rogers, females were affected more than males (3:2) and less than 5% of cases had bilateral involvement.[104,110] The acquired progressive nature of hemifacial atrophy differentiates it from the congenital nonprogressive spectrum of Goldenhar's hemifacial microsomia and the branchial arch syndromes.[48,49,84]

The etiology of PHA remains unclear. Various hypotheses have been proposed that can be largely grouped into four general categories: neurotrophic, vascular, exogenous insult, and autoimmune mediated. Neurotrophic theories implicate a trigeminal neuritis,[80,101] a cerebral deregulation of the peripheral and sympathetic nervous systems through a heredodegenerative process,[128] or a sympathetic nerve loss or interruption.[84,89] The vascular theory, which itself relates to the trigeminal nerve, stems from work with electron microscopic and cytoimmunological techniques showing the possible role of a "lymphocytic neurovasculitis" deleteriously affecting endothelial regeneration of vessels in close proximity with the trigeminal nerve. This process, in turn, leads to facial atrophy.[104] Case studies of PHA with either uveitis and retinal vasculitis, or retinal vascular malformation, suggest that a mechanism for PHA is related to a disruption in the normal angiogenic process.[82,100] Possible exogenous insults include a slow virus, which initiates atrophy, as well as other infectious agents and/or trauma, which serve to "trigger" the atrophic process.[48,49] *Borrelia* infection (or Lyme disease) has also been implicated in a case of PHA, the atrophic progression of which was halted with treatment using penicillin.[121] An autoimmune mechanism has also been proposed because both linear alopecia (a focal variant of scleroderma) and PHA share many features. However, unlike immune-related scleroderma, PHA is not associated with an elevated antinuclear antibody (ANA) titer, hyperglobulinemia, or circulating immune complexes.[73]

Ocular Findings

Ocular findings are present in approximately 40% of cases of PHA.[84] They may also be grouped into four general categories (Table 11-1). The first, and most clinically evident, involves structural abnormalities. Enophthalmos is the most prominent ocular finding in PHA and is secondary to orbital, lid, and brow atrophy. In rare cases, there is a "monostotic form fruste" with pure maxillary bone atrophy and maxillary sinus implosion.[47,57,138] Lid atrophy with madarosis and pseudocolobomatous changes, ptosis, ectropion, blepharophimosis, and extraocular motility disturbances can occur. Ipsilateral upper lid retraction, with subsequent corneal exposure, has also been reported as a late finding.[42] A variety of nonspecific abnormalities, including a case of ophthalmoplegia,[65] is thought to result from connective tissue atrophy and fibrotic-like changes in the orbit.[17,40,124]

A second constellation of features is consistent with involvement of sympathetic and trigeminal innervation. The sympathetic features include pupillary disturbances (miosis and

three types of *Arnold–Chiari malformations* (ACM) describe a gradient of anatomic distortion; the fourth type is structurally different.

Type I ACM involves a partial caudal herniation of the cerebellar tonsils and medial lobes through the foramen magnum with a normally positioned fourth ventricle. Although the foramen magnum is usually normal, type I ACM may incorporate acquired defects of the foramen magnum as seen with basilar impression syndromes, and with defects more commonly associated with type II ACM, such as meningomyelocele.[8]

Type II ACM includes type I anomalies plus a descent of the pons and fourth ventricle via an enlarged foramen magnum. Virtually all ACM type II patients also have a meningomyelocele, or dysraphism of the spine, as well as clinical findings associated with subsequent hydrocephalus. There is typically an outflow obstruction of cerebrospinal fluid (CSF) at the foramina of Luschka and Magendie, an increase in intracranial pressure, and, in turn, a characteristic kinking (in approximately 70% of patients) of the cervicomedullary region.[94] The fourth ventricle may become isolated secondary to aqueductal stenosis and diminished CSF outflow; when this occurs, there is a high incidence of associated syringohydromyelia.[8] Hindbrain molding around the dens of the axis, rostral cervical nerve deviation, and stretching of cranial nerves is also typical.[62] In effect, the cerebellum becomes compressed between a small posterior fossa and a low tentorial attachment (Fig. 11-2).

A Chiari type III defect is much rarer and more severe. The cerebellum and lower brainstem herniates through the foramen magnum and becomes squeezed over a widely cystic fourth "*ventriculocele*." This defect presents as a low occipital or high cervical (C1–C2) encephalocele[87] and secondary cerebellar parenchymal damage is common. The fourth type of Chiari malformation is distinctly different and actually resembles the cystic ventricular Dandy–Walker anomaly. In type IV ACM, the malformation is contained within the posterior fossa; under conditions of raised intracranial pressure, the dilated fourth ventricle becomes cystic in nature and the brainstem and cerebellum become compressed and degenerated respectively.

Ocular Findings

The neurological and neuro-ophthalmic changes in ACM are primarily due to structural anomalies (cerebellar and brainstem dis-

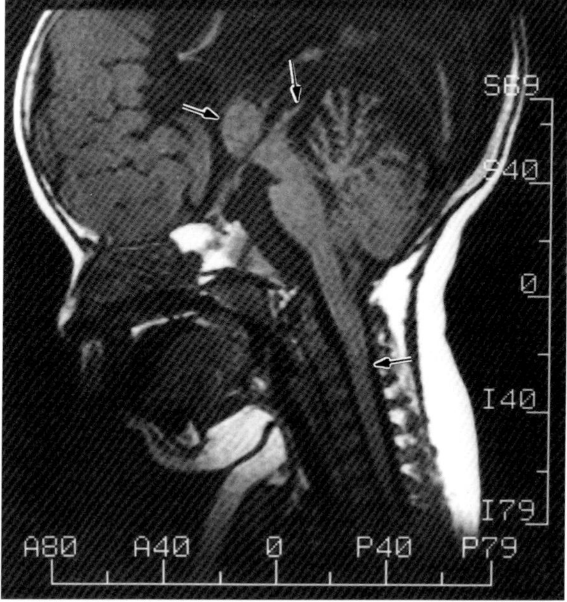

FIGURE 11-2. Sagittal MRI of a patient with type II Arnold–Chiari malformation shows cerebellar atrophy, a small posterior fossa, and inferior vermian displacement to the level of C3 with an inferiorly displaced cervicomedullary junction (*bottom arrow*). Other anomalies present include massive cortical loss, agenesis of the corpus callosum, beaking of the tectum (*top arrow*), and a large massa intermedia (*middle arrow*).

tortion) and the dynamics of CSF flow (hydrocephalus). Because of the close association between hydrocephalus and ACM, many ocular findings can be attributed to one or both entities. These findings most typically include optic atrophy, Parinaud's syndrome, horizontal and downbeating nystagmus, diplopia, and strabismus.[127]

A classic finding of advanced hydrocephalus in the setting of ACM is vertically downbeating nystagmus (DBN). DBN is associated with craniocervical lesions, most often with basilar impression/platybasia or ACM.[28,137] ACMs usually do not directly effect rostral structures associated with vergence movements (midbrain and pretectal areas), although cases have been reported with abnormal convergence and retraction nystagmus.[90,130] The authors postulate that convergence nystagmus is caused by mechanical brainstem and cerebellar distortion, combined with abnormal transmission of cerebrospinal fluid to the aqueductal region.

Duane's retraction syndrome has also been found in association with Arnold–Chiari malformation type I.[136] Authors postulate a common early embryogenic mechanism between Duane's and Arnold–Chiari malformation involving aberrant brainstem innervation[35,86] and incomplete neural tube closure, causing suboptimal distension of the developing ventricular system.[79,83]

Attempts have been made to correlate motility disorders with the level of CNS distortion in patients with ACM and meningomyelocele.[72] In a clinical series by Lennerstrand, strabismus and nystagmus generally correlated with hydrocephalus and secondary higher cerebral changes more than with lower brainstem structural deformities.[72] Oblique muscle motility disorders, horizontal and vertical gaze difficulty, and saccadic control correlated with lower brainstem lesions (tectal plate and medulla oblongata). Convergence defects related to upper brainstem deformities and the level of herniation.[70,72]

The strabismus most commonly seen with ACM is largely comitant and seldom caused by cranial nerve paralysis.[77] It is frequently associated with "A" or "V" patterns, and a possible supranuclear origin has been postulated (see section on Meningomyelocele).[72] Acquired esotropia, often with other motility anomalies, may present as an early sign of Arnold–Chiari malformation I. Some authors suggest divergence palsy as a mechanism for which neurosurgical suboccipital and upper cervical decompression is utilized.[75] Strabismus surgery may then be performed should proper realignment not be achieved.[129] Other associated motility disturbances include horizontal and vertical gaze paresis, saccadic defects, cogwheel pursuits, optokinetic nystagmus (OKN) abnormalities, convergence insufficiencies, and partial sixth nerve palsies,[14] which are often attributed to altered CSF dynamics.[72] Bilateral and unilateral internuclear ophthalmoplegia (INO),[5,96,135] upbeating nystagmus, torsional nystagmus (associated with syringomyelia),[16] see-saw nystagmus,[139] periodic alternating gaze and skew deviations, saccadic dysmetria, and inappropriate vestibular ocular reflex (VOR) gain have also been reported.[44,87,123] "Nystagmus of skew," whereby one eye demonstrates an upward vertical jerk nystagmus while the other eye has a simultaneous downward beating jerk nystagmus, has also been seen with Arnold–Chiari malformation.[106] It has been suggested that the presentation of nystagmus of skew should prompt an MRI study to rule out Arnold–Chiari malformation. Autonomic dysfunction, including sinus arrhythmia, Horner's syndrome, and anisocoria (at a greater rate than healthy controls), have also been reported, which suggests a sympathetic lesion at the T1 level of the cord in association with Arnold–Chiari malformation type I.[122]

Other CNS anomalies associated with ACM appear unrelated to CSF dynamics. These defects include a dysgenetic corpus callosum with absence of the splenium and rostrum,[7] defects in the septum pellucidum and falx cerebri, enlargement of the caudate heads and massa intermedia,[93] and stenogyria, multiple small gyri of the medial regions of the occipital lobes.[133] Recent genetic studies link *renal-coloboma syndrome* (an autosomal dominant disorder that includes colobomatous eye defects, vesicoureteral reflux, and kidney anomalies) in a patient with hydrocephalus associated with platybasia and Arnold–Chiari malformation. Genetic studies demonstrate the renal-coloboma syndrome results from mutations in PAX 2. The homoguanine tract in PAX 2 is a "hot spot" for spontaneous expansion or contraction mutations and demonstrates the importance of homonucleotide tract mutations in human malformation syndromes.[116]

Diagnosis

Currently, the best method available for the diagnosis of ACM is magnetic resonance imaging (MRI). Although cranial nerve nuclei and specific CNS pathways may not be imaged, brainstem, cerebellar, and spinal anomalies are clearly visualized.[11,16,71,74,115,137] Sagittal imaging provides the most information and allows an overview from ventricular contour, to mid- and hindbrain placement, down to spinal and vertebral anomalies. Sagittal MRI can also demonstrate the presence of stenogyria, as well as the presence of a "trapped" fourth ventricle, which are both difficult to evaluate on axial sections.[8] Axial sections highlight defects that violate the midline as in the corpus callosum, septum pellucidum, and falx cerebri.[8,133]

Cysternography has been the radiographic gold standard for evaluating CSF flow; however, cine-mode MRI is an alternative for accurate noninvasive assessment of CSF dynamics.[126] Computed tomography (CT) also has a role because of its ability to image particularly bony regions. For example, with axial CT slices, one can appreciate the posterior concavity and scalloped shape of the petrous bones underlying areas of chronic cerebellar pressure often present with ACM.[95]

Treatment

The treatment of Arnold–Chiari malformation and associated hydrocephalus traditionally has been neurosurgical. Although the severity of anatomic defect does not always correlate with an individual's clinical presentation,[71] patients may require decompression of the deformity and a subsequent valved shunting procedure. Suboccipital craniotomy with sharp dissection into the foramen of Magendie has been described for ACM I with associated hydrosyringomyelia and syringobulbia in the left pons in a case presenting with acute left gaze paralysis.[66]

In patients with largely dorsal compression, a standard laminectomy with or without resection of the posterior margin of the foramen magnum is performed. Soft tissue excision is also needed when constricting dural bands are present.[21] Alternatively, anterior (transoral) decompression may be the method of choice for patients with ventral compression at the cervicomedullary junction in ACM and basilar impression.[126] Placement of a ventricular shunt is usually a concomitant or secondary procedure required for patients with ACM and hydrocephalus.

MENINGOMYELOCELE

Failure of the embryologic neural groove to form an intact neural tube results in a spectrum of neurological defects. Lack of vertebral closure is spina bifida, herniation of meninges is a meningocele, and involvement of the spinal cord itself is termed meningomyelocele (MMC).[103] MMCs are most commonly located in the mid- to caudal groove (i.e., lumbar region). More rostral defects in the skull, such as with a midline cleft, may result in protrusion of brain tissue or encephalocele, the majority of which are over the occipital region[118] and may occasionally cause cortical blindness.[12] Alternatively, if the sacral area is involved, neurogenic bladder and associated urinary tract infections, hydronephrosis, and renal calculi may ensue.[119]

The incidence of MMC is approximately 1 in 1000 in the United States, and is slightly greater in whites than in African-Americans; the risk of recurrence for parents with one affected child is approximately 4%.[118] The etiology is unclear, and polygenetic inheritance, environmental conditions, and maternal malnutrition have all been implicated.[88,98] Prenatal diagnosis during the 14th to 20th week of gestation is accomplished through amniocentesis by the detection of alpha-fetoprotein and acetylcholinesterase liberated via a leaky neural tube defect.[3,56]

Ocular Findings

Modern neurosurgical, urosurgical, and medical management have increased the quality and lifespan of patients with MMC; as a result, there is a greater opportunity for neuro-ophthalmic anomalies to manifest themselves and require proper care. Although the majority of neuro-ophthalmic findings associated with MMC are motility disorders,[71] other findings, such as optic atrophy,[112] are intimately linked with CSF dynamics and generally increase in proportion to the severity of hydrocephalus. Hydrocephalus has been reported in up to 90% of patients with MMC.[13]

Hydrocephalus results in ventricular dilation, chiasmal and optic nerve compression with secondary ischemia, midbrain distortion, and hindbrain herniation. Most MMCs, particularly in the lumbosacral region, are associated with some degree of ACM; in turn, more than 90% of children with MMC develop hydrocephalus secondary to aqueductal stenosis and the associated ACM.[114,120] Nearly all patients with ACM type II or worse have an associated MMC[12,115]; conversely, almost all patients with MMC have an ACM.[58]

Papilledema (and eventual optic atrophy), cortical blindness, sixth nerve palsy, vertical gaze palsy, and downbeat nystagmus may all develop when intracranial pressure (ICP) rises acutely.[12,71] In younger patients, before fusion of the fontanelles, the head often expands rather than progress to clinical papilledema. If a sixth nerve palsy from hydrocephalus does occur, the eventual level of binocular development and realignment is often poor.

Early comprehensive ophthalmic examination for optic nerve anomalies, nystagmus, and motility disorders, combined with appropriate amblyopia therapy and surgical intervention, have led to excellent visual outcomes (90%–95% have greater than or equal to 6/12 visual acuity)[12] in patients with MMC. Fortunately, there is a low rate of decreased visual function from amblyopia in these patients[26,44,77,107] because early occlusion treatment yields good results.[12] However, causes responsible for decreased visual acuity include amblyopia, latent nystagmus, optic atrophy, and cortical blindness, as well as apparently unassociated or "independent" reasons such as refractive errors, cataracts, and keratoconus.[12] Generally, in patients with MMC and ACM, visual difficulty seems to be more often related to refractive errors and strabismus than to optic atrophy.[71]

Approximately 60% of patients with MMC are found to have some form of strabismus.[23] Even without hydrocephalus, 50% of patients with MMC also develop strabismus.[26] Of the many types of strabismus found, "A" patterns, with overacting superior oblique and superior recti muscles[23,39] and esotropia,[113] are the most frequent, although "V" patterns and exodeviations can occur.[12,23,38,71,77] A patterns have also been more commonly seen with exodeviations than with esodeviations (Fig. 11-3).[13]

The A-pattern strabismus associated with spina bifida is most likely acquired and related to hydrocephalus.[13] Skew deviation, with supranuclear origins, is generally considered a sign of posterior fossa disease, and can clinically mimic superior oblique over-action. In turn, some cases of superior oblique over-

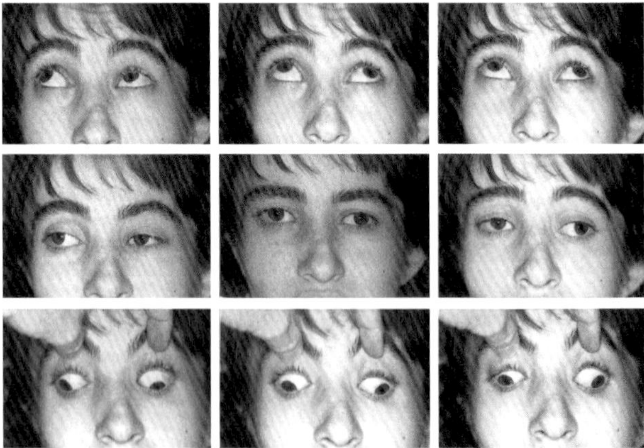

FIGURE 11-3. "A" pattern exotropia in a patient with Klippel–Feil syndrome (KFS).

action can represent a form of skew deviation.[58] This relationship is consistent with the finding that children with superior oblique overaction have a significantly higher incidence of concurrent neurological diseases than control subjects.[58] A classic "setting-sun" sign, with the eyes deviated downward and outward in the presence of increased ICP, may actually represent a severe A pattern superimposed on a hydrocephalus-induced vertical gaze palsy. Lid retraction commonly seen in hydrocephalic infants may accentuate this sign. Theories surrounding A-pattern esotropias implicate inherently weak lateral recti, partial sixth nerve palsies, primary midbrain pathology (a supranuclear defect in the brainstem),[77] and fluctuating ICPs.[12,71,77] Both the deficiency of upward gaze and the lid retraction may be secondary to dilation of the posterior portion of the third ventricle and possibly the cerebral aqueduct.[127] MRI studies demonstrate that beaking of the rostral area of the brainstem is associated with an A-pattern strabismus, which correlates with defects in the vertical gaze pathways.[13,22]

Treatment

Bilateral superior oblique tenotomies have had greater success for A-pattern deviations in patients with MMC than infraplacement of the lateral recti (A-pattern exotropia) or supraplacement of the medial recti (A-pattern esotropia).[13] A tenotomy of the superior oblique muscle, nasal to the medial border of the superior rectus muscle, has been recommended for larger A-pattern deviations; a tenotomy lateral to the superior rectus muscle has been recommended for smaller A-patterns.[13]

ABNORMALITIES OF THE CRANIAL–VERTEBRAL BORDER: PLATYBASIA AND BASILAR IMPRESSION

Malformation of the base of the occipital bone (forming the base of the skull) and of the cervical spine may be manifested as *platybasia* and/or *basilar impression*. Other malformations of this region include defects of the atlas and axis, cervical fusional syndromes, such as the *Klippel–Feil* syndrome and the Arnold–Chiari malformation. Each of these entities may occur singly or within the scope of a larger syndrome, and may exist as a primary maldevelopment or as a secondary change from a systemic/bony disease.

Although the terms *platybasia* and *basilar impression* are often used interchangeably and are conditions that frequently occur together, they can each be distinctly defined. The condition of a flat skull base, or platybasia (from the Greek; *platys*, flat, and *basia*, base),[41] exists when the angle formed by a line connecting the nasion, tuberculum sella, and anterior margin of the foramen magnum is greater than 143°.[81] Normally this angle ranges from 110 to 140°.[103] Essentially, the basal angle of the skull, made by the intersection of the plane of the sphenoid with that of the clivus, is flattened. The effect is that the anteroposterior (AP) diameter of the foramen magnum is decreased and the depth of the posterior fossa becomes shallow, thereby allowing less space for the cerebellum and brainstem to properly align themselves along the axis of the spinal column.

Basilar impression, or invagination, occurs when the margins of the foramen magnum are variably indented into the base of the skull. The foramen magnum contours become distorted and narrowed, more so in the AP dimension, by upward displacement of the odontoid process above Chamberlain's line (hard palate to the posterior border of the foramen magnum) and into the foramen magnum.[18,30,81] Localized thickening of the dura at the cranial vertebral junction is frequently associated, which further constricts the brainstem.[62]

As primary developmental anomalies, platybasia and basilar impression are relatively rare, and are more commonly associated with a systemic condition. When they are secondary to a systemic/bony disease, the cranial bones are usually softened so that the weight of the skull causes the cranial vertex to approach the occiput as the occiput and cervical spine press into the posterior fossa. This configuration may result from mucopolysaccharidoses (Hurler's), Paget's disease of the bone, rickets (osteomalacia), osteogenesis imperfecta, osteitis deformans, fibrous dysplasia, hyper- and hypoparathyroidism, hypo- and achondroplasia, cleidocranial dysostosis, histiocytosis X, rheumatoid arthritis, Conradi's disease, and Klippel–Feil syndrome.[32,61,125,134]

The clinical findings may be attributed to mechanical forces, such as direct compression or hydrocephalus, or to associated CNS defects. Clinical manifestations are proportional to the anatomic extent of the defect, and frequently to the degree of resultant hydrocephalus. Both platybasia and basilar impression lead to a diminished capacity of the posterior fossa. The pons, medulla, and cervical cord may be compressed, and the posterior cranial nerves may become stretched as the occipital bone and cervical spine rise and the foramen magnum narrows. The cerebellum may also be compromised from above as it is pressed against the resistant tentorium cerebri.[103] Hydrocephalus, often dependent upon head position about the atlanto-occipital junction, is a frequent complication due to obstruction of CSF at the level of the crowded posterior fossa.[106] A coincident vertebral basilar vascular insufficiency, also positionally dependent, has been implicated in producing clinical findings such as transient dizziness, hemiparesis, and bilateral blurring of vision, which may occur with platybasia and basilar impression.[64,125]

Atlantoaxial dislocation is a significant structural anomaly of the spine that often accompanies platybasia and basilar impression; this may lead to compression of the upper cervical cord (between the odontoid process and posterior arch of the atlas), and compromise of the lower medulla, which becomes distorted at its junction with the posteriorly displaced spinal cord.[30] A variant of this dislocation, which requires surgical correction, is "odontoideum" in which the odontoid is separated from the body of the axis. The effect of this can range from mild transient neck discomfort to the extreme presentation of quadriplegia.[1]

Clinical and Ocular Findings

Platybasia and basilar impression often remain relatively asymptomatic until adult life, when they are aggravated by minor trauma. However, they may cause more severe clinical problems as a primary structural anomaly or as part of a progressive systemic disease (Table 11-2). Symptoms may be grouped in rela-

TABLE 11-2. Systemic Conditions Leading to Platybasia.
Mucopolysaccharidoses (Hurler's)
Paget's disease
Osteomalacia (rickets)
Osteogenesis imperfecta
Osteitis deformans
Fibrous dysplasia
Hyperhypoparathyroidism
Achondroplasia
Histiocytosis X
Rheumatoid arthritis
Conradi's disease
Klippel–Feil syndrome

tion to the areas affected (such as cerebellum, medulla and pons, posterior and lower cranial nerves, upper cervical nerves, musculoskeletal system), and according to those that are associated with hydrocephalus.[127]

Cerebellar changes may cause atonia, ataxia, and poor coordination. Impingement of the pons and medulla by the clivus can induce pyramidal tract symptoms such as abnormal reflexes, spasticity, lateral spinothalamic tract impairment with dissociated sensory pain loss, weakness, and general paresthesias.[127] Such a patient may also have loss of position sense, bladder dysfunction, and neuromuscular atrophy.[30] Lower cranial nerves are typically affected, which causes descending trigeminal tract (facial) sensory loss and palatal and vocal cord weakness.[30] Cervical nerve involvement may be detected by the dermatomal distribution of sensory loss, whereas musculoskeletal symptoms reflect the extent of malformation and include pain, shortening, and rigidity of the neck, in addition to torticollis and a sensation of heavy pressure.[46]

A syringomyelic syndrome may develop with hindbrain herniation and subsequent cavitation of the lower medulla and cervical cord. These patients typically exhibit spinal features such as upper limb neuromuscular atrophy early in their clinical course and often require a surgical laminectomy to decompress the expanding cord.[30,33]

Ocular findings reflect direct posterior fossa compression in addition to hydrocephalic changes. Nystagmus is often present and is usually horizontal, but, as seen with posterior fossa lesions, it also becomes vertical with upgaze and occasionally with downgaze.[27,127] Hydrocephalus may lead to papilledema, secondary optic atrophy and decreased vision, ptosis and anisocoria, paralysis of convergence, and corneal anesthesia.[54]

Diagnosis

Clinical diagnosis requires recognition of early symptoms such as transient dizzy episodes seen with vertebral-basilar insufficiency,[125] spastic weakness, ataxia, and focal neurological complaints. In addition, symptoms consistent with an elevated intracranial pressure such as nausea, vomiting, and headache may occur. Downward nystagmus, which is dependent on head position, and other neurological changes are followed by eventual signs of a bullneck appearance with decreased head movement and loss of the normal cervical lordosis.[1] Syringomyelia, demyelinating disease, and posterior fossa tumors must be ruled out in patients exhibiting the progressive and diverse findings of cerebellar, brainstem, and cervical cord syndromes.[81]

Confirmatory diagnosis is imperative and has traditionally been demonstrated with lateral X-ray studies; however, MRI is superior. With sagittal sections, one can see Chamberlain's line (described earlier) intersect Bull's line (an extended line drawn through the spine and body of the first cervical vertebrae), instead of parallel each other, as in the normal configuration.[1] Some authors believe that posterior inclination of the odontoid, with respect to the foramen magnum, is the best radiographic indicator to determine if the patient is at risk for basilar impression.[50]

Treatment

Cases with minor cervical vertebral anomalies may simply require neck immobilization; however, worsening posterior fossa and cord compression or CSF obstruction require surgical decompression and possible shunting. Radiologic studies demonstrating the direction of compressive force on the cervicomedullary junction show the need for anterior or posterior decompression. If atlantoaxial dislocation is a concurrent condition, then skeletal traction is required for performing surgery and stabilization of the spine by bony fusion is recommended.[30,63]

KLIPPEL–FEIL SYNDROME

Klippel–Feil syndrome (KFS), also known as congenital brevicollis, was described in 1912. It is typified by a no-neck or head-on-shoulders appearance resulting from a congenital synostosis of the upper cervical vertebrae, limitation of neck movement, and a low posterior hairline[68] (Fig. 11-4). This appearance is exaggerated by "pterygium colli" or webbing of the neck similar to the Turner's syndrome patient. Although the primary skeletal defect is fusion of the atlas and axis, three types of KF dysostosis have been described according to their anatomic extent.[10,31,52] Type I involves fusion of cervical and upper thoracic vertebrae, type II is solely a cervical fusion, and type III includes an associated fusion of lower thoracic and lumber vertebrae (Fig. 11-5). In addition to the variable degree of cervical fusion, there are

KFS patients is "mirror movement" usually involving the hands.[9] These contralateral mimicking motions seem to result from abnormally branched, fast-conducting, corticospinal tract fibers projecting through motorneuron pools on each side of the spinal cord.[36]

Various syndromes incorporate KFS as part of their collection of features.[105] KF dysostosis combined with sensorineural deafness and Duane's syndrome is called cervico-oculo-acoustic or "Wildervanck's syndrome."[31,131] Wildervanck's syndrome and KFS both show a female preponderance,[105] and their incidence has seemed predominantly sporadic.[24] Wildervanck's syndrome is typically lethal in males,[53] and it has been postulated that Wildervanck's syndrome is a clinical variant of Klippel–Feil syndrome. The case study reporting this theory also reported severe growth and bony delays, renal abnormalities, and mild mental retardation, suggesting that the primary developmental defect is part of a larger disruption sequence.[31,36]

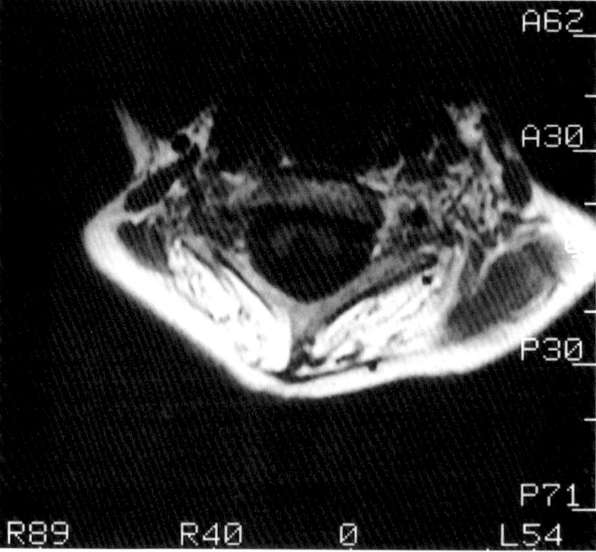

FIGURE 11-6. Same KFS patient demonstrating enlarged foramen magnum and splitting of the cord at the cervicomedullary junction (with caudal reuniting of the cord below the level of C2). No frank diastematomyelia is present.

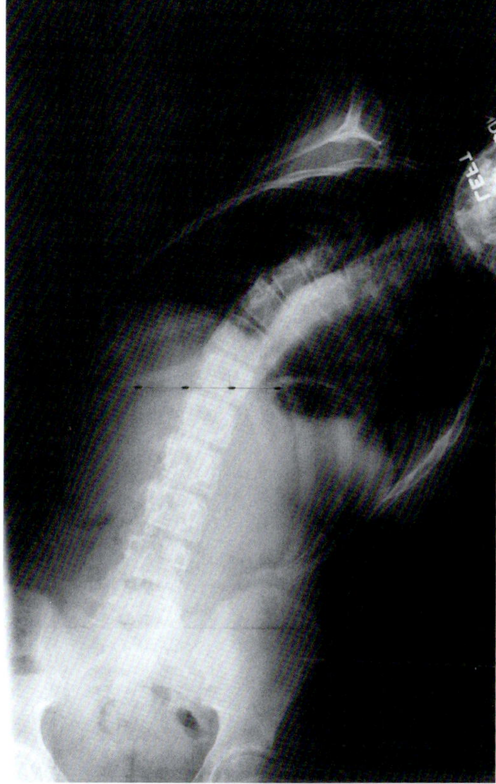

FIGURE 11-7. Preoperative severe thoracolumbar kyphoscoliosis (with right-sided rib fusion, mild Sprengel's deformity, and pelvic obliquity) in the same KFS patient.

Ocular Findings

Ophthalmic findings specifically found with KFS include congenital esotropia and nystagmus, Duane's syndrome (not necessarily with deafness), paralysis of conjugate lateral gaze, and external ophthalmoplegia[31,92] (Table 11-4). Pseudopapilledema has also been reported in patients with Wildervanck's syndrome.[67] Crocodile tears (paradoxical gustatory-lacrimal reflex)

TABLE 11-4. Ocular Findings in Klippel–Feil Syndrome.

Esotropia	Lateral gaze paralysis
Nystagmus	Crocodile tears
Duane's syndrome	Pseudopapilledema
External ophthalmoplegia	

has also been reported in patients with KFS.[15,55] MRI confirmed that one of these cases included a posterior fossa malformation complex with brainstem hypoplasia, which was consistent with the multiple clinical lower cranial neuropathies.[15] Other authors describe crocodile tears in a patient with Wildervanck's syndrome, Dandy–Walker syndrome, and lateral thoracic meningocele.[55] Patients with KFS frequently exhibit overlapping components of basilar impression and ACM. When this occurs, any associated neuro-ophthalmic finding with these other latter conditions may also develop (see Fig. 11-3).

References

1. Adams RD, Delong GR. Harrison's principle of internal medicine. 10th edn. New York: McGraw-Hill, 1983.
2. Albert DM, Nordlund JJ, Lerner AB. Ocular abnormalities occurring with vitiligo. Ophthalmology 1979;86:1145–1158.
3. Allen LD, Ferguson-Smith MA, Donald I, et al. Amniotic-fluid alpha-fetoprotein in the antenatal diagnosis of spina bifida. Lancet 1973; 2:522–525.
4. Aracena T, Roca FP, Barragan M. Progressive hemifacial atrophy (Parry–Romberg syndrome): report of two cases. Am J Ophthalmol 1979;11:953–958.
5. Arnold AC, Balon RW, Yee RD, et al. Internuclear ophthalmoplegia in the Chiari type II malformation. Neurology 1990;40:1850–1854.
6. Arnold J. Myelocyste, transposition von Gewebskeimen und sympodie. Beitr Pathol Anat Allg Pathol 1894;16:1–28.
7. Barkovich AJ, Norman D. Anomalies of the corpus callosum: correlation with further anomalies of the brain. AJNR 1988;9:493–501.
8. Barkovich AJ. Pediatric neuroimaging. New York: Raven Press, 1990.
9. Bauman GI. Absence of the cervical spine: Klippel–Feil syndrome. JAMA 1932;98:129–132.
10. Beighton P. Inherited disorders of the skeleton. 2nd edn. Edinburgh: Churchill Livingstone, 1988.
11. Bewermeyer H, et al. MRImaging of familial basilar impresson. J Comput Assist Tomogr 1984;8:953–956.
12. Biglan AW. Ophthalmic complications of meningomyelocele: a longitudinal study. Trans Am Ophthalmol Soc 1990;88:389–462.

13. Biglan AW. Strabismus associated with meningomyelocele. J Pediatr Ophthalmol 1995;32:309–314.
14. Bixenman WW, Laguna JF. Acquired esotropia as initial manifestion of Arnold–Chiari malformation. J Pediatr Ophthalmol Strabismus 1987;24:83–86.
15. Brodsky MC, Fray KJ. Brainstem hypoplasia in the Wildervanck (cervico-oculo-acoustic) syndrome. Arch Ophthalmol 1998;116:383–385.
16. Břonstein AM, Miller DH, Rudge P, Kendall BE. Down beating nystagmus: magnetic resonance imaging and neuro-otological findings. J Neurol Sci 1987;81:173–184.
17. Calmettes L, Amalric P, Bessou P. L'hemiatrophie faciale (maladie de Romberg) eses manifestations oculaires. Riv Oto-Neuro Oftalmol 1959;31:215.
18. Chamberlain WE. Basilar impression (platybasia). A bizarre developmental anomaly of the occipital bone and upper cervical spine with striking and misleading neurologic manifestations. Yale J Biol Med 1938–39;11:487–496.
19. Chiari H. Ueber die pathogenese der sogenannten Syringomyelia. Z Heilkd 1888;9:307–336.
20. Chiari H. Ueber veranderungen des kleinhirns, des pons und der medulla oblongata in folge von congenitales hydrocephalie des gross hirns, denkschr. Akad Wiss Wien 1896;63:71.
21. Chopra JS, Sawhney IM, Kak VK, Khosla VK. Craniovertebral anomalies: a study of 82 cases. Br J Neurosurg 1988;2:455–464.
22. Christoff N. A clinicopathologic study of vertical eye movements. Arch Neurol 1974;31:1–8.
23. Chu A, Seaber JH, Buckley EG. "A" pattern strabismus in myelomeningocele. Association for Research in Vision and Ophthalmology 1987;28.
24. Clarke RA, Catalan G, Diwan AD, Kearsley JH. Heterogeneity in Klippel syndrome: a new classification. Pediatr Radiol 1998;28:967–974.
25. Cleland J. Contribution to the study of spina bifida, encephalocoele, and anencephalus. J Anat Physiol 1883;17:257–259.
26. Clements DB, Kaushal K. A study of the ocular complications of hydrocephalus and meningomyelocele. Trans Ophthalmol Soc UK 1970;60:383–390.
27. Cogan DG, Barrows LJ. Platybasia and Arnold Chiari malformation. Arch Ophthalmol 1954;52:13–29.
28. Cogan DG. Downbeat nystagmus. Arch Ophthalmol 1968;80:757–768.
29. Collier M. Hemiatrophic faciale progressive avec megalocornea, micropapille et dysrophie naugeuse centrale du la cornea. Acta Ophthalmol 1971;49:946.
30. Collins WF, et al. Neurologic surgery. In: SI S (ed) Principles of surgery. New York: McGraw-Hill, 1984:1819–1820.

31. Corsello G, Carcione A, Castro L, Giuffre L. Cervico-oculo-acusticus (Wildervanck's) syndrome: a clinical variant of Klippel–Feil sequence? Klin Padiatr 1990;202:176–179.
32. Dolan KB. Cervicobasilar relationships. Radiol Clin North Am 1977; 15:155–166.
33. Duthie RB, Hoagland FT. Manifestations of musculoskeletal disorders. In: SI S (ed) Principles of surgery. New York: McGraw-Hill, 1984.
34. Eulenburg A. Lehrbuch der functionellen Nervenkrankheiten. Berlin: S. Karger, 1871.
35. Everberg G, Ratjen E, Sorenson H. Wildervanck's syndrome. Klippel–Feil's syndrome associated with deafness and retraction of the eyeball. Br J Radiol 1963;36:562–567.
36. Farmer SF, Ingram DA, Stephens JA. Mirror movements studies in a patient with Klippel–Feil syndrome. J Physiol 1990;428:467–484.
37. Ford JG, Busbee B, Reed JW, Yu D. Hemifacial atrophy and primary corneal endothelial failure. Arch Ophthalmol 1998;116: 1246–1248.
38. France TD. Strabismus in hydrocephalus. Am Orthopt J 1975;25: 101–105.
39. France TD. The association of A-pattern strabismus with hydrocephalus. In: Moore SMJ, Stockbridge L (eds) Orthoptics past, present and future. 1976.
40. Franceschetti A, Koenig H. L'importance du facteur hegeredodegeneratif dans l'hemiatrophie faciale progressive (Romberg): etude des complications oculaires dans ce syndrome. J Genet Hum 1952;1: 27–64.
41. Friel JP. Dorland's illustrated medical dictionary, 25 edn. Philadelphia: Saunders, 1974.
42. Galanopoulas A, McNab AA. Hemifacial atrophy: an unusual case of upper eyelid retraction. Ophthalmic Plast Reconstr Surg 1995;11: 278–280.
43. Gardner WJ. The dysraphic states from syringomyelia to anencephaly. Amsterdam: Excerpta Medica, 1973.
44. Gaston H. Does the spina bifida child need an ophthalmologist? Z Kinderchir 1985;40:46–50.
45. Gilmour JR. The essential identity of the Klippel–Feil syndrome and iniencephaly. J Pathol Bacteriol 1941;53:117–131.
46. Goldberg MF. Waardenberg's syndrome with fundus and other anomalies. Arch Ophthalmol 1966;76:797–810.
47. Goldhammer Y, Kronenberg J, Tadmor R, et al. Progressive hemifacial atrophy (Parry–Romberg's disease), principally involving bone. J Laryngol Otol 1981;95:643–647.
48. Gorlin RJ, Pindborg JJ. Syndromes of the head and neck. New York: McGraw-Hill, 1976.
49. Gorlin RJ, Pindborg JJ, Cohen MM. Hemifacial atrophy. Syndromes of the head and neck. New York: McGraw-Hill, 1976.

50. Gosian AK, McCarthy JG, Pinto RS. Cervicovertebral anomalies and basilar impression in Goldenhar syndrome. Plast Reconstr Surg 1994;93:498–506.
51. Gumerlock MK, Belshe BD, Madsen R, Watts C. Cervical neurenteric fistula causing recurrent meningitis in Klippel–Feil sequence: case report and literature review. Pediatr Infect Dis J 1991;10:532–535.
52. Gunderson CG, Geenspan RH, Glaser GH, Lubs HA. The Klippel–Feil syndrome: genetic and clinical reevaluation of cervical fusion. Medicine (Baltim) 1967;46:491.
53. Gupte G, Mahajan P, Shreenivas VK, Kher A, Bharucha B. Wildervanck syndrome (cervico-oculo-acoustic syndrome). J Postgrad Med 1992;38:181–182.
54. Gustafson WA, Oldberg E. Neurologic significance of platybasia. Arch Neurol Psychiatry 1940;44:1184–1198.
55. Hacryakupoglu G, Pelit AA, Altunbasak S, Soyupak S, Ozer C. Crocodile tears and Dandy–Walker syndrome in cervico-oculo-acoustic syndrome. J Pediatr Ophthalmol Strabismus 1999;36:301–303.
56. Haddow JE, Macri JN. Prenatal screening for neural tube defects. JAMA 1979;242:515–516.
57. Hakin KN, Yokoyama C, Wright JE. Hemifacial atrophy: an unusual cause of enophthalmos. Br J Ophthalmol 1990;74:496–497.
58. Hamed LM, Fang EN, Fanous MM, et al. The prevalence of neurologic dysfunction in children with strabismus who have superior oblique overaction. Ophthalmology 1993;100:1483–1487.
59. Hensinger RN, Lang JE, Macewan GD. Klippel–Feil syndrome. A constellation of associated anomalies. J Bone Joint Surg 1974;56:1246.
60. Hoang-Xuan T, Foster CS, Jakobiec FA, et al. Romberg's progressive hemifacial atrophy: an association with scleral melting. Cornea 1991;10:361–366.
61. Hurwitz LJ, Shepard WH. Basilar impression and disordered metabolism of bone. Brain 1966;89:223–240.
62. Huttenlocher PR. The nervous system. Nelson's textbook of pediatrics, 13 edn, vol 23. 1987:1357–1358.
63. Jagjit SC, et al. Craniovertebral anomalies: a study of 82 cases. Br J Neurosurg 1988;2:455–464.
64. Janeway R, Toole JF, Leinbach LB, Miller HS. Vertebral artery obstruction with basilar impression. Arch Neurol 1966;15:211.
65. Johnson RV, Kennedy WR. Progressive facial hemiatrophy (Parry–Romberg syndrome): Contralateral extraocular muscle impairment. Am J Ophthalmol 1969;67:561–564.
66. Kaney PM, Getch CC, Jallo J, Faerber EN. Cerebral syrinx with Chiari I malformation. Pediatr Neurosurg 1994;20:214–216.
67. Kirkhan TH. Cervico-oculo-acousticus syndrome with pseudopapilledema. Arch Dis Child 1969;44:504–508.
68. Klippel M, Feil A. Un cas d'absence des vertebres cervicales. Nouv Iconogr Salpet 1912;25:223.

69. La Hey E, Seerp Baarsma G. Fuchs' heterochromic cyclitis and retinal vascular abnormalities in progressive hemifacial atrophy. Eye 1993;7: 426–428.
70. Leigh RJ, Zee DS. The neurology of eye movements. Philadelphia: Davis, 1983.
71. Lennerstrand G, Gallo JE. Neuro-ophthalmological evaluation of patients with myelomeningocele and Chiari malformations. Dev Med Child Neurol 1990;32:415–422.
72. Lennerstrand G, Gallo JE, Samuelsson L. Neuro-ophthalmological findings in relation to CNS lesions in patients with myelomeningocele. Dev Med Child Neurol 1990;32:423–431.
73. Leroy EC. Scleroderma (systemic sclerosis). In: Kelley WN (ed) Textbook of rheumatology. Philadelphia: Saunders, 1985.
74. Lewis MA, Goldstein S, Baker RS. MRImaging of the posterior fossa in ocular motility disorders-four case studies. J Clin Neuroophthalmol 1987;7:235–240.
75. Lewis AR, Kline LB, Sharpe JA. Acquired esotropia due to Arnold–Chiari I malformation. J Neuroophthalmol 1996;16:49–54.
76. Lucchese NJ, Goldberg MF. Iris and fundus pigmentary changes in tuberous sclerosis. J Pediatr Ophthalmol Strabismus 1981;18:45–46.
77. Maloley A, Weber S, Smith DR. A and V patterns of strabismus in meningomyelocele. Am Orthopt J 1977;27:115–118.
78. McLay K, Maran AGD. Deafness and the Klippel–Feil syndrome. J Laryngol 1969;83:175–184.
79. McLone DG, Knepper PA. The cause of Chiari II malformation: a unified theory. Pediatr Neurosci 1989;15:1–12.
80. Mendel. Uber hemiatrophia facialis. Dtsch Med Wochenschr 1888; 14:321.
81. Merritt HH. A textbook of neurology. Philadelphia: Lea & Febiger, 1979.
82. Miedziak AL, Stefanyszyn M, Flanagan J, Eagle RJ. Parry–Romberg syndrome associated with intracranial vascular malformations. Arch Ophthalmol 1992;116:1235–1237.
83. Mikulis DJ, Diaz O, Egglin TK, Sanchez R. Variance of the position of the cerebellar tonsils with age: preliminary report. Radiology 1992;183:725–728.
84. Miller MT, Sloane H, Goldberg MF, et al. Progressive hemifacial atrophy (Parry–Romberg disease). J Pediatr Ophthalmol Strabismus 1987;24:27–36.
85. Miller MT, Spencer MA. Progressive hemifacial atrophy: a natural history study. Trans Am Ophthalmol Soc 1995;93:203–217.
86. Miller MT, Stromland K. Ocular motility in thalidomide embryopathy. J Pediatr Ophthalmol Strabismus 1991;1:47–54.
87. Miller NR. Walsh and Hoyt's clinical neuro-ophthalmology, vol 2. Waverly Press, 1985.
88. Milunsky A, Jick H, Jick S, et al. Multivitamin folic acid supplementation in early pregnancy reduces the prevalence of neural tube defects. JAMA 1989;262:2847–2852.

89. Moss ML, Crikelair GF. Progressive facial hemiatrophy following cervical sympathectomy in the rat. Arch Oral Biol 1959;1:254–258.
90. Mossman SS, Bronstein AM, Gresty MA, et al. Convergence nystagmus associated with Arnold–Chiari malformation. Arch Neurol 1990;47:357–359.
91. Muchnick RS, Aston SJ, Rees TD. Ocular manifestations and treatment of hemifacial atrophy. Am J Ophthalmol 1979;88:889–897.
92. Nagib MG, Maxwell RE, Chou SN. Klippel–Feil syndrome in children: clinical features and management. Child's Nerv Syst 1985;1: 255–263.
93. Naidich TP. Cranial signs of the Chiari II malformation. J Neuroradiol 1981;8:207–227.
94. Naidich TP, McLone DG, Fulling KH. The Chiari II malformation. Part IV. The hindbrain deformity. Neuroradiology 1983;25:179–197.
95. Naidich TP, Pudlowski RM, Naidich JB. Computed tomographic signs of the Chiari II malformation. Part II. Midbrain and cerebellum. Radiology 1980;134:391–398.
96. Nishimura H, Okamoto N. Congenital malformations of the brain and skull, part I. In: Vinken PJ, Bruyn GW (eds) Iniencephaly: handbook of clinical neurology, vol 30. Amsterdam: North-Holland, 1977.
97. Nishizak T, et al. Bilateral internuclear ophthalmoplegia due to hydrocephalus: a case report. Neurosurgery 1985;17:822–825.
98. Noetzel MJ. Myelomeningocele: current concepts of management. Clin Perinatol 1989;16:311–329.
99. Ofodile FA, Woods JE. Progressive hemifacial atrophy. Surg Clin North Am 1977;57:621–627.
100. Ong K, Billson FA, Pathirana DSJ, Clifton-Bligh P. A case of progressive hemifacial atrophy with uveitis and retinal vasculitis. Aust NZ J Ophthalmol 1991;19:295–298.
101. Oppenheim H. Lehrbuch der nervenkrankheiten. Berlin: Karger, 1923.
102. Parry CH, Wartenberg R. Collection from unpublished medical writing of the late Calet Hillier. London: Underwood, 1825.
103. Peele TL. The neuroanatomic basis for clinical neurology. New York: McGraw-Hill, 1977.
104. Pensler JM, Murphy GF, Mulliken JB. Clinical and ultrastructural studies of Romberg's hemifacial atrophy. Plast Reconstr Surg 1990; 85:669–674.
105. Pfeiffer RA, Rott HD, Angerstein W. An autosomal dominant facioaudio symphalangism syndrome with Klippel–Feil anomaly: a new variant of multiple synostoses. Genet Counsel 1990;38:133–140.
106. Pieh C, Gottlob I. Arnold-Chiari malformation and nystagmus of skew. Neurol Neurosurg Psychiatry 2000;69:124–126.
107. Rabinowicz IM. Visual function in children with hydrocephalus. Trans Ophthalmol Soc UK 1974;94:353–365.
108. Rees TD. Facial atrophy. Clin Plast Surg 1976;3:637.
109. Rhaney K, Barclay GPT. Alimentary and spinal abnormalities. J Pathol Bacteriol 1959;77:457.

110. Rogers BO. Progressive facial hemiatrophy (Romberg's disease): a review of 772 cases. In: Transactions of third international congress of plastic surgery. International Congress Series No. 66. Washington: Excerpta Medica Foundation, 1963.
111. Romberg HM. Cited in Wartenberg R. Trophoneurosen. Klinische Ergenbnisse. Berlin: Forstner, 1846.
112. Rothstein TB, Romano P, Shoch D. Meningomyelocele-associated ocular abnormalities. Trans Am Ophthalmol Soc 1973;LXXI:287–293.
113. Rothstein TB, Romano PE, Shoch D. Meningomyelocele. Am J Ophthalmol 1974;77:690–693.
114. Russel D, Donald C. The mechanism of internal hydrocephalus in spina bifida. Brain 1935;58:203–215.
115. Samuelsson LG. Meningomyelocele: a neuro-orthopedic and radiologic assessment. Dissertation. Stockholm: Karolinska Institutet, 1988.
116. Schimmenti LI, et al. Homonucleotide expansion and contraction mutations of PAX2 and inclusion of Chiari I malformation as part of renal-coloboma syndrome. Hum Mutat 1999;14:369–376.
117. Segal P, Jablonska S, Mrzyglod S. Ocular changes in linear scleroderma. Am J Ophthalmol 1961;51:807–813.
118. Smith DW. Recognizable patterns of human malformation. Philadelphia: Saunders, 1982.
119. Smith ED. The urinary trait in meningomyeloceles. In: Ed S (ed) Spina bifida and the total care of spinal myelomeningocele. Springfield: Thomas, 1965.
120. Stein SC, Schut L. Hydrocephalus in myelomeningocele. Child's Brain 1979;4:413–419.
121. Stern HS, Elliot LF, Beegle PH. Progressive hemifacial atrophy associated with lyme disease. Plast Reconstr Surg 1992;90:479–483.
122. Stovner LJ, Kruszewski P, Shen J. Sinus arrhythmia and pupil size in Chiari I malformation: evidence of autonomic dysfunction. Funct Neurol 1993;8:251–257.
123. Straudenmaier C, Buncic JR. Periodic alternating gaze deviation with dissociated secondary face turn. Arch Ophthalmol 1983;101:202–205.
124. Sugar HS, Banks TL. Fuchs' heterochromic cyclitis, associated with facial hemiatrophy (scleroderma en coup de sabre). Am J Ophthalmol 1964;57:627–632.
125. Taylor AR, Chakravorty BC. Clinical syndromes associated with basilar impression. Arch Neurol 1964;10:475.
126. Tominaga T, Koshu K, Ogawa A, Yoshimoto T. Transoral decompression evaluated by Cine-Mode magnetic resonance imaging: a case of basilar impression accompanied by Chiari malformation. Neurosurgery 1991;28:883–885.
127. Walsh FB, Hoyt WF. Clin Neuroophthalmol 1969;1:707–724.
128. Wartenberg R. Progressive facial hemiatrophy. Arch Neurol Psychiatry 1945;54:75–96.

129. Weeks CL, Hamed LM. Treatment of acute comitant esotropia in Chiari I malformation. Ophthalmology 1999;106:2368–2371.
130. Weintraub MI. Ophthalmoplegia and Arnold Chiari malformation without hydrocephalus. Dev Med Child Neurol 1990;32:929.
131. Wildervanck LS. The cervico-acusticus syndrome. In: Vinken PJBG, Myrianthopoulos NC (eds) Handbook of clinical neurology, vol 32. Amsterdam: North-Holland, 1978.
132. Widgerow AD. Klippel-Feil anomaly, cleft palate, and bifid tongue. Ann Plast Surg 1990;25:216.
133. Wolpert SM, Anderson M, Scott RM, et al. The Chiari II malformation: MR imaging evaluation. AJNR 1987;8:783–791.
134. Wong VCN, Fung CF. Basilar impression in a child with hypochondroplasia. Pediatr Neurol 1991;7:62–64.
135. Woody RC, Reynolds JD. Association of bilateral internuclear ophthalmoplegia and meningomyelocele and Arnold Chiari malformation type II. J Clin Neuroophthalmol 1985;5:124–126.
136. Yamanouchi H, Iwasaki Y, Sugai K, Mukono K. Duane retraction syndrome associated with Chiari I malformation. Pediatr Neurol 1993;9:327–329.
137. Yeow YK, Tjia TL. The localizing value of down beating nystagmus. Singapore Med J 1989;30:273–276.
138. Zafarulla MYM. Progressive hemifacial atrophy: a case report. Br J Ophthalmol 1985;69:545–547.
139. Zimmerman CF, Roach ES, Troost BT. See-saw nystagmus associated with Chiari malformation. Arch Neurol 1986;43:299–300.

12

Management of Common Pediatric Neuro-Ophthalmology Problems

James W. McManaway III and Dean J. Bonsall

The purpose of this chapter is to provide guidelines for the management of pediatric neuro-ophthalmic problems commonly seen in a general or pediatric ophthalmology practice. The most common neuro-ophthalmic entities encountered include functional visual loss, headaches, the "swollen" disc, and anisocoria. Neonatal blindness, although less common, is also discussed. Evaluation of nystagmus, paralytic strabismus, and nuclear or supranuclear eye movement disorders is discussed in other chapters. With this information, the ophthalmologist should be able to separate real from functional problems and benign from malignant disorders. This chapter is designed to be self-contained, although additional information is available in other chapters in this volume.

FUNCTIONAL VISUAL LOSS

Functional (psychogenic) visual loss is a fairly common problem in a pediatric ophthalmology practice. Patients need to be divided into binocular blindness, monocular blindness, binocularly decreased visual acuity, and monocularly decreased visual acuity because the testing strategies differ for each group. Monocular functional visual loss is more common, and must be distinguished from amblyopia; some patients have a component of amblyopia in addition to their functional component. Bilateral functional visual loss is less common. Children with functional visual loss nearly always have some sort of secondary gain; this may be something as simple as a need for attention or a desire for glasses or may be as complicated as a presenting symptom of child abuse or of a psychiatric disorder.

Testing Methods

There are many ways to assess the visual acuity of a patient with suspected functional visual loss.[9,15] It is not necessary that all these tests be utilized; rather, learn a few tests and learn to use them well. The testing methods can be classified into four different categories: (1) observation, (2) indirect measurement of visual acuity, (3) direct measurement of visual acuity, and (4) supportive findings. Following the discussion of the testing techniques, the best tests for a given patient presentation are recommended.

Observation of the patient with binocular blindness or decreased visual acuity can be very helpful. A truly blind person will bump gently into things; a patient with functional visual loss will either avoid the object or strike the object in an exaggerated manner. The patient's attitude toward his blindness may also support the diagnosis of functional visual loss.

Pupillary function testing is one of the most useful indirect measures of visual function. Intact, direct, and consensual pupil responses exclude severe and moderate unilateral or asymmetrical visual pathway disorders anterior to the chiasm. Conversely, an afferent pupillary defect clearly supports the claim of a patient with monocular blindness or decreased acuity.

An optokinetic nystagmus (OKN) drum can be utilized to demonstrate visual function. However, some patients can suppress the OKN reflex. A better test utilizes a large mirror placed very close in front of the patient's face. The mirror is then slowly rocked back and forth (Fig. 12-1). This visual stimulus is almost impossible to suppress if the mirror is large enough to prevent the patient from looking around it. The examiner should observe the patient's eye following the movement of the mirror from above. If the patient can see, the eyes will move in the same direction as the rocking mirror. A ridiculous facial expression or humorous cartoon may also trick the child into making some sort of response.

The 4-prism diopter base-out prism test is very useful for the patient complaining of monocular blindness. In this test, the prism is placed base out in front of the suspect eye. The normal response is a rapid saccade of both eyes to the side opposite the

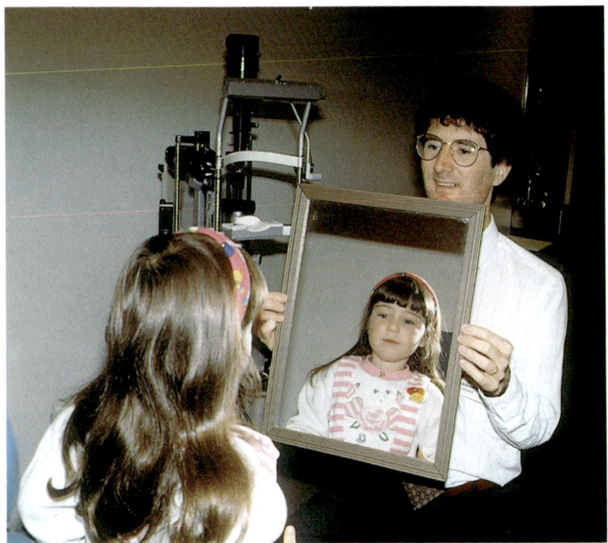

FIGURE 12-1. Use of the rocking mirror test in a patient with suspected functional visual loss.

prism, followed by a convergence movement of the uncovered eye 1 to 2 s later. The prism is then placed in front of the good eye as a control. Observing a saccade with the prism in front of the suspect eye rules out acuity less than light perception on that side. Absence of a response suggests but does not prove an organic problem.

A normal response to the Worth four-dot test rules out monocular blindness. Even more useful is stereo-acuity testing. The Wirt circles are large enough to be readable by patients complaining of monocular or binocular decreased visual acuity. The patients do not realize that a stereo-acuity of 40 arc seconds correlates with 20/20 visual acuity in both eyes.[23]

The last indirect measure of visual acuity is visual evoked response (VER) testing. A recordable response to a flash stimulus rules out absolute blindness of the suspect eye. A correlation also exists between check size and level of visual acuity. Unfortunately, some patients can consciously suppress the response to pattern reversal stimulation. An electroretinogram should be performed in patients with suspected functional visual loss before making that diagnosis if they cannot be tricked into reading normally or at least substantially better than initially claimed.

After using indirect measures to assess the patient's acuity, then proceed with direct measures. Children desiring a pair of glasses will frequently read the 20/20 line through a plano lens. I frequently perform a quick, noncycloplegic retinoscopy to look for significant myopia, astigmatism, or anisometropia. Having ruled these things out, I put up the plano lens with the comment that "this is the lens that is measured to be just right for your eye." More stubborn children can sometimes be cajoled with a combination of +0.25 sphere and −0.25 sphere lenses back to back in a trial frame. The child is told that this is a "telescope" to improve their vision. Keep in mind that the child's visual acuity may significantly improve once his parents leave the room.

When testing acuity of a child with suspected functional acuity loss, it is best to start with the 20/10 or 20/15 line and express disbelief that such "large" letters cannot be seen. Slowly move through six 20/20 lines with the instructions that each line is twice as large as the one before. With patience and persistence, the child will frequently read 20/20 to 20/30. Testing the consistency of the visual acuity either with different type targets or by maintaining a constant visual angle at different testing distances is very useful and often shows significant inconsistencies in functional patients.

Fogging techniques can be used to blur the vision of the good eye of patients who present with monocularly decreased visual acuity. Three major methods are used. The first method involves secretly slipping a high plus lens in front of the good eye while rapidly performing a subjective distance refraction of the suspect eye. The patient can be confused by all the activity going on around the suspect eye and not realize that the high plus lens has made the good eye quite myopic. The best acuity obtained by the suspect eye is recorded. As a check, the patient should have the suspect eye occluded and then should have the acuity of the previously fogged good eye recorded.

A second *fogging* method involves placing two high-power cylinders of equal and opposite sign in a trial frame in front of the good eye. So long as the cylinder axes are parallel, the net lens power lens is plano. As the axes are secretly made nonparallel, a large cylinder power results, fogging the good eye. As the patient is reading the acuity chart, the examiner reaches up and adjusts the lens axis dial as if he is making a minor adjustment, fogging the good eye. Any subsequent lines read are performed with the suspect eye.

A third *fogging* method involves instilling a drop of 1% Tropicamide solution into the good eye during applanation tonometry. The patient's near visual acuity in both eyes needs to be recorded beforehand. After 30 min, check the patient's near visual acuity with both eyes open. The smallest line read is recorded as the visual acuity of the suspect eye at near. For conformation, check the patient's acuity at near with the eye that received Tropicamide. The suspect eye reads any lines smaller than that read by the cyclopleged eye.

Two final, direct measures of visual acuity utilize different visual inputs to each eye. The duochrome test utilizes a red-green projector slide with a patient wearing a pair of red-green glasses. The eye behind the red eyeglass lens can see letters on the red and the green side of the chart. The letters on the green side will appear dimmer to the eye behind the red glass. The eye behind the green eyeglass lens can only read the green side of the chart. A useful mnemonic is to remember to place the red lens over the "injured" (red) eye. If the patient can read the entire line of letters, the suspect eye has that level of visual acuity. The vectograph chart utilizes a special slide to project a line of letters; some letters are 45° right polarized, some are 45° left polarized, and some are unpolarized. With the child wearing special polarized glasses, some letters are visible only to the right eye, some only to the left eye, and some to both eyes. If the child reads the entire line of letters, the suspect eye has that level of visual acuity.

Patients with functional visual loss may also give functional responses to other types of tests. The most common example is the *tubular visual field* that can be documented by tangent screen visual field testing at 1- and 2-m testing distances. Functional patients may also claim that they are unable to read the numbers on the color vision testing plates. The numbers displayed are so large that the patient's acuity must be worse than approximately finger counting at 1 foot to have difficulty reading them.

Patient Evaluation

Important historical points include how the visual loss was discovered, the time course and duration of the visual loss, previous evaluations of the visual loss, results of eye examinations in the past, any history of recent or remote ocular trauma, and any significant past ocular and past medical history. While obtaining the history, observe the affect of the child and their interaction with the parents. Inquiries into the social situation can be obtained after the parents and the child are separated.

The patient with claimed binocular blindness can best be assessed using pupillary function testing and the rocking mirror. The OKN drum is less effective as it may be suppressed. Observation of how the patient navigates in his environment is also very useful. The patient presenting with monocular blindness should be tested using the same techniques with the good eye patched.

Patients with binocularly decreased visual acuity seem to be the most difficult because there is no good eye to fog or to isolate using the vectograph or duochrome tests. Stereo acuity testing is helpful in this situation. Persistent visual acuity testing starting at the bottom of the chart and working upward with use of plano lenses will often give results.

Patients with monocularly decreased visual acuity are best evaluated using the vectograph chart, the duochrome test, or the crossed cylinder fogging technique. Some intelligent patients can be observed intermittently closing the suspect eye to prevent the examiner from secretly fogging the good eye. Computerized video acuity testers utilizing high-speed liquid crystal shutter glasses are often helpful in this particular situation. As mentioned, any patient thought to have functional visual loss who cannot be tricked into reading normally should have a normal electroretinogram before making the diagnosis of functional visual loss.

Differential Diagnosis

The major factor to be ruled out in the pediatric age group is amblyopia. The ocular examination must show that strabismus, media opacities, bilateral ametropia, or anisometropia are not present. Keratoconus should be diagnosed by retinoscopy, although keratometry is also helpful. Retinal and macular dystrophies also may present with bilateral acuity loss, or sometimes as monocular acuity loss if the process is asymmetrical. A normal electroretinogram with normal scotopic, photopic, and flicker waveforms rules out these possibilities.

Treatment

Once normal visual acuity in the suspect eye(s) has been documented, one must decide what to tell the patient and what to tell the parents. If the patient wanted a pair of glasses, reassurance that the eyes are normal and that she sees excellently without glasses is all that is necessary. Patients with less identifiable secondary gain should also be reassured. A 1-month trial of multiple vitamins often will allow the patient to give up her functional behavior. Patients with claimed significant visual acuity loss, who do not improve, can frequently be cured with retinal rest.[15] This test involves hospitalization with bilateral eye patching. No radio or television is allowed, and visitors are kept to an absolute minimum. The patient's visual acuity nearly always becomes normal within 2 to 3 days. Psychiatric consultation is frequently helpful in this situation as well.

HEADACHES

Children are frequently referred to ophthalmologists for evaluation of headaches despite the admonition that the eyes are infrequently the cause of headaches. It seems that some pediatricians refer children with headaches to the ophthalmologist to make sure that the eyes are not the cause of headaches before proceeding with a more detailed evaluation. Possible ocular causes of headaches include significant hyperopia, anisometropia, a poorly controlled heterophoria or intermittent heterotropia, convergence insufficiency, and accommodative insufficiency. Ocular disease including glaucoma, uveitis, and corneal disease may give rise to eye pain that may be described as a headache. If ocular examination can rule out these conditions, the search should lead elsewhere.

The difference between a successful and an unsuccessful headache evaluation depends on the history. The headaches should be described as to frequency, duration, severity, location at onset, exacerbating or precipitating factors, and associated signs and symptoms. The patient's past medical history is important, as is a family history of migraine headaches. Using the history, one should attempt to classify the headaches as (1) an acute single episode, (2) acute recurrent episodes, (3) subacute, and (4) chronic.[20]

Etiologies

Acute Severe Headache

The child presenting with the first episode of an acute severe headache poses somewhat of a diagnostic dilemma. These patients usually present to the Emergency Room and do not initially see the ophthalmologist. Possible causes include (1) intracranial processes such as meningitis, encephalitis, or bleeding from an arterovenous malformation; (2) extracranial causes such as sinusitis or head trauma; (3) systemic diseases such as vasculitis or hypertension; (4) environmental causes such as solvent or lead exposure or hypoxia; (5) assorted causes including hypoglycemia or ingested medications; and (6) the first episode of a migraine headache. Evaluation, generally done in the Emergency Room, includes an adequate history, appropriate laboratory studies, and probably CT scan followed by lumbar puncture. Although headaches are rarely caused by hypertension, children with hypertension frequently complain of headaches that are made worse by stooping or lifting heavy objects.

Migraine Headaches

Children presenting with acute recurrent episodic headaches generally have migraine. One should keep in mind that migraine describes a spectrum of disease that includes visual auras, anorexia, nausea, vomiting, and sensitivity to noise and light. Headache is the most commonly considered symptom, but is not necessary to make the diagnosis of migraine.[28]

Migraine can be classified as common, classic, and complicated.[34] Common migraine begins with a poorly defined prodrome of psychic or gastrointestinal disturbances, which precede the attack from hours to days; there are no premonitory visual symptoms. The headache usually begins unilaterally but often spreads to involve the entire head. Nearly all patients have nausea; vomiting occurs frequently, and may signal the end or exacerbation of the attack. The duration of the headache is variable and ranges from several hours to several days. About 80% of patients have a family history of common migraine.[84]

Classic migraine describes a well-defined syndrome, which begins with a visual aura or other sensory disturbance and is followed by an intense, pounding headache. The episodes of classic migraine are shorter than those of common migraine and tend to last 2 to 4 h although occasionally longer. The visual aura of classic migraine has been well described.[6,27,28] It consists of scintillating lights surrounding a scotoma, which begins near central fixation and then gradually expands to move into the peripheral visual field and away from central fixation. The scintillations surrounding the scotoma often form angled lines that mimic the appearance of fortifications around a medieval town; hence the name *fortification scotoma*.[21] The pathophysiology of the migraine scotoma is thought to be a wave of activation, which is generated in the occipital cortex after the initial event of ischemia secondary to vasoconstriction. This wave of activation starts at the macular occipital pole and then gradually spreads anteriorly to the cortex that represents the peripheral visual field. Children may find it difficult to describe their visual symptoms, but often do have visual impairment, or binocular scotomas. Children may also have visual field defects, distortions of vision such as micropsia, an impairment of time sense, or even hallucinations.[12]

Complicated migraine describes migraine with associated neurological phenomena that are generally transient but can occasionally become permanent. This group includes cerebral migraine, ophthalmoplegic migraine, retinal migraine, and migraine equivalents. Patients with cerebral migraine may have hemiplegia, hemianopia, sensory defects, and even aphasia. Ophthalmoplegic migraine is particularly common in children and usually starts before the age of 10 years. The oculomotor nerve is most commonly involved, followed by the abducens and trochlear nerves. The term retinal migraine should probably be expanded into anterior visual pathway migraine to describe a monocular visual disturbance accompanying an episode of migraine or in a patient with a strong history of migraine. The key distinction in this case is the monocular nature of the visual disturbance. Anterior visual pathway migraines do not have a preceding fortification spectrum, are not associated with headache, and rarely last more than 10 min. *Migraine equivalent* describes episodic conditions that are believed to be migrainous in origin but do not have the typical headache history. The most common example in children is abdominal migraine, which consists of episodic nausea, vomiting, or abdominal pain.

Other Causes of Recurrent Headaches

Recurrent headaches, very similar to migraine, can be associated with preceding head trauma. The head trauma does not have to be severe or associated with loss of consciousness. Patients with a seizure disorder may complain of postictal headaches; this usually does not cause diagnostic confusion. Additional causes of recurrent headaches include episodes of elevated intracranial pressure from intermittent hydrocephalus or small recurrent subarachnoid hemorrhages from aneurysms or arteriovenous malformations.

Subacute Headaches

Subacute headaches are headaches of moderate intensity that have been present for days to weeks. The head pain is present nearly all the time, although exacerbations of severe, intense pain are frequent. Because most of these headaches are associated with elevated intracranial pressure, the headaches are often progressive. It is very important to recognize the patient with the subacute headache, as they usually have a life-threatening or vision-threatening process as the cause of the headaches. The two basic causes are (1) expanding intracranial tumor or subdural hematoma and (2) pseudotumor cerebri.

Fifty percent of patients with an intracranial mass lesion consider headache to be their chief complaint.[26] The headache results from traction on pain-sensitive structures within the skull. The headache has a nonthrobbing quality and is worsened by physical activity. Like migraine headaches, the headache often has associated nausea and vomiting. The sudden exacerbations are an important finding. More than half of children with brain tumors are awakened from sleep by their headache. The intracranial mass lesion produces papilledema; focal neurological signs are frequently present. Thus, any child with papilledema or focal neurological sings must have a CT or MRI scan of the head immediately.

Pseudotumor cerebri has an ophthalmoscopic picture nearly identical to the patient with an intracranial mass lesion, the only difference being the lack of focal neurological signs. Four criteria are required to make the diagnosis of pseudotumor cerebri: (1) increased intracranial pressure, (2) normal to small-sized ventricles on CT scan, (3) normal cerebrospinal fluid composition, and (4) optic disc edema. Patients may also have a sixth nerve palsy or visual field changes, but with rare exceptions no other focal neurological deficits are present. Pseudotumor cerebri is not rare in childhood and can be associated with an extensive list of conditions including steroid withdrawal, tetracycline ingestion, vitamin A intoxication, dural sinus thrombosis, polycythemia, and systemic lupus erythematosus.[3] Unfortunately, many cases occur without an obvious precipitating cause. The headaches are typically moderate to severe in intensity, nonpounding, and may be localized to the frontal area. The children frequently have visual obscurations from the associated disc edema; this often occurs when the child stands up. The child may describe these obscurations as transient blurring of vision rather than visual loss.

All patients with a clear history of subacute headaches need to have a cranial neuroimaging to rule out an intracranial mass lesion. If the scan is normal, a lumbar puncture should be performed to measure the cerebrospinal fluid composition and the intracranial pressure. Patients with an intracranial mass lesion need appropriate neurosurgical intervention. Patients with pseudotumor cerebri need to have any possible precipitating factor removed. The elevated intracranial pressure can be treated with Diamox or Lasix. Steroids can be used in the acute setting, although chronic long-term steroid use often worsens the situation due to the associated weight gain. Repeated lumbar punctures are effective, but have some risk and should be reserved for patients unresponsive to medical therapy. If progressive vision or visual field loss is occurring, surgical intervention is warranted. Ventriculoperitoneal shunting and optic nerve sheath decompression are the methods most commonly used.[14]

Chronic Nonprogressive Headaches

Patients with chronic nonprogressive headaches fortunately do not have life- or vision-threatening conditions. A long list of potential causes exists. The most important ones are (1) the tension or stress headache, (2) eyestrain, and (3) functional complaints, psychiatric disorders, and school avoidance.

Tension or stress headaches are classically thought to be the result of sustained contraction of muscles in the scalp and neck, which leads to the typical complaints of "tightness" or "head in a vise." The head pain is dull, diffuse, and nonthrobbing. One may find tenderness in the scalp or neck muscles. Tension is an important precipitating factor. Unfortunately, the distinction between migraine headaches and tension headaches may be somewhat blurry, and patients with tension headache symptoms may respond to therapy for migraine headaches. It is often difficult to control external stressors, although modifying the patients' response to those stressors often improves the headache symptoms.

Patients with eyestrain may complain of headache. The ophthalmologist can best benefit the patient by carefully ruling out the few ocular disorders that cause eyestrain; these include (1) significant hyperopia, (2) anisometropia, (3) heterophoria or intermittent heterotropia, (4) convergence insufficiency, and (5) accommodative insufficiency. Hyperopia and anisometropia can be reliably excluded by an accurate cycloplegic refraction. Heterophorias or intermittent heterotropias can be ruled out using alternate prism cover testing on an accommodative target at distance and near. Convergence insufficiency and accommodative insufficiency seem to be the most commonly overlooked factors. Patients should have their fusional convergence amplitudes measured at near using a 20/30 target. Normal patients should be able to overcome a minimum of 25 prism diopters base out before subjective diplopia or an objective exotropia is noted. Patients should also have their amplitudes of accommodation measured using a device such as the Royal Air Force near point rule. A 20/30 near target is utilized and the patient's subjective observation of visual blur is used as the endpoint. Because the subjective endpoint is rather soft, the test should be repeated using +3 sphere, plano, and −3 sphere lenses to check for consistency. Plano lenses frequently cause a significant improvement in the near point of accommodation in functional patients. One can consult Duane's table to determine the normal near point for a patient of a given age.

A very common cause of chronic, nonprogressive headaches in children is on a functional basis. Children may complain of headaches for various reasons including unhappiness with the teacher, unhappiness with the subject, or unhappiness with school altogether. Children with psychiatric or behavioral disturbances may complain of these headaches as well.

Patient Evaluation

As discussed previously, the history is the most important factor in the evaluation of a patient with headaches. At least 90% have normal neurological and ophthalmologic examination findings.

Once sufficient history is obtained to classify the symptoms into one of the four headache types, proceed with directed questioning appropriate to the causes within each group. For example, ask the parents of a child with subacute headaches if the headaches awaken the child at night, if projectile vomiting has been noted, and if any changes in balance or coordination have been observed.

A complete ophthalmologic and ocular motility examination should be performed. Particular attention should be paid to cycloplegic retinoscopy, ocular motility testing, measurement of fusional convergence amplitudes and near point of accommodation, and assessment of the optic nerve. If the child has normal strength, symmetrical deep tendon reflexes, and normal gait and balance, neurological consultation is probably not necessary. If there is any question regarding focal neurological designs, the patient should see a pediatric neurologist as soon as possible. Patients with subacute headaches, as well as the patient presenting with a first episode of an acute severe headache, should have cranial neuroimaging. If the scan does not show an intracranial mass lesion, lumbar puncture with cerebrospinal fluid analysis and measurement of intracranial pressure should be performed. Patients with a good history for migraine who have normal ocular and neurological examinations can be given the clinical diagnosis of migraine. Any atypical features warrant neuroimaging followed by a lumbar puncture. Patients with chronic, nonprogressive headaches do not require evaluation beyond that discussed.

Headache Treatment

The following discussion assumes that treatable causes of headaches such as pseudotumor cerebri have been ruled out. Patients with significant hyperopia or convergence insufficiency need appropriate eye care. Functional patients need reassurance and possibly psychiatric consultation.

Once the foregoing specific causes have been excluded, treatment has four phases: (1) reassurance, (2) exclusion of precipitating factors, (3) abortive treatment, and (4) preventive treatment. Many patients will have a significant improvement once they have been reassured that their headaches are not the sign of a brain tumor or other life-threatening problem. A common precipitating factor of headaches is stress. Unfortunately, stress is almost impossible to avoid in modern society.

Rather than avoiding the stress, the patient needs to learn to modify his response to it. Some patients may have their headaches triggered by a variety of foods including chocolate, red wine, caffeine, nitrates, and certain cheeses. Patients should initially exclude these foods from their diet. Once the headaches are controlled, they can restart these items one at a time to see if they exacerbate the headaches. Oral contraceptives may exacerbate headaches, and a trial off these medications is warranted.

If the patient's headaches are not frequent or incapacitating, treatment can be initiated when the first symptoms of headache appear. Patients should be instructed to lie down in a dark, quiet room and to take an appropriate dose of aspirin, acetaminophen, a nonsteroidal antiinflammatory agent, or Fiorinal. An antiemetic such as Tigan or Compazine is often helpful to keep the preceding medications in the stomach. Ergot preparations are poorly tolerated in children because these produce nausea.[34]

If the patient has frequent or incapacitating headaches or if abortive treatment is not satisfactory, then prophylactic treatment should be initiated in children 7 years of age and older. The three most commonly used medications are (1) Inderal, a beta-blocker, (2) Verapamil, a calcium channel blocker, and (3) Elavil, a tricyclic antidepressant. Inderal is started at 10 to 20 mg orally once daily, and is gradually increased to 40 to 80 mg/day. If a satisfactory response is not obtained in 6 weeks at the higher dose, discontinue the medication gradually over several weeks. Verapamil is used at 40 to 80 mg orally twice daily. Elavil is started at 10 to 20 mg orally at bedtime; the dose can be increased to 40 mg/day.

"SWOLLEN" OPTIC DISC

Pediatricians, pediatric neurologists, pediatric neurosurgeons, and ophthalmologists examine optic discs of children for various reasons including complaints of headache or history of ventriculoperitoneal shunt placement. Occasionally, the optic disc appears abnormal, and the patient is then referred to rule out optic disc edema or papilledema.

To start, some definitions are necessary. Optic disc edema and papilledema have essentially identical ophthalmoscopic features. The increased intracranial pressure transmitted to the optic nerves by the cerebrospinal fluid causes papilledema.

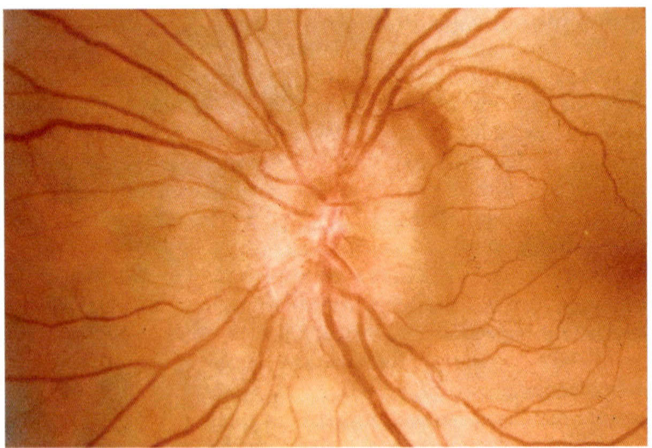

FIGURE 12-2. Papilledema demonstrating obscuration of the retinal vessels, disc hyperemia, hemorrhages, and exudates.

Optic disc edema can be caused by a variety of optic and systemic conditions including pseudotumor cerebri, hypertension, juvenile diabetes, uveitis, anemia, lymphoma, and papillitis.[11] Unilaterality is not particularly helpful, as localized processes can cause unilateral optic disc edema, and optic atrophy on the contralateral side can be associated with unilateral papilledema. The characteristic ophthalmoscopic features of papilledema and disc edema include opacification of the peripapillary nerve fiber layer and consequent haziness or obscuration of the retinal vessels at the disc margin, disc hyperemia, as well as exudates, splinter hemorrhages, and cotton wool spots (Fig. 12-2). One should carefully observe the retinal veins for spontaneous venous pulsations. If venous pulsations can be visualized, the cerebrospinal fluid pressure is typically less than 200 mm of water.[41]

Pseudopapilledema can be defined as any disc appearance that can be confused with papilledema. The distinction is obviously important because of the profound implications associated with papilledema. The most frequently encountered causes of pseudopapilledema include (1) hyperopia, (2) hyaloid remnants, (3) optic disc drusen, (4) congenital disc elevations without visible drusen, and (5) myelinated nerve fibers.[31]

Ophthalmoscopic Characteristics of Pseudopapilledema

In making the distinction between papilledema and pseudopapilledema, a critical evaluation of the optic disc appearance is necessary. Magnification and stereoscopic examination of the optic nerve utilizing the slit lamp with a 90 diopter lens should be routinely used. Using these aids, the ophthalmologist should be able to arrive at a definitive diagnosis in most patients.[31]

Optic Disc Elevation

Elevation of the optic disc is typically seen with pseudopapilledema. The most common cause of disc elevation is *optic disc drusen,* in which calcium accumulates at varying depths in the prelaminar disc tissue. The most superficial drusen appear as highly refractile yellowish-white masses (Fig. 12-3). Deeper drusen are not visible, although illuminating the optic disc with the slit beam through a 90 diopter lens may show a glowing appearance of the buried drusen. Drusen of the optic disc tend to become more visible with age. Other modalities such as CT scan, brain ultrasound, and fundus photography can aid in the diagnosis of drusen. Drusen appear calcified on CT scan and show autofluorescence when photographed with red-free light.

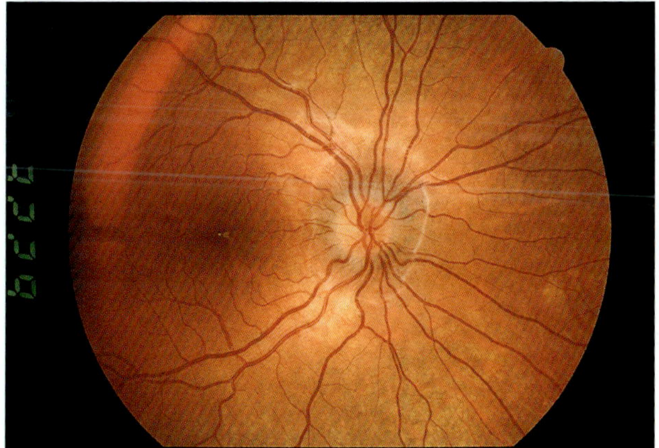

FIGURE 12-3. Optic disc drusen causing pseudopapilledema.

Blurred Disc Margins

The optic disc can have blurred margins from a variety of causes. Myelinated nerve fibers obscure the disc margins but should not pose a diagnostic dilemma. Myelinated nerve fiber layers can be a component of neurofibromatosis. Drusen may also give blurring of the disc margin. Drusen are more commonly found in the nasal disc tissue. A peripapillary halo of pigment epithelial loss and hyperplasia may be noted in association with buried drusen. In pseudopapilledema, the outline of subsurface retinal vessels is not obscured; additionally, one does not see wrinkling of the peripapillary internal limiting membrane around the disc (Paton's lines).

Optic Cup

The optic disc with pseudopapilledema has no central optic cup. The optic disc with papilledema still has a cup unless the papilledema is advanced and obvious. Because optic disc characteristics are often similar among family members, examining the patient's parents for anomalous discs provides useful evidence in favor of pseudopapilledema.

Venous Pulsations

Venous pulsations occur spontaneously in most normal eyes. Increased intracranial pressure causes congestion of the veins and loss of venous pulsation. The presence of venous pulsations indicates that the intracranial pressure is below 200 mm of water.[41] The absence of venous pulsations yields little information unless they have been previously documented to be present.

Vascular Abnormalities

Anomalies of disc vasculature are characteristic of pseudopapilledema. The vessels exit the disc centrally and show a pattern of anomalous branching or trifurcations of the arterioles or venules.

Hemorrhage

Although splinter hemorrhages in the nerve fiber layer are characteristic of papilledema, patients with pseudopapilledema may also rarely have nerve fiber layer hemorrhages as well as preretinal hemorrhages and subretinal hemorrhages. These hemorrhages may be caused by contact between blood vessels and the drusen. An infarct of the nerve fiber layer along with hemorrhages strongly suggests papilledema.

Patient Management

As discussed, differentiating papilledema from pseudopapilledema requires careful biomicroscopic evaluation of the optic disc. Patients whose optic discs show pseudopapilledema can be reassured although patients with optic nerve drusen are at risk of retinal hemorrhage, as well as development of an arcuate scotoma in the inferior nasal quadrant of the visual field.[31] Patients with disc edema need a CT scan followed by a lumbar puncture to distinguish between papilledema and pseudotumor cerebri. Despite careful examination, some patients elude definitive diagnosis. In this situation, remember to look at the optic disc of other family members, as well as to perform serial evaluations including photography of the patient's optic discs. One should also keep in mind the general health status of the patient. The existence of neurological signs or symptoms demands further evaluation. Given the relative safety of today's CT and MRI scanners, as well as the lack of radiation exposure with the MRI scan, we are encouraged to err on the side of conservatism and order a head scan in patients where the diagnosis cannot be obtained by ophthalmoscopy.

ANISOCORIA

Neuroanatomy

Evaluation of patients with anisocoria requires a good understanding of the relevant neuroanatomy. The pupillomotor system can be divided into the sympathetic and parasympathetic systems. The sympathetic nervous system fibers, which cause pupillary dilation, form a three-neuron system (Fig. 12-4). The first-order neurons originate in the hypothalamus and travel downward in the brainstem to the C8–T2 level of the spinal cord called the ciliospinal center of Budge. They synapse with the second-order neurons in the *ciliospinal center of Budge*. The second-order neurons exit the spinal cord, enter the paravertebral sympathetic chain, and run upward to the superior cervical ganglion. These preganglionic second-order neurons then

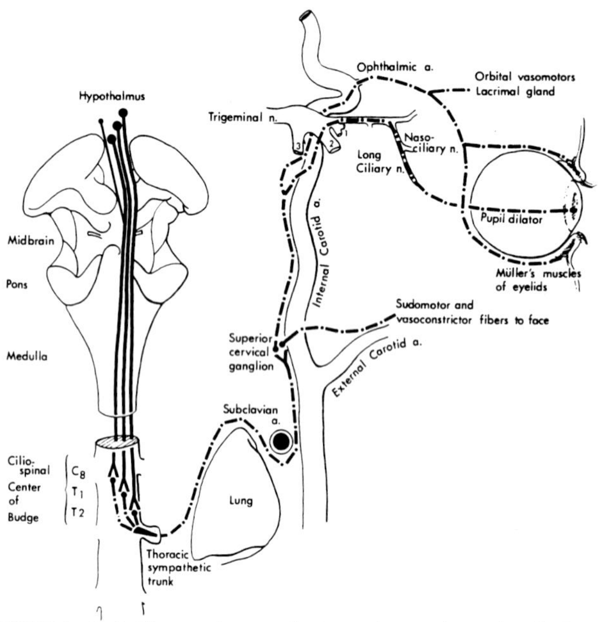

FIGURE 12-4. The oculosympathetic pathway. (Reproduced from Slamovits TL, Glaser JS. The pupils and accommodation. In: Glaser JS (ed) Neuro-ophthalmology, 2nd edn. Philadelphia: Lippincott, 1990:464, with permission.)

synapse with the postganglionic third-order neurons in the *superior cervical ganglion*. The third-order neurons travel upward along the internal carotid artery. The pupillomotor fibers of the third-order neuron travel with the nasociliary nerve and then the long ciliary nerves and eventually reach the dilator muscle of the iris. The sympathetic fibers of the third-order neuron to Muller's muscle and the inferior tarsal muscle travel with branches of the ophthalmic artery. Sudomotor and vasoconstrictor fibers to the facial skin travel along branches of the external carotid artery.

The parasympathetic fibers cause pupillary constriction. Preganglionic fibers leave the Edinger–Westphal nucleus and travel along the third cranial nerve. The preganglionic fibers then enter the ciliary ganglion in the orbit, where they synapse with postganglionic fibers. The postganglionic fibers are then distributed to the iris sphincter and the ciliary body via the short ciliary nerves.

Causes

Simple Anisocoria

Up to 20% of normal children have measurable anisocoria. Most of these patients have simple anisocoria in which the degree of anisocoria is equal in dim and bright conditions or the anisocoria is greater in dim light. Intermittancy or variability is also a hallmark of simple anisocoria. There are no associated findings suggestive of a sympathetic or parasympathetic lesion.

Sympathetic Lesions

A lesion somewhere in the three-neuron sympathetic chain characterizes Horner's syndrome. The classical findings include a small pupil on the involved side with more anisocoria being measured in the dark. There is an associated ptosis of the upper lid on the involved side due to the lack of Mueller's muscle function. An "upside-down" or "inverse" ptosis of the lower lid also occurs secondary to lack of inferior tarsal muscle function. Additionally, there is anhydrosis due to involvement of the sudomotor fibers to the skin of the face. Patients with a long-standing Horner's syndrome may show cool, blanched skin as a result of denervation supersensitivity to circulating catecholamines. Patients with a congenital Horner's syndrome show these findings as well as iris heterochromia, with the involved iris being lighter (Fig. 12-5). Depending on the location of the lesion, fewer signs may be present, or additional signs may be present, reflecting other cranial nerve involvement. For example, a lesion at the base of the skull will affect only the fibers to the pupil and the lids. There would be no anhydrosis. On the other hand, a lesion at the apex of the thorax (Pancoast's tumor) would present with anhydrosis. Alternatively, a lesion in the cavernous sinus might present with a Horner's syndrome as well as evidence of a third nerve palsy.

Because the sympathetic fibers are not functioning properly in Horner's syndrome, the anisocoria is largest under conditions requiring the sympathetic pupillomotor fibers to be working, that is, in the dark. This dilation lag is extremely characteristic of Horner's syndrome, but cannot always be reliably treated in

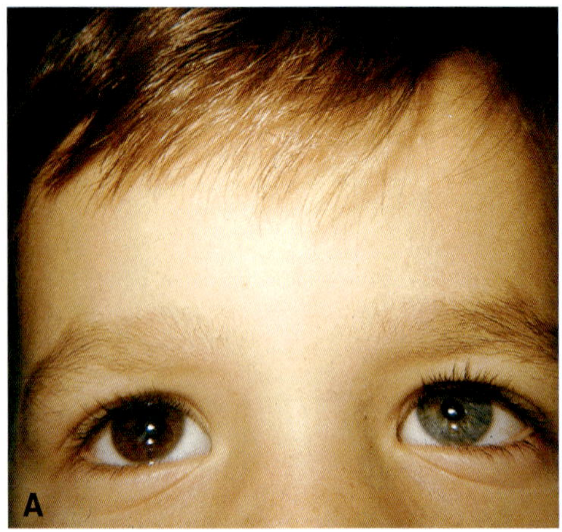

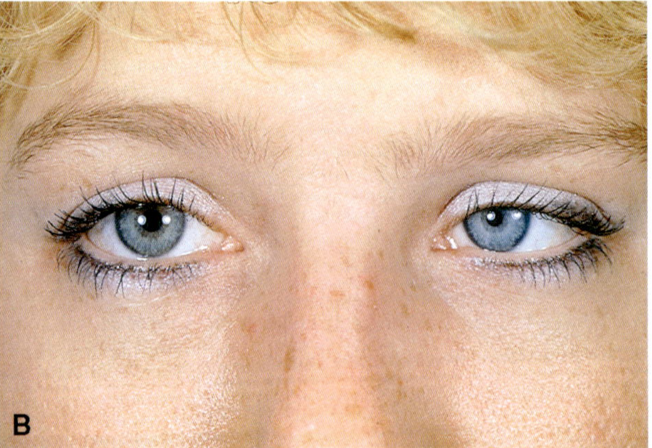

FIGURE 12-5A,B. **(A)** Iris hypochromia, left eye, due to congenital Horner's syndrome. **(B)** Left congenital Horner's syndrome showing ptosis, miosis, and iris heterochromia. (Courtesy of Dr. R. Kardon.)

children. Cocaine testing and Paredrine (hydroxyamphetamine) testing are more reliable and useful. Cocaine has a sympathomimetic effect by blocking the reuptake of norepinephrine from the synaptic junction. Topical cocaine solution will dilate a normal pupil, but fails to dilate a Horner's pupil. It fails to dilate the pupil because norepinephrine is not released from the sympathetic neuron in Horner's syndrome. Paredrine has a sympathomimetic effect by releasing norepinephrine from vesicles at the end of an intact third-order neuron. Paredrine will dilate a normal pupil as well as the pupil of a first- or second-order Horner's syndrome. Paredrine will not dilate the pupil of a third-order Horner's syndrome because the neuron is not intact. Paredrine has been unavailable in the past, but now can be obtained by contacting Allergan Pharmaceuticals.

Parasympathetic Lesions

Parasympathetic lesions are all characterized by loss of the pupillary constricting action of the oculomotor nerve. The pupillomotor fibers travel in the outer aspect of the third nerve and are therefore more sensitive to compression, but are less likely to be involved by microvascular disease. Depending on the site of the lesion, one may see a complete third nerve palsy or may only see a dilated, poorly reactive pupil. The anisocoria is largest under conditions requiring the parasympathetic pupillomotor fibers to be working, that is, in the light.

Third Nerve Palsy

The signs of a complete third nerve palsy—a fixed, dilated pupil, an incomitant exotropia, hypotropia, and ptosis—are easily recognized and do not cause diagnostic confusion. Expanding intracranial mass lesions result in uncal herniation with resultant compression of the third nerve. The pupillomotor fibers travel in the outer aspect of the nerve, and thus are sensitive to compression. Pupillary dilation (the Hutchinson pupil) is an early sign of an expanding, supratentorial mass lesion. Most patients with an expanding mass lesion show other signs of third nerve involvement or worsening mental status by the time the ophthalmologist arrives, making the pupillary examination moot. The Hutchinson pupil does not have denervation supersensitivity, and will not constrict to 0.1% pilocarpine solution, but will constrict to 1% pilocarpine.

Adie's Tonic Pupil

This condition may occur in children[37] but is more commonly seen in young women. Children present because of the anisocoria, photophobia, or difficulty reading at near. The Adie's pupil is generally the result of a viral-mediated ciliary ganglionitis with disruption of the accommodative and the pupillomotor fibers. The process is usually unilateral, but may be bilateral with an asymmetrical onset. Segmental iris involvement occurs, and may vary from a small sector to near total iris involvement. Initially, both accommodation and pupil constriction are lost, but accommodation generally recovers within 3 months due to the large proportion of parasympathetic fibers that innervate the ciliary body (97%) as compared to the iris sphincter (3%). The dilated pupil remains poorly reactive to light, but develops a tonic, slow constriction to a near stimulus as a result of aberrant regeneration. Because of the tonic nature of the accommodative response, the pupil dilates slowly once the accommodative stimulus is removed. The vermiform movements seen at the slit lamp represent "hippus" of the iris sectors still connected to the original pupillomotor fibers. The Adie's pupil has denervation supersensitivity, and constricts to dilute 0.1% pilocarpine, whereas a normal pupil will not constrict.[2] Patients with Adie's syndrome have diminished deep tendon reflexes, reflecting a generalized ganglionitis affecting dorsal root ganglia.[32] One other potential complication of Adie's pupil in children is the development of amblyopia in the involved eye. The authors have also seen an intermittent exotropia made worse by an Adie's pupil. This condition was treated successfully with dilute pilocarpine 0.125% three times a day.

Atropine Mydriasis

Dilated, nonreactive pupil(s) may result from ingestion or topical application of atropine or other parasympatholytic substances. Children may accidentally gain access to a parent's or grandparent's eyedrops, but environmental exposure to the seeds of jimson weed, or the berries of deadly nightshade and henbane, is also possible. A pupil dilated with atropine will not constrict to 0.1% or 1% pilocarpine solutions. Children with systemic atropine poisoning have bilateral dilated pupils that may constrict to 1% pilocarpine solution.

Other Causes

Pilocarpine, phospholine iodide, and other miotics may occasionally be instilled in one eye only and will give unilateral miosis. Phenylephrine or cocaine may get in one eye and cause unilateral mydriasis. Anisocoria may result from localized processes such as iris sphincter damage, iritis, or prior intraocular surgery.

Patient Evaluation

Important historical points include the date the anisocoria was first noticed, any associated neurological dysfunction, and any possible exposure to atropine-like compounds. Patients appearing to have a Horner's syndrome need to be questioned regarding birth trauma or early cardiothoracic surgery. Many patients can have their pupillary abnormality diagnosed by careful observation of the pupillary reactions and the amount of anisocoria in the dark as compared to in the light. Sympathetic lesions have more anisocoria in the dark; parasympathetic lesions have more anisocoria in the light and the involved pupil is poorly reactive to light. Thompson's flowchart for evaluating anisocoria is the gold standard guide to pharmacological pupillary testing and is reproduced in Figure 12-6.[38]

Patient Management

Once the cause of the anisocoria is diagnosed, parents want to be given information regarding the prognosis, further workup, and possible treatment of the problem. Patients with a con-

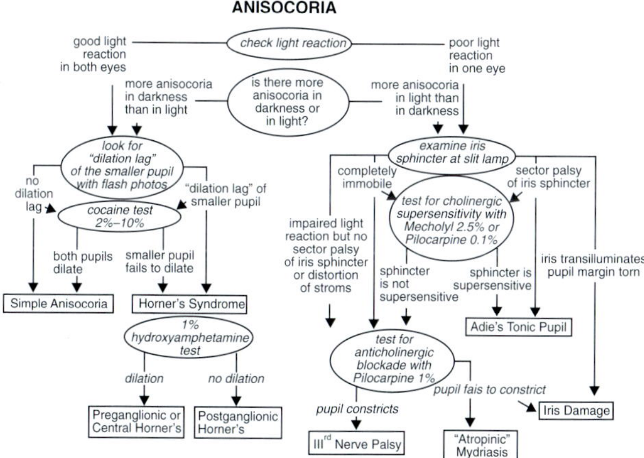

FIGURE 12-6. Anisocoria flowchart. (Reproduced from Thompson HS, Pilley SEJ. Unequal pupils. A flowchart for sorting out the anisocorias. Surv Ophthalmol 1976;24:45–48,[38] with permission.)

genital Horner's syndrome with a history of birth trauma or cardiothoracic surgery need no further workup.[22] The iris heterochromia could be treated with a cosmetic contact lens when the child reaches adolescence. Patients with a congenital Horner's syndrome with no obvious cause may need to be investigated with a chest radiograph, an MRI scan or CT scan of the head, neck, and upper thorax, as well as a 24-h urine catecholamine assay to rule out an occult neuroblastoma.[42] Patients with an acquired Horner's syndrome must be evaluated with chest radiograph, MRI or CT scan of the head, neck, and upper thorax, as well as a 24-h urine catecholamine assay. Sauer and Levinsohn have emphasized the seriousness of an acquired Horner's syndrome in children.[30]

Patients with a Hutchinson's pupil need urgent neurosurgical intervention to treat their brain herniation. The management of patients with a congenital or acquired third nerve palsy is beyond the scope of this chapter. Children with Adie's tonic pupil do not require further evaluation, but the parents should be warned that the other eye may become affected in the future. The photophobia and accommodative paresis may be improved with pilocarpine 0.1% solution in the affected eye several times daily. Young children should be carefully observed for the development of amblyopia or strabismus in the affected eye. Patients with atropine mydriasis need to be evaluated for signs of atropine poisoning. The mnemonic "hot as a hare, blind as a bat, dry as a bone, red as a beet, mad as a hen" provides a useful way of recalling the associated symptoms.[36] If the child has no signs of atropine poisoning, the parents can be reassured that the pupils will return to normal within 2 weeks.

NEONATAL VISUAL IMPAIRMENT

The causes of neonatal visual impairment can be grouped into four major categories: (1) disorders of the media, (2) disorders of the retina, (3) disorders of the optic nerve, and (4) disorders of the visual pathways and cortex. Some causes in each category are easily diagnosed such as congenital cataracts, optic nerve colobomas, or macular toxoplasmosis. The disorders that present with an essentially "normal" ocular examination provide the real diagnostic confusion and are the topic of this section. One must take care to distinguish between poor vision from birth and acquired visual loss. Patients with near-normal vision in infancy that develop progressive visual loss are beyond the scope of this section.

Causes of Visual Impairment with a "Normal" Ocular Examination

Delayed Visual Maturation

Delayed visual maturation (DVM) is characterized by visual inattention during infancy, which improves significantly by 3 to 9 months of age. Fielder et al. divided DVM into three groups: an isolated finding, in association with neurological abnormalities, and in association with ocular abnormalities.[8] Patients with isolated DVM show a normal flash electroretinogram (ERG) and also an essentially normal flash and pattern visual evoked potential (VEP).[18] These patients generally have normal visual attention by 6 months of age; their prognosis for normal intellectual development is good. Patients with DVM in association with neurologic defects often have mental retardation and seizures. These children appear to see better when their seizures are controlled; their vision is often variable and is better when sound or tactile means also stimulates them. These children have a slower and less complete recovery of vision. Patients with DVM in association with ocular disease will have acuity worse than expected for the ocular disease alone. Their acuity will likely recover to the expected level by 9 to 12 months of age.

Saccade Palsy

Disorders such as oculomotor apraxia or bilateral type III Duane's syndrome may mimic blindness because the child cannot fix or follow objects in the horizontal plane. Patients with type III Duane's syndrome can follow objects moving vertically; patients with oculomotor apraxia can be diagnosed by the characteristic head thrusts.

High Ametropia

Occasionally infants with very high refractive errors may present with visual inattention, which probably represents delayed visual maturation in association with ocular disease. A cycloplegic refraction should be performed on every infant with neonatal visual impairment. These children should be followed to assure normal visual development.

Infantile Retinal Dystrophies

This group represents a heterogeneous group of disorders that have a rod/cone dystrophy as a common factor. Some patients have no associated systemic disease, while others with diseases such as Zellweger syndrome will die in the first year of life. The most important disorders include Leber's congenital amaurosis, Joubert's syndrome, infantile Batten disease, and peroxisomal disorders including Zellweger syndrome, Refsum's disease, and neonatal adrenoleukodystrophy.

Leber's Amaurosis

Children with Leber's amaurosis present with poor vision and nystagmus from birth. The pupils are minimally reactive to light. Eye poking—the digitoocular sign of Franceschetti—is common. Cycloplegic retinoscopy may show high hyperopic or myopic refractive errors.[40] The fundus examination is often normal early, but will eventually show disc pallor, arteriolar narrowing, and retinal pigmentary changes. The scotopic and photopic electroretinograms are extinguished. Inheritance is autosomal recessive. Many patients with Leber's amaurosis are otherwise healthy, but some patients may have mental retardation[19] or renal disease.[7,24,33] Low-vision services should be offered to the patient.

Joubert's Syndrome

Patients with Joubert's syndrome[13] present in a manner similar to Leber's amaurosis. These infants have a variety of oculomotor abnormalities including saccade palsies and nystagmus, cerebellar vermis hypoplasia, and breathing difficulties in addition to their retinal dystophy.[17] Similar to Leber's amaurosis, the fundus examination is normal in infancy, but will eventually show disc pallor, arteriolar narrowing, and retinal pigmentary changes. The ERG is markedly attenuated, but the VER is preserved, indicating the better visual prognosis for this disorder. Inheritance is autosomal recessive. Diagnosis is by an attenuated ERG, a preserved VEP, and cerebellar vermis hypoplasia on MRI scan.

Infantile Batten Disease

This disorder is not strictly a cause of neonatal blindness, as the children present at 9 to 18 months with loss of developmental milestones, seizures, and visual failure. Death occurs by 4 years of age.[29] The pathogenesis is neuronal storage of lipopigments of the ceroid-lipofuscin type with secondary neuronal destruction and phagocytosis. The fundus is similar to Leber's amaurosis. The ERG and VEP are both markedly attenuated or absent. Inheritance is autosomal recessive. Diagnosis is by histopathological study of rectal neurons or conjunctiva.

Peroxisomal Disorders

The peroxisome is a subcellular, single membrane-bound organelle that harbors a large number of important biochemical reactions, including the catabolism of long chain fatty acids such as phytanic acid and pipecolic acid. Absence of peroxisomes gives rise to three important disorders: Zellweger syndrome, neonatal adrenoleukodystrophy, and infantile Refsum's disease. All three disorders are characterized by poor vision, a pigmentary retinopathy, retinal arteriolar attenuation, an extinguished ERG, optic atrophy, elevated serum long chain fatty acids, and autosomal recessive inheritance. Zellweger syndrome is further characterized by facial dysmorphism, hypotonia, seizures, psychomotor retardation, renal cysts, and hepatosplenomegaly. Most patients die within 1 year of age. Neonatal adrenoleukodystrophy is additionally characterized by adrenal cortical atrophy, patchy brain demyelination, and seizures. The disease is milder than Zellweger syndrome, and patients live an average of 4 years. Infantile Refsum's disease is the least severe of these three disorders, and is further characterized by deafness. Further information can be obtained in the excellent review by Folz and Trobe (see also Chapter 54).[10]

ACHROMATOPSIA

Achromatopsia (rod monochromatism) is a stationary retinal dystrophy characterized by a lack of functioning cones in the retina. It can be divided into complete (no functioning cones), incomplete (some functioning cones), and blue cone (no functioning red or green cones). All three disorders are characterized by marked photophobia, nystagmus, paradoxical pupil responses (constriction in the dark), poor color vision, reduced central visual acuity, and a normal scotopic (rod) response with an absent photopic flicker response on electroretinography. Complete rod monochromatism is the most severe, and adults have 20/200 acuity and no color vision. Incomplete rod monochromatism is less severe, and adults have 20/50 to 20/200 acuity with abnormal color vision.[4] Patients with both forms have decreased photophobia and decreased nystagmus as adults. The fundus examination is usually normal, although complete rod monochromats may show a nonspecific or bull's-eye maculopathy as adults. Complete and incomplete rod monochromatisms are inherited in an autosomal recessive manner; blue cone monochromatism differs with X-linked recessive inheritance. Specialized psychophysical tests can be used to diagnose blue cone monochromatism.[1]

ALBINISM

Patients with ocular albinism and oculocutaneous albinism have reduced vision, nystagmus, iris transillumination, foveal hypoplasia, and defective fundus pigmentation. Oculocutaneous albinism type 1 (OCA1) is due to a defect in the tyrosinase gene located on chromosome 11q. Oculocutaneous albinism type 2 (OCA2) results from a defect in a transmembrane protein necessary for melanogenesis. Patients with tyrosinase-negative oculocutaneous albinism (OCA1) are easy to diagnose, but those with tyrosinase-positive oculocutaneous albinism (OCA2) and ocular albinism (OA) may provide diagnostic confusion. The key to diagnosis is to suspect ocular albinism (OA) in any male child with congenital nystagmus, especially in darkly pigmented races. There are three types of ocular albinism, called OA1, OA2, and OA3. OA1 is the classic X-linked variety (Nettleship–Falls) mapped to chromosome Xp22.3. OA1 results from the formation of abnormal macromelanosomes. These abnormal macromelanosomes can be detected on skin biopsy. OA2 has been defined in a series of patients from the Aland Islands. OA3 is an autosomal recessive type that has an unknown genetic defect. Slit lamp examination in the classic type will show iris transillumination, and the fundus will be lightly pigmented with macular hypoplasia. Female carriers (the patient's mother) have normal vision with iris transillumination (Fig. 12-7) and hypopigmented areas in the peripheral retina. The ERG is normal in all varieties of albinism, and may be supranormal due to light scatter in these lightly pigmented fundi.[5] Tinted lenses and low-vision aids are recommended for these patients.

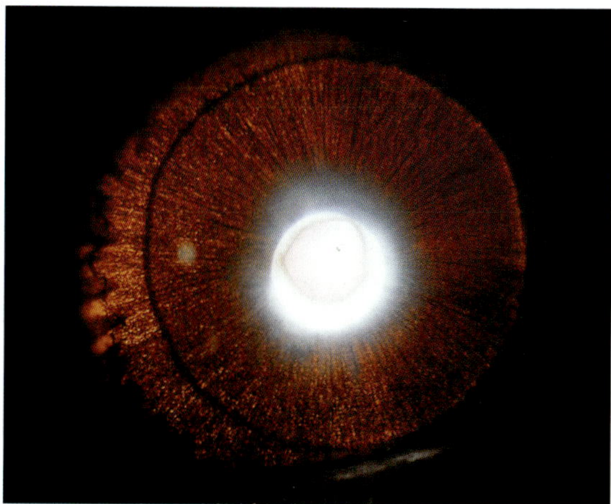

FIGURE 12-7. Slit lamp photograph of patient with ocular albinism demonstrating iris transillumination.

OPTIC NERVE HYPOPLASIA

Optic nerve hypoplasia is discussed in detail in Chapter 49, Congenital Optic Nerve Abnormalities. Children with severe bilateral optic nerve hypoplasia (Fig. 12-8) will present with

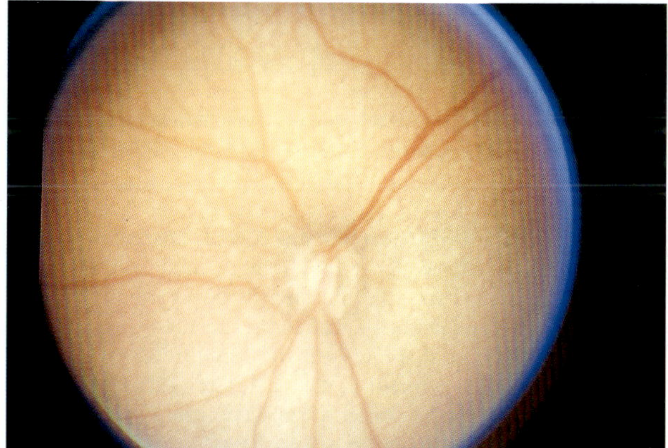

FIGURE 12-8. Fundus photograph of optic nerve hypoplasia.

poor vision and nystagmus from birth. Lesser degrees of bilateral hypoplasia may result in milder visual defects. All patients with optic nerve hypoplasia should be referred for a pediatric endocrinology evaluation. Clinical diagnosis is based upon careful observation of the optic disc size in relation to the exiting vessels; accuracy is improved with the direct ophthalmoscope and the use of the slit lamp with a 90 diopter lens, but few children are cooperative for this unless under anesthesia.

CEREBRAL VISUAL IMPAIRMENT

Cerebral visual impairment describes poor vision resulting from injuries to either the optic radiations or to the visual cortex. These injuries are generally hypoxic and occur as a result of hypotension, birth asphyxia, or cardiac surgery; other causes include hydrocephalus, stroke, and direct trauma. Children with cortical visual impairment have bilateral poor visual acuity and loss of optokinetic nystagmus with brisk pupillary reactions, clear media, and normal fundi. Other associated neurological defects are common. Children with cortical visual impairment may have some gradual visual recovery over months to years. An MRI scan of the visual pathways and cortex may aid in providing an ultimate visual prognosis; changes in the visual cortex do not correlate well with the final visual acuity, but changes in the optic radiations do correlate well.[16]

Patient Evaluation

In evaluating the child with neonatal visual impairment, one should question the parents about the child's visual behavior and if things seem to be stable or improving. Observations of photophobia (achromatopsia) or eye-poking (Leber's) are quite useful. Determine if the pregnancy was complicated, or if perinatal asphyxia occurred. Assess the infant's medical history for hydrocephalus, head trauma, meningitis, developmental delay, failure to thrive, and seizures. The family history is often negative, as most of these disorders are autosomal recessive.

Visual acuity assessment in young children is frequently difficult. Fixation on the examiner's face is commonly used in children under 6 months of age. The optokinetic nystagmus drum is quite useful, and can be used in an attempt to superimpose a vertical nystagmus on an existing horizontal nystagmus. Teller acuity cards are also helpful, but have limited use in very young children and in children with neurological deficits with a limited attention span.

Ocular examination should focus on the pupillary reactions and the existence of a paradoxical pupil, iris transillumination, macular hypoplasia, retinal arteriolar attenuation, optic atrophy, or optic nerve hypoplasia. Sluggish pupillary reactions suggest one of the retinal dystrophies. A paradoxical pupil is found in achromatopsia, Leber's congenital amaurosis, optic nerve hypoplasia, and albinism.[25] If the ocular examination is truly normal, the child has either delayed visual maturation or cortical visual impairment; the past medical history should distinguish between the two possibilities.

Electrophysiological Testing

If albinism and optic nerve hypoplasia have been ruled out, electrophysiological testing will often give useful results. The VEP is useful in diagnosing disease of the visual pathways and cortical visual impairment, and will help to distinguish Joubert's syndrome from Leber's congenital amaurosis; on a practical basis, however, patients with a consistent wince to a bright light stimulus will also have a recordable flash VEP. If a VEP needs to be performed, we perform it first and then dilate, sedate, and dark-adapt the child in preparation for the ERG. The scotopic and photopic ERG will be extinguished or nearly extinguished for all the retinal dystrophies. Rod monochromatism has a normal scotopic (rod) response with an absent photopic flicker response on electroretinography. We perform a scotopic white (rod) ERG, photopic white (cone) ERG, and photopic flicker (cone) ERG on all patients, with additional testing as deemed necessary.

Patient Management

Once the diagnosis has been made, the parents need to be given a visual prognosis. Patients with an extinguished ERG need to be evaluated for renal disease (Senior–Loken syndrome). Those with an extinguished ERG and developmental delay need to be evaluated for a peroxisomal disorder or infantile Batten disease. Patients with optic nerve hypoplasia need to have an MRI scan of the brain to rule out associated structural abnormalities, and

40. Wagner RS, Caputo AR, Nelson L, Zanoni D. High hyperopia in Leber's congenital amaurosis. Arch Ophthalmol 1985;103:1507–1509.
41. Walsh TJ, Garden JW, Gallagher B. Obliteration of retinal venous pulsations. Am J Ophthalmol 1969;67:954–956.
42. Woodruff G, Buncic JR, Morin JD. Horner's syndrome in children. J Pediatr Ophthalmol Strabismus 1988;25:40–44.

Index